HANDBOOK OF SCHOOL HEALTH

THE MEDICAL OFFICERS OF SCHOOLS ASSOCIATION

EIGHTEENTH EDITION
1998

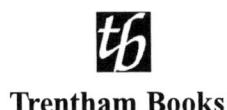

Trentham Books

First published in 1998 by Trentham Books Limited

Trentham Books Limited
Westview House
734 London Road
Oakhill
Stoke on Trent
Staffordshire
England ST4 5NP

British Cataloguing in Publication Data
A catalogue record for this book is available from the British Library
ISBN 1 85856 081 0

Designed and typeset by Trentham Print Design Ltd., Chester and printed in Great Britain by Bemrose Shafron (Printers) Ltd., Chester

CONTENTS

Chapter 6

Chapter 7

Chapter 8

FOREWORD

"For when I was a babe and wept and slept, time crept;
When I was a boy and laughed and talked, time walked;
Then when the years saw me a man, time ran;
But as I older grew, time flew".

(Epitaph in Chester Cathedral).

It is not just the flow of time that astonishes, but also the acceleration. That acceleration has continued in the six years since the last edition of this handbook, with many changes in society, health and health care. Some members of the Association will look back to their early years when they saw in one week more children with measles than are seen now in the whole of the UK in one winter. (I saw 24 new cases of measles in my first weekend of duty in the 1960's as a newly appointed School Medical Officer/GP). There have been great improvements both in health and in the delivery of health care, yet significant problems remain.

Mortality rates for school children have continued to decrease. Even the main killer – accidents – has been accompanied by a 30% reduction in mortality in the last four years; but the *morbidity* continues to be high. Much of the decrease in mortality is the result of more effective treatment, yet at the cost of permanent handicap. Death from other chronic disorders, for example cystic fibrosis, malignant disease and renal failure, has decreased spectacularly, but a large population of surviving children lead uncomfortable and, at times, precarious lives with intensive chemotherapy, dialysis, parenteral nutrition and repeated major surgery. In earlier decades such children would not have been attending normal schools, but now with the continued drive for integration, school doctors encounter a full range of healthy and unhealthy children.

As death from natural diseases has continued to decrease, death from *unnatural* behaviour increases – suicide has become a significant problem, death from misuse of drugs is not uncommon, and the morbidity from both recreational drugs and tobacco continues to pose serious problems. The nutritional deficiencies of the first half of this century have been replaced by nutritional excess and unhealthy eating, leading to more obesity and associated ill health and unhappiness in the next generation. Not all fat babies become fat adults, but there is increasing evidence of the strong link between obesity in 10 year olds and obesity and ill health in adult life.

The delivery of healthcare is influenced by many factors including government legislation. At the time of the previous edition, the Children Act 1989 was coming into full operation. Since then there has been extensive experience of both its good features and its limitations. The legislation provides a framework for the protection of children from abuse, and it has clarified the responsibilities of doctors working with other agencies when children are disadvantaged or at risk. Many Department of Health guidelines have changed, not least in relation to immunisation, and the expanded chapter on immunisation reflects those changes. Newer immunisation policies have had an immediate impact on the incidence of infectious diseases: Haemophilus influenzae infection has become a thing of the past. Other diseases have gone, only to be followed by troublesome substitutes. Rheumatic fever may have disappeared, but Kawasaki disease has emerged as the commonest cause of acquired heart disease in childhood. Changes in our lifestyle and overseas travel mean that today's School Medical Officers have to consider a much larger range of unusual infective organisms and parasites as possible causes for illness than did our predecessors.

The last decade has seen a further increase in the delivery of care by multidisciplinary teams, and recognition of the important contributions made to the health of school children by many specialists other than Medical Officers. It is appropriate that, for the first time, the handbook should have a separate chapter on school nursing.

All medical work is influenced not only by the changing pattern of disease in a changing society, but also by the expectations that society has of its doctors; and those expectations can be most difficult to fulfil. Older children and their parents expect the doctor to be an expert at diagnosis, treatment and management, and to be a wise friend and sympathetic counsellor. This book is a valuable aid to the many doctors who by their work and dedication to school medicine are providing a specialist service for children and their families.

"When I was a boy and laughed and talked, time walked" – School years may occupy only 15% of the life expectancy of today's school child, but they are impressionable years when time merely walks and there is space and potential for learning and benefit, as well as suffering and disadvantage. School Medical Officers are amongst those in the best position to help and to influence today's children to be fit for the future.

Sir Roy Meadow
Professor of Paediatrics and Child Health
St James's University Hospital, Leeds

PREFACE TO THE EIGHTEENTH EDITION

As the President of M.O.S.A. I am delighted to introduce a new edition of this essential handbook, for all medical staff working in schools. This is both an everyday source of reference and an up-to-date view on medical and administrative issues. We are indebted to Dr Peter McWilliam and his Committee who have put in so much hard work in collating this authoritative handbook as well as the countless people who have contributed to its enduring success.

11, Chandos Street,
Cavendish Square,
London W1   Giles R. Smith,
January 1998   President of MOSA 1997—1999

PREFACE TO THE FIRST EDITION

In bringing this code of rules before the general public and the Medical and Scholastic professions in particular, the Medical Officers of Schools Association desire to say a few words as to its compilation.

On the formation of the Association in 1884 one of the most urgent matters which forced itself to the front, as claiming immediate attention, was the need for the general adoption of more definite rules for guarding our great educational establishments from the outbreak and spread of preventable infectious diseases.

With this object an attempt was made to ascertain the rules and customs which are at present enforced in such cases, by circulating to every school of importance in the country an elaborate series of questions covering the ground of this enquiry.

The replies they obtained proved very interesting, and contained much valuable material;at the same time they revealed wide differences of procedure in different institutions when dealing with the same conditions of disease, and, in some cases, a considerable laxity of precaution. Nothing could more clearly demonstrate the necessity for some definite and generally recognised standard of School Hygiene than the curiously divergent character of many of the answers furnished in response to our paper of questions on the commoner epidemic diseases.

In the course of their deliberations on the information thus collected, the Association have embodied opinions and suggestions from many authorities on the several questions dealt with. It is hoped that the result of these labours may prove no less useful to parents and guardians, who deal with the home life of the children, than to the school authorities, since without the sympathy and the intelligent cooperation of the former no real progress can be made in this great department of preventive medicine, which is fraught with so much benefit to the community at large.

The Medical Officers of Schools Association cannot allow this Code to go forward to the public without placing on record the great debt of gratitude which they owe to their indefatigable secretary, Dr. Aldersmith, the Medical Officer of Christ's Hospital. This code is to a very large extent based on the valuable paper on 'The Preventive Treatment of Infectious Diseases in Public and High Schools' read by him at the Conference of School Hygiene, at the International Health Exhibition. The extensive correspondence involved in communicating with a large number of schools and of individuals in all parts of the Kingdom has been entirely in his hands; upon him devolved the heavy labour of comparing and collating the replies from the various authorities consulted; and upon him, too, has fallen the duty of preparing this work for the press.

G. J. H. Evatt, MD
Surgeon Major (later Surgeon-General) Army Medical Staff
President MOSA

Woolwich
January 1885

CONTRIBUTORS TO THE HANDBOOK

P. Bosworth,* BSc, MB ChB, FRCS, MRCGP. Medical Officer to Bryanston School, Dorset, and MOSA Council Member

R. W. E. Harrington, MB BS, MRCGP, DFFP, D Obst RCOG. Medical Officer to Stowe School, MOSA Council Member and former Hon. Secretary of MOSA.

T. W. Hoskins, MA MB B Chir, DCH., D Obst RCOG. Fellow of MOSA, formerly Medical Officer to Christ's Hospital, Horsham. Past President and Hon Secretary of MOSA.

Mrs. B. Lawder, * RGN. School Nurse, Edgarley Hall School, Glastonbury. Somerset.

D. M. Layton, MB BS, FRCP, MRCPCH. Senior Lecturer and Consultant Haematologist, Kings College Hospital and Dental School, London. SE5. Honorary Medical Adviser to the Sickle Cell Society.

P. K. A. McWilliam, *MB ChB, DCH (Lond), DCH (Glasg). Former Medical Officer to Ackworth School. Council Member and Honorary Life Member of MOSA. (Honorary Editor)

P. T. Penny, MB BS, MRCS, LRCP, AFOM (RCP). Former MOSA Council Member, and former Medical Officer to Taunton School and King's College, Taunton. Somerset. Honorary Medical Adviser to the Institute of Swimming Teachers and Coaches.

J. O. B. Rosedale, MB BS, D Obst. RCOG, DCH, DTM and H. Hon. Life Member of MOSA and former MOSA Council Member. Medical Officer to the British Everest Expedition, 1972.

Margaret E. M. Williams*, MB BS, MRCS, MRCP, D Obst RCOG. MOSA Council Member. Consultant Community Paediatrician, East Surrey Health Authority.

Ann M. Wood* MB ChB, MRCPsych. MOSA Council Member and Medical Officer to Benenden School, Kent.

* Members of the Handbook Committee.

EDITORIAL

This, the 18th Edition of the Handbook of School Health is much bulkier than its predecessors, reflecting some of the many changes which have taken place in school medicine in the last six years.

Now, school doctors have to know more about the day-to-day management of the rarer conditions from which increasing numbers of school children are surviving, so as to ensure minimal disruption of their schooling. In recent years, MOSA Members have attended meetings and conferences and, for example, have learned of children having been successfully treated for neoplastic disease now resuming their schooling, perhaps with the aid of some special provisions.

During the next four or five years, whilst this handbook will be current, it is likely that more immunocompromised children will be attending school suffering from a variety of underlying conditions, together with children suffering from, for example, antibiotic resistant infections and from the haemoglobinopathies. Perusal of all these eleven chapters will give some idea of the potential challenges for us which lie ahead.

A significant feature of this edition of the Handbook is the inclusion for the first time, of a chapter on 'School Nursing' written by Mrs Bridget Lawder, RGN, who is the School Nurse at Millfield Preparatory School, Glastonbury, Somerset. School nurses of all grades have not always received their due recognition, but now, they are rightly considered to be autonomous practitioners working 'with' rather than 'for' school doctors, with the aim of providing a better service for the children in our schools.

I thank Mrs Lawder, who also served on the Handbook Committee, devised the 'Job Description for The School Nurse', and undertook the writing of the chapter on 'Child Protection Policies and the Children Act'. I was anxious to include in this edition some information on child protection and The Children Act from a practical point of view, now that the latter has been in operation for a few years and Mrs Lawder was able to accomplish this task by using information taken from the Somerset Child Protection Policy and the Somerset Child Protection Handbook. Permission to enable her to use this material was readily and kindly given by Mr Tony May, Policy Development Manager and Child Protection Register Custodian for Somerset Child Protection Committee, to whom I extend my thanks. My thanks too, go to Mr Simon Cummins, Headmaster of Millfield Preparatory School, Glastonbury Somerset, for permission to use The Policy on Child Protection, currently in use at the school.

Before leaving details of the 'nursing input' to this Handbook I must thank Ms Hilary Fairford, Primary Care Facilitator, Wiltshire NHS Trust (1994), and the Trust, for permission to use 'Levels of Competence for Immunisation and Vaccination', the 'School Nurse Self Assessment Form' which she adapted from the Policies and Standards Group Document of the Nurses, Midwives and Health Visitors Advisory Council, to which Council I also record my thanks.

In addition to being centres of learning. all schools are places of employment and, necessarily, must observe their legal obligations under the Health and Safety at Work Act and related legislation. For guidance in these matters, I thank Dr. P.T. Penny, formerly Medical Officer to Taunton School, now an Occupational Physician and Miss Morag McWilliam BSc, MIOSH, a Safety and Hygiene Adviser. Dr Penny also advised on tuberculosis and swimming and swimming pools, since he is also Honorary Medical Adviser to The Institute of Swimming Teachers and Coaches.

I am grateful to The Child Growth Foundation for kindly giving permission for the free reproduction of the 4yr-18yr Height/Weight Growth charts for Boys and Girls. (These are part of the range of 9 centile charts produced for the UK, obtainable from Harlow Printing). I am also indebted to Blackwell Science Ltd., Osney Mead, Oxford, for permission to publish The diagrams of 'Sequences of Events at Adolescence and the Stages of Genital Development, for Boys and Girls', taken from 'Growth at Adolescence' (1962) by J.M. Tanner.

Two criticisms of the 17th. Edition of the Handbook were the paucity of information regarding dental matters and the inadequacy of the information on the haemoglobinopathies. Attempts have been made in this Edition to rectify these shortcomings and I am very grateful to The British Association for the Study of Community Dentistry, Mr G.H.Choyce, BChD, DGDP, and Mr.J Page, BDS, MScD, for dental advice and to Professor A.S. Blinkhorn for dental publications. I thank Dr. D.M. Layton of Kings College Hospital NHS Trust London and his very helpful secretaries for the contribution on the haemoglobinopathies.

Dr. M.D. Peake, Consultant Physician, Pontefract General Infirmary, advised about HIV infection and drew my attention to the British Thoracic Society's updated Asthma Guidelines and I acknowledge the help from these sources. Miss Jane Smethurst, BA, ALA, Librarian at Pontefract Post Graduate Centre was most helpful, especially in tracking down elusive references. My 'local' MOSA colleague, Dr Ivan Hanney, kindly advised on the management of asthma in general practice and updated my knowledge about the recent changes in general practice. Dr. R.S. Thiagarajah, Consultant Community Paediatrician at Pontefract Infirmary, also gave me some helpful advice. I record my thanks to all of these colleagues.

I thank The Society of Optometrists for kindly updating their appendix on 'Colour Vision and Eye Care in Sports', which includes some practical advice with regard to choices of careers.

I am indebted to The Copyright Unit of Her Majesty's Stationery Office for permission to quote extensively from the HMSO publication 'Immunisation against Infectious Disease 1996', in the compilation of the chapters on Immunisation and to a lesser extent, Communicable Diseases. I also acknowledge with gratitude, the help from Dr. David Salisbury of The Department of Health and Dr. Norman Begg of the Communicable Disease Surveillance Unit of The Public Health Laboratory Service, co-editors of 'Immunisation against Infectious Disease 1996'. MOSA is of course, entirely committed to following the policy of Her Majesty's Government with regard to immunisation and I thought it right and helpful to school doctors, especially from the medico-legal standpoint, to have the information on immunisation relevant to children and adolescents at school, actually in the Handbook.

Also, I thank Her Majesty's Stationery Office for permission to include material from 'Education (School Premises) Regulations, 10/96 1996, Part 111 – Accommodation Boarding Schools: Sleeping accommodation for boarding pupils, and from 'First Aid in Educational Establishments (1986)'.

My predecessor in the office of Honorary Editor, Dr. Trevor Hoskins, also past President, former Honorary Secretary and now Fellow of MOSA, kindly provided helpful criticism and, from his recent coign of vantage as a Medical Officer with Minbank Medical Services in Lusaka, Zambia, for the last five or six years, also provided information about HIV infection.

MOSA Members at the Annual Clinical Meeting at Sevenoaks School in January 1996, heard Dr. Adrienne Rievely, Consultant in Adolescent Psychiatry at the Maudsley Hospital, Denmark Hill, London, talk about 'Adolescent adjustment and mental illness' and I am very grateful to her for her permission to reproduce notes taken during her talk on this most important branch of adolescent medicine.

I thank Professor Michael Levin and his erstwhile colleague, Dr. Jennifer Evans, of the Department of Paediatrics, St. Mary's Hospital, Paddington, for permission to quote from their lectures to MOSA Members, on 'Meningococcal Disease' and 'The Care of HIV infected Children in School,' respectively.

The other contributions have been 'in house', from current (or only recently) retired MOSA Council Members, most of whom are (or were) school doctors. Thus, Dr. Margaret Williams, Consultant Community Paediatrician, East Surrey Health Authority, updated the Chapter on Child Abuse, to be read in close conjunction with the next Chapter on Child Protection policies and The Children Act. Dr.Ann Wood (MO to Benenden School) contributed the information on Eating Disorders and on Menstrual Difficulties. Dr. Philip Bosworth (MO to Bryanston School) provided Chapter 9 on Sports Injuries, the medical examination forms for boys and girls, the information on allergy to peanuts and other foods and, with the aid of Professor Jonathan Brostoff, Professor of Clinical Immunology at the Middlesex Hospital,(whom we thank), has set up an Anaphylaxis Helpline.(See Chapter 6). 'The Doctor', Dr Barry Brewster MBE, recently MO to Giggleswick School, kindly provided the specimen Medical Report and Examination Forms for staff members and Dr. J.O.B. Rosedale, formerly MO to Marlborough College and Medical Officer to the 1972 British Everest Expedition, updated the section on Adventure Training in Schools. It is a great pleasure to thank all these colleagues.

The indefatigable erstwhile Honorary Secretary of MOSA, Dr Roger Harrington, (MO to Stowe School) provided the sections on Consent, Confidentiality, Contraception and Drug Misuse, including alcohol and tobacco, and the MOSA Policy of Drug Testing in Schools, plus the specimen contract in Appendix K. To him, I owe a tremendous debt of gratitude.

I thank the Members of the small but hardworking Handbook Committee, identified elsewhere, for their expert advice and for submitting their contributions on time. However, I have undertaken the writing of the Handbook, thereby incurring sole responsibility for errors, inaccuracies and any other deficiencies. 'He' has been used to indicate a pupil of either sex unless the context indicates otherwise.

Proof reading has been undertaken by Dr. R.J.R. Moffat, Fellow of MOSA and former Senior Medical Officer to Whitgift Educational Foundation, Croydon, who also, kindly provided forensic guidance and Dr. J.H.D. Briscoe LVO, who recently retired from the post of Senior Medical Officer to Eton College. I greatly appreciate the painstaking thoroughness with which Dr. Moffat and Dr. Briscoe accomplished this task.

Finally, I thank Stuart McWilliam, BSc, for occasional computer 'trouble shooting', my wife for her constant support and inexhaustible patience and our publishers, Trentham Books Limited for their understanding and forbearance.

11, Chandos Street,   Peter McWilliam.
Cavendish Square, London W.1.   HonoraryEditor.
January 1998.   Medical Officers of Schools
                                  Association.

CHAPTER I

RESPONSIBILITIES OF SCHOOL MEDICAL OFFICERS

Introduction

The school doctor should be appointed by the Governing Body of the school or the Local Health Authority and he should be directly responsible to them. The doctor must, however, respect the jurisdiction of the headmaster who has the ultimate responsibility for the whole school.

There are considerable differences in medical organisation between maintained and independent schools, and between day and boarding schools. However, more boarding schools are now taking increasing numbers of day pupils. In maintained schools, there is a division of responsibility between the school medical officer and a senior medical officer of the employing authority, generally the Consultant Community Paediatrician. In independent schools, the school doctor should be responsible for advising on all matters relating to the health of the school. This includes not only the pupils but everyone who is concerned with the working of the school, e. g. teaching, nursing, domestic, clerical and maintenance staff and visitors to the school premises. There is an obligation to provide medical care for any emergency or injury which might occur to members of visiting games teams, for example, and to report details to the patient's own doctor very soon afterwards. There should, of course, be sound communications with the parents and general practitioners of day children concerning any treatment given to them whilst they are at school.

The school doctor should carry out medical examinations on pupils as necessary and ensure that regular screening of vision, hearing, height and weight is performed.

Epidemiological control is very important in a school community. The independent school doctor should strongly advise that all pupils are fully immunised in accordance with current Department of Health recommendations and it is for him to decide, on medical grounds, when a pupil can be allowed to return to school. Generally, he should have the power to act as an epidemiologist for the prevention and control of communicable diseases. He should, however, realise that the school is part of a larger community for which the Consultant in Communicable Diseases and (ultimately) the Director of Public Health of the Area Health Authority have overall responsibility, with whom he should work in close collaboration. The school doctor has a statutory duty to notify certain specified diseases to the Consultant in Communicable Diseases of the Area Health Authority. (See Appendix A).

When an outbreak of communicable disease occurs the school doctor should communicate with the school doctor of any other school with which sports fixtures or social events are planned. If care is taken to see that members of the teams or other groups of pupils are healthy on the day of the match or social occasion, then only rarely should it be necessary to cancel fixtures or other arrangements.

The school doctor should actively concern himself with the hygienic conditions of the school premises, and, where necessary, call upon the services of the Environmental Health Officer from the Area Health Authority. Some doctors like to make annual inspections of the school premises: others like to keep them under less formal, but equally rigorous review. At least, *annually* and more frequently at the request of the school Governing Body, a report should be made to them on the general health of the pupils, the incidence of illness, the level of prophylaxis and the environmental health of the school premises, detailing any alterations or improvements necessary for promotion of health and well-being of the school community.

Administration in Maintained Schools
The School Health Service was first established in 1907 as a result of the poor physical condition noted in young men medically examined for military service for the Boer war. In 1973, the NHS Reorganisation Act transferred responsibility for the Service from Local Education Authorities to the National Health Service. Following further NHS reorganisation in 1981, the Service in England and Wales became the responsibility of the District Health Authorities which have now become Area Health Authorities. These bodies manage all community health services for the population within their areas. They employ school medical officers, community medical officers, who are on the staff of the Consultant Community Paediatrician, on behalf of the Director of Public Health. In day schools, community medical officers do not prescribe treatment, but should maintain close contact with the pupils' general practitioners, either direct with the doctors or via the Consultant Community Paediatrician. The school nursing service is managed and administered by the Director of Nursing (Community Services). The policy whereby named school doctors and nurses are responsible for individual schools is good.

Administration in Independent Schools
The doctor appointed to an independent school is usually a general practitioner who is contracted both to the Governing Body of the school and also to the Area Health Authority for the provision of general medical services. The boarding pupils and such staff and dependents who elect to do so, register with him under the National Health Service and he is therefore responsible for providing general medical services during term time and during school holidays provided they remain resident in the school medical officer's practice area. For children and staff, who have holiday addresses outside the school doctor's practice area, necessary medical services required during the holiday period may be obtained, as NHS temporary residents, from

any medical practitioners offering general medical services under the National Health Service in whose practice areas the holiday addresses of the pupils or members of staff are situated.

Many general practitioners are now 'Fundholding' and are primary care providers and secondary care purchasers. They contract with selected hospitals for the provision of secondary care for their registered patients, and since they hold budgets out of which they pay the hospitals for these contracted services, at a preferential rate, they are in a position to exert a greater degree of influence than before, over the care of their patients, by these selected hospitals. The fundholding practitioners have a greater say, for example, in the size of hospital waiting lists, hospital OPD waiting times and the accessibility of consultants. All NHS GP practices however, fundholding or not, are responsible to the Local Health Authority .

Fundholding general practitioners have a financial disincentive to refer their NHS list patients to hospitals other than those with which they have contracts. However, in cases of clinical need, 'extra-contractual referrals' are permitted and this may be of relevance to boarding pupils.

'Outreach clinics' are another feature of fundholding, whereby the doctor contracts with individual consultants to hold clinics for practice patients, in his or her specialty, on the practice premises, thus short-circuiting the normal process of out-patient clinic referral.

Lastly, separate prescriptions for vaccines from the general practitioners of day children are not now required, so that in residential schools, day scholars may be included in the vaccination and immunisation sessions for boarding children.

Day Surgery sessions have increased in the last few years for minor procedures in general surgery, (herniae), gynaecology (tubal ligation, TOP, D&C) and some ENT procedures, thus reducing or even dispensing with overnight stays in hospital, with consequent financial savings.

As implied above, pupils attending residential schools are there for the greater part of the year and the school address is their permanent address as far as the NHS is concerned.

The school medical officer is not always the doctor of the parents' or the childrens' choice, and in order to gain their confidence, the doctor should do everything that he can do to build up good relations with the teaching staff, pupils and parents, and communicate closely with the general practitioners of the families concerned when the need arises, so that there is continuity of care.

The school doctor must be the person responsible for the administration of the services necessary for the treatment and nursing of sick and injured pupils and staff during term time. In co-operation with the headmaster and the sanatorium and teaching staff, the school doctor should provide for the full medical care of all needy day pupils and staff, not on his NHS list, during the time they are within the precincts of the school, i. e., until they are able to return home to the care of their parent or guardian and to the supervision of their family doctor, with whom he will communicate regarding the treatment of the pupil or staff member whilst under his temporary care.

The school doctor is strongly advised to enter into a contract with his employers for services which are outside and additional to his NHS obligations for the provision of general medical services. (A specimen contract is set out in Appendix K)

An independent school medical officer has many duties which are outside his National Health Service contractual obligations, for which he is remunerated by the school. They include the following;

(a) Advising the Headmaster and the Governing Body on matters of health.

(b) Discussions with housemasters, housemistresses and other staff concerning the physical and mental fitness of individual pupils, subject to the constraints of confidentiality.

(c) The medical supervision of the sanatorium or sick bay(s) . Advice on the appointment of nursing staff, and the general direction of their professional duties. (A specimen job description for a school nurse is set out in Appendix H.)

(d) The periodical medical examination of pupils, including supervision of the testing of vision and hearing and the measuring of weight and height.

(e) The establishment of epidemiological surveillance, including the maintenance of sickness and injury records additional to clinical notes which form part of the National Health Service records.

(f) The maintenance of separate immunisation records and arranging immunisation programmes to ensure that all pupils having the necessary parental consent where applicable, and all other pupils giving their consent, are immunised in accordance with current practice recommended by the DOH.

(g) The maintenance of communication with parents in respect of their sons and daughters, subject of course, to the restraints of confidentiality; obtaining their informed consent, where applicable, to medical investigations, treatment and immunisations and informing them of subsequent outcome and progress. Advising them on the procedure to be followed in the case of communicable diseases occurring at home, and advising them of any necessary immunisations and medication in connection with overseas travel. (Note: in cases where parental consent is not required the doctor should, especially on request from the pupil, be willing to communicate with the parents on the above matters although legally he is not obliged to do so.)

(h) To collaborate with the Headmaster and the Governing Body and, where applicable, the Environmental Health Officer, to advise on the hygiene of the school premises.

(i) The giving of advice on the prevention of accidents and sports injuries, including being aware of The Health and Safety at Work Act (1974), which is the 'enabling' piece of legislation, under which all other UK Health and Safety legislation is made. Other relevant pieces of legislation are:

(i)   Control of Substances Hazardous to Health (COSHH) Regulations, 1997. In schools, this would be applicable particularly to science laboratories, craft, design and technology workshops and to art rooms.

(ii)   Reporting of Injuries, Diseases and Dangerous Occurrences Regulations, 1995 (RIDDOR).

(iii) Display Screen Equipment Regulations, 1992. This affects the use of Visual Display Units in information technology departments and also in school offices.

(iv) The Management of Health and Safety at Work Regulations, 1992. This governs general risk assessment and would be applicable to all departments.

(v)   The Noise at Work Regulations, 1989. Applicable to craft, design and technology and also maintenance departments.

(vi) The Workplace Health, Safety and Welfare Regulations, 1992. General application.

(j)   To offer and provide regular dental inspections and arrange any necessary treatment for which consent has been obtained, either in or nearby school or through parents or guardians, and to implement a school dental policy. (See Appendix E).

(k)   To arrange for pre-employment medical examinations of teaching and non-teaching staff, and advising the headteacher and governing body accordingly. (See appendix G).

(l)   The provision or discussion, as seems appropriate, of certificates of incapacity required by the school in respect of employees.

(m) The provision of certificates of freedom from infection, e. g. for Combined Cadet Force camps, travel and employment, and the provision of international vaccination certificates where appropriate.

(n)   The provision of reports to university or college medical officers and issuing certificates of fitness to attend a university or college of further education.

(o)   The completion and signing of certificates required to support claims from a provident association.

(p)   The demonstration and explanation, to eligible pupils, of their medical records held since 1st November 1991 on request, or, at the request of the pupil, after due notice, the provision of written copies of the same records. (See later in this chapter.)

Although the school authorities may exercise some selection in the duties which the school doctor may be asked to undertake, it is thought that the best practice is for the doctor to provide the fullest services.

Medical Services in Boarding Schools
School Sanatoria

With the decline in boarding education and the consequent rise in provision for day pupils together with the current practice of having small sick bays in boarding houses, the need for sanatorium accommodation has diminished and now, in many of the older, smaller boarding schools, the original capacious sanatorium buildings have been allocated for other purposes.

However, if possible, it is desirable to have some dedicated medical premises, staffed by trained personnel and under the direction of the school doctor, to act as a focus for most of the medical needs of the school.

The design of such premises inevitably will be individual. No two schools will be alike, nor will they have identical requirements. The number of beds required will vary from school to school and will depend on:

The number of boarders in the school.

The age range of the pupils.

Whether or not it is a single sex or a co-educational establishment.

What sick room facilities are available in the boarding houses and how these are utilised.

The proximity of hospitals and their willingness to provide care.

In view of the continuing fall in bed occupancy in most school sanatoria and the financial burden of maintaining large numbers of under used beds, which would always be insufficient to cope with significant epidemics, a provision of one bed per fifty boarders could be sufficient.

All schools should realise that when epidemics occur, boarding house sick rooms and dormitories shall have to be used to accommodate sick pupils, and pre-planning for this will pay dividends. Each house would do well to have a panel of volunteers who are willing to come in during epidemics. At these times it shall be necessary to recruit extra nursing staff. The compilation and maintenance of a register of local nurses and familiarisation with the details of nearby Nursing Agencies should be part of the contingency plans for the management of epidemics.

Government Regulations on accommodation for the sick are included in **Education (School Premises) Regulations, 10/96, 1996, Part 111 – Accommodation in Boarding Schools.**

Sleeping accommodation for boarding pupils

33 Any school with boarding pupils—whether or not it has day pupils—must provide sleeping accommodation for all boarding pupils.

34 Pupils age 8 years and over (Y4 and above) must not share sleeping accommodation with pupils of the opposite sex.

35 There are minimum floor areas for pupils' dormitories, cubicles and bedrooms.

Dormitories

36 To find the minimum floor area which must be provided:

* multiply the number of pupils sleeping in the dormitory by **4. 2 m squared** and

* add **1.6 m squared** to the result.

37 There should be a distance of at least **0.9m** between any two beds in a dormitory.

Bedrooms and cubicles

38 A cubicle for a single pupil must have its own window and a minimum floor area of **5.0m squared.**

39 A bedroom for a single pupil must have a minimum floor area of **6.0 m squared.**

Washrooms for boarding pupils

40 Boarding schools must have water closets, washbasins, baths and showers which are reasonably accessible to the sleeping accommodation. There must be at least one water closet for every five pupils, and at least one washbasin for every three of the first 60 boarding pupils, for every four of the next 40 boarding pupils and for every five further boarding pupils. The number of pupils should always be **rounded up** to the next multiple of three, four or five as appropriate.

41 For example, a school with 30 boarding pupils would need six water closets and 10 washbasins. But a school with 31 boarding pupils would need seven water closets and 11 washbasins.

42 The minimum number of baths or showers is one for every 10 boarding pupils: the number of pupils being **rounded up** to the next multiple of 10 if it is not a multiple of 10. **At least** 25% of that number must be baths (so, if 25% of the minimum number does not produce a whole number, the answer should again be rounded **up**.)

43 A school with 30 boarding pupils would therefore need three fittings, at least one of which must be a bath, while a school with 31 boarding pupils would need four fittings, at least one of which must be a bath.

Living accommodation for boarding pupils

44 All boarding schools must include living accommodation for the boarding pupils with a total floor area of at least **2. 3 m squared for** each pupil. Any social areas such as common rooms, games rooms and TV rooms should be included in the calculation, as should areas set aside for private study outside school hours. Other areas in which pupils socialise also count as living accommodation. These will vary from school to school, but may include kitchens where pupils can prepare hot drinks and snacks; and other, informal meeting areas.

45 The following rooms or spaces are also taken into account in calculating the minimum area:

* study bedrooms/cubicles; and

*   any part of the school adjacent to the boarding accommodation, which pupils can appropriately use for social purposes or private study outside school hours.

Accommodation for cooking and eating

46   All boarding schools should have somewhere to prepare meals for boarding pupils (see paragraph 32 above) and also somewhere for them to eat. This does not have to be within the boarding accommodation, providing it is part of the school **and** is adjacent to the boarding accommodation.

Sick rooms

47   A boarding school must have one or more sick rooms —and if the school has more than 40 boarding pupils, one or more separate isolation rooms and associated facilities such as baths, washbasins and water closets.

48   The minimum floor areas of sick rooms and isolation rooms are larger than those in ordinary dormitories, and so is the minimum distance between the beds. There should be at least **7.4m squared** of floor area for each bed, and a distance of at least **1.8m** between any two beds. If **cubicles** are provided within sick rooms, each cubicle should have its own window. The requirement to have associated facilities 'by way of baths, washbasins and water closets' does not of course, prevent schools from providing *additional* facilities, such as showers for their sick rooms.

Accommodation for residential staff

49   Accommodation for residential staff, whether teachers or otherwise, must be separate from accommodation for boarding pupils. The staff accommodation should include somewhere for the staff to eat, somewhere for them to sleep and an appropriate number of baths, showers, washbasins and water closets.

Storage facilities

50   A boarding school shall include adequate storage facilities for pupils' belongings and adequate storage facilities for the storage and care of linen.

Statutory Regulations

As in all school buildings

   (a)   Environmental Health Regulations

   (b)   Safety at Work Regulations

   (c)   Fire Regulations

   (d)   C.O.S.H.H. Regulations

   (e)   R.I.D.D.O.R. Regulations must be observed

In co-educational schools there must be facilities to nurse boys and girls in separate rooms, but it is a mistake to earmark individual rooms to be used by each sex. It is better to have an adaptable arrangement and allow the nurse in charge to manipulate the placement of beds as is most fitting.

A large proportion of rooms should be in one bed units which can be used for isolation and observation but it should be borne in mind that many children prefer to be in a room with someone else with whom they can talk and, for this reason, two-bedded rooms are useful. Secondary or cross infection can be minimised by adequate bed spacing.

In school sanatoria which are being purpose built, toilet facilities should be located adjacent to the bedrooms. In all cases where girls are catered for there must be adequate provision for the disposal of soiled sanitary towels, preferably within each female toilet.

Near bath and shower rooms, there must be provision for the patients to undress and dress and they should be allowed to bathe or shower in privacy.

In all schools which provide a variety of sporting activities, there should be a room close to the treatment room available for patients with acute injuries and for injured patients who have received attention, who are awaiting transport home or to their house. As well as being near the treatment room it should be borne in mind that the nearer to the entrance this room is situated, the smaller is the amount of mud which will be introduced into the sanatorium.

There should be a room near to the staff quarters where patients who have been concussed, or who for any other reason, require observation can be nursed and observed over night.

If X-ray facilities are provided in the sanatorium, and this can save both time and expense in cases where the school is some distance from a hospital, the X-ray department should be situated near to both the treatment room and the doctor's consulting room. Care should be taken to see that the unit complies with regulations governing the use of X-ray apparatus and does not contravene Safety at Work or COSHH Regulations. The treatment room should be properly equipped and allow sufficient space to permit more than one patient to be examined or treated at any one time, with of course, adequate screening between patients.

There should be a well equipped consulting room for the doctor which, ideally, will have been designed by him, or her. For sight testing the patient must be able to stand 6 metres from the chart.

Within the sanatorium there should be recreation rooms and a dining room for convalescent patients, and where possible, there should be access to a balcony or garden. Television points should be in every room.

Medical Records

A questionnaire should be completed before the entry of each pupil giving the medical history. Where there has been significant illness, an accompanying letter from the family doctor or the hospital consultant is helpful. The form should be signed by the parent or guardian and sent to the school before the pupil's acceptance, which in rare instances may have to be postponed or even refused. (The sample questionnaire printed in Appendix L, will serve as a guide.)

In the case of pupils moving from preparatory schools to independent schools, it is of great help to the doctor of the latter if a card is sent on ahead of the pupil bearing his name, date of birth, NHS number and immunisation status, together with details of any allergies, drug sensitivities and current treatment. In the maintained schools, this information is recorded on Form 19M which should be forwarded without delay to the doctor of the new school, via the Consultant Community Paediatrician or the Consultant in Public Health Medicine, under the National Health Regulations. The private school medical officer has the normal responsibilities for maintaining records on Forms FP7 and 8. Also, it is desirable that special records shall be kept for each pupil, recording the data on the entrance questionnaire, the findings at the initial medical examination and such events of medical importance as occur during the school life of the pupil. Records must be conspicuously marked with details of any drug allergies or sensitivities and haemoglobin abnormalities and the information should be immediately available to medical and nursing staff. All this can be incorporated in an A4 file, wherein all correspondence and hospital reports and the like can be filed and which is retained after the pupil has left school. The alternative is a school medical record card which can be placed in the pupil's FP5 or 6 on leaving school. Whatever method is used, it is imperative that a summary is placed in the NHS card or envelope and a rubber stamp, worded as follows, on the FP7 or 8, can be useful. i. e.

This patient was a pupil at...School from.................to....................

If further details are required, please write to the Medical Officer, ... School..

The Access to Medical Records Act (1990) came into effect on 1st November 1991 in England, Scotland and Wales, but not Northern Ireland. The Act affords patients the right of access (subject to some exceptions) to their manually held records. Under the provisions of the Data Protection Act (1984), access to computerised records has been available since 1985. School doctors need to be aware that the Act applies to all the medical records appertaining to any pupil in their care, i. e. the NHS records on Forms FP7 and FP8 and other medical details recorded elsewhere during the pupil's stay at the school. The Act applies to medical details recorded after 1st, November 1991. Ordinarily, there is no right of access to medical records constructed before that date unless this is necessary to clarify the meaning of the accessible records. Health records are made in respect of a person by any health professional. Thus, in addition to records made by doctors the Act applies equally to records made by dentists, nurses, psychologists, speech therapists, optometrists, etc.

Children of 16 and 17 and even younger children, provided they can convince the school doctor or the other health professional concerned, that they are capable of understanding the nature of their request, will be able to apply to see their records. The school doctor or other professional concerned should accede to the pupil's request provided, having regard to the contents of the records, that to do so would be in the best interests of the pupil. Access may be declined for example, if, in the opinion of the record holder, such disclosure would be injurious to the pupil's physical or mental health.

When pupils see the notes, it is preferable that the school doctor should be available at the time in order to explain medical terminology or any other points which may be unclear to the pupil. Alternatively, the eligible pupil may request a written copy of the records after giving due notice, for which service a fee may be charged, subject to the doctor's contract with the school.

After perusal of the records, the pupil may consider that there should be some amendment or correction, which, if agreed, should be inserted without removing or obscuring the original entry. If the amendment or correction is not agreed, there is a statutory obligation to note it in the appropriate part of the records. The supplying of the amended or corrected version of the records attracts no further fee. Full, objective and accurate notes, legibly written, about all clinical dealings with pupils and their parents would be most helpful, not only in the implementation of the above Act, but in all school medicine.

Medical Regulations.

Medical regulations should be formulated so that parents are properly informed about the school's requirements. The need for quarantine and isolation has now almost disappeared in respect of diseases commonly acquired in the United Kingdom, but in contrast, greater vigilance is needed in respect of some pupils returning from abroad, to prevent the spread of enteric and other infections.

A clear statement should be obtained from the parents or guardians about medical insurance, especially in respect of boarding school pupils. It is important for the school doctor to know if the family subscribes to a provident association and prefers private treatment from consultants. Also, it is important to encourage all parents to participate in an insurance scheme. Details of such schemes are discussed in the chapter on Sports Injuries.

Confidentiality

For both doctors and nurses, clear guide lines are laid down regarding their obligation to maintain professional confidentiality. In essence, a duty of confidentiality is owed to all patients from birth to death and beyond, although there are clearly defined situations where a doctor or nurse may break that confidence. The General Medical Council (GMC) on behalf of doctors and the United Kingdom Central Council (UKCC) for nurses are responsible for maintaining professional standards and a breach of confidence by either a doctor or a nurse may render them liable to disciplinary proceedings by their respective professional body.

Some situations where confidential information may be disclosed to a third party may include:

when the patient gives informed consent or a person properly authorised to act on the patient's behalf gives consent.

when the information is passed between members of a health care team caring for that patient. In schools, the team might consist of the school doctor and his/her partners, school nurses, physiotherapists, chiropodists, psychologists and counsellors. Additionally, some individuals outside the health care professions might be involved in looking after pupils e. g. house matrons and other lay staff providing pastoral care. It is the doctor's responsibility to ensure firstly, that pupils and their parents understand why and when information might be disclosed to any team member and secondly, that all the other team members understand and observe confidentiality, as noted below.

When a medical emergency means a patient's consent cannot be obtained e. g. serious accident or unconsciousness.

When it is considered that disclosure, without the patient's consent, is in their medical interests. The doctor may judge that because of immaturity, illness or mental incapacity the patient is unable to give valid consent. If the patient will not allow the involvement of an appropriate third party to represent their interests, the doctor may disclose relevant information. The patient must be informed before disclosure and it should be recognised that the judgment of whether a patient is capable of withholding consent to treatment or disclosure must be based on their ability to under stand the situation, and not solely on their age; this is important in boarding schools because of the wide age range encountered.

When it is believed that the patient is a victim of neglect or physical or sexual abuse and in schools doctors should be aware of any statutory obligations they may have in connection with child protection matters.

When the information is required or requested for medical teaching, research or audit.

When it is judged that disclosure is in the public's interests and failure to disclose may expose a patient, or others to risk of death or serious harm.

When satisfying a specific statutory requirement. e. g. notification of a communicable disease.

When ordered to do so by a judge or the presiding officer of a court or if summoned to assist a coroner, procurator fiscal or other similar officer in connection with an inquest or comparable judicial investigation.

In any school there is much information available regarding any one pupil and this information travels in different directions between various members of staff. Most of the information is not sensitive or controversial but the recipient of the information makes his or her own value judgment about whether it is kept confidential or passed on to a third party. A number of factors help to make that particular judgment and there also has to be a framework within the school itself for handling personal information about pupils.

Certain subjects may be judged more sensitive than others e. g.

bereavement

parental separation or divorce

serious physical or mental illness

suicide or attempted suicide

physical abuse—bullying, sexual abuse and actual rape

substance misuse including alcohol and tobacco, and illegal substances e.g. cannabis, ecstasy, heroin or LSD

sexual problems—contraception, pregnancy and abortion

eating disorders—anorexia nervosa and bulimia nervosa

serious academic problems

disciplinary matters

Knowledge about any of these may come from any source and the school doctor or nurse may or may not be involved. Medical confidentiality does not distinguish between the various conditions and situations and the doctor owes the same duty of confidentiality to a pupil consulting because of a cold as to one seeking an abortion. In the same way that there must be no distinction between the reasons for the consultation. Confidentiality must be maintained regarding the treatment given and even the fact that the consultation had taken place at all. Similarly, age is not a consideration and the duty of confidentiality owed to a pupil under 16 is as great as that owed to any other person.

However, in practice, it is obvious that the doctor will take different actions according to the nature of the presenting problem and part of his or her management might involve informing a third party. Ideally, if disclosure of information is judged to be necessary, it will be with the pupil's consent but should not be made without first discussing it with the pupil whose co-operation is being sought. In any situation where confidentiality is breached, the doctor must be prepared to justify his decision, possibly before the General Medical Council.

The doctor and nurse in any school are in both a privileged and difficult position with regard to matters of confidentiality. On the one hand they are contracted to the school to provide a range of medical and nursing services, yet on the other they have their own professional obligations and standards to observe and uphold. The latter requirements are the greater and difficulties can and do arise where the doctor and nurse, as the recipients of much varied, and often delicate, information have to balance their obligations to the pupils with the school's 'need to know.' This is particularly pertinent in the boarding situation where the governing body, head teacher, academic and non-academic staff are acting in *loco parentis* and are expected to be in possession of certain information about the pupils for whom they have responsibility. Through discussion with the various parties, it should be possible to strike this balance and it is incumbent on the doctor and nurse to make the school aware of the ethical responsibilities they have.

Every school, should have a medical policy which sets down the way in which medical care will be provided in that particular institution. This policy should reflect the philosophy of the school and the needs of the parents and pupils. It should also refer to the doctor's professional and ethical obligations. and it is recommended that a paragraph about confidentiality is included, in the School's Prospectus. e. g.,

'In accordance with the school doctor's professional obligations, medical information about pupils, regardless of their age, will remain confidential. However, in providing medical care for a pupil, it is recognised that on occasions the doctor may liase with parents or guardians, the head teacher or other academic staff and house staff, and that information, ideally with the pupil's prior consent, will be passed on as appropriate. With all matters, the doctor will respect a pupil's confidence except on the very rare occasions when, having failed to persuade a pupil, or his or her authorised representative, to give consent to divulgence, the doctor considers it in the pupil's better interests, or necessary for the protection of the wider school community, to breach confidence and pass information to a relevant person or body.'

Note. This specimen paragraph may be amended according to the ages of the pupils and the type of school e. g. preparatory or senior, day or boarding, co-educational or single sex and state or independent.

School Closure

Even in the days when poliomyelitis was common, MOSA argued forcefully against the practice of school closure as a preventive measure. In today's conditions, it is hard to envisage any situation which would justify it and such a move should certainly never be contemplated without prior discussion with the Director of Public Health.

Advisory Responsibilities of the School Doctor
Diet

School catering is increasingly managed by professionally qualified staff. The school meals service is generally controlled and subject to financial restraint by the education authorities, and the individual school doctor can have little influence over it. In independent schools his responsibilities are greater and he should be concerned to see that the diet is nutritionally balanced, sufficiently varied, attractively served and adequate for the energy needs of the growing child.

The school doctor should use his influence to encourage a diet high in fibre, low in animal fat and sugar, and to discourage excessive and frequent intake of foods and drinks which lead to dental caries, for the number of times that sugar enters the mouth is the most important factor in determining the rate of dental decay.

Bran-containing breakfast cereals should be encouraged, together with the consumption of whole meal bread and fresh fruit, with the active disapproval of the consumption of sucrose rich drinks. Liaison with the tuck- shop manager over the hours of opening and the types of food sold there can be helpful. The doctor should take an interest in the type of cooking oils used in the kitchens, in order to encourage the use of polyunsaturated fats such as corn oil rather than the cheaper substitutes.

It is important to have a policy on diet and nutrition in schools, which follows H.M. Government Guidelines, of which everyone in the school should be aware. The headteacher and all the teaching staff, the school doctor and dental surgeon, the catering staff and the bursar should know about it and do what they can to implement it enthusiastically, in discussions with parents and children. To this end, it would be helpful if school doctors and dental surgeons could establish contact with their local health promotion service, or the Health Education Authority, in order to obtain up to date literature and other resource material. No doubt effective health education in schools will adhere to the requirements of the National Curriculum. (No5.)

Obesity is a common condition in growing children today and the school doctor should consult with the catering staff on the provision of a satisfactory low-calorie diet. He should also advise about the diet for diabetic pupils and other pupils with special dietary needs.

Nowadays, many young people are attracted to the vegetarian way of life and schools are having increasing numbers of requests from pupils for vegetarian diets. These requests should receive sympathetic consideration but before acceding to them it would seem prudent, where applicable, for the doctor to obtain informed, written parental permission and to ensure that the pupil has a clear understanding of his or her dietary needs. The doctor should enlist the co-operation of the catering staff to ensure that the vegetarian meals are correctly and willingly supplied.

Rest and Exercise

In the last century, MOSA has been concerned to prevent the erosion by boarding schools of the hours of sleep needed by pupils. In the light of present knowledge, it is not possible to be dogmatic and the subject does not appear to have merited much attention of recent years. A fifteen year old study, which measured the inclusive duration of sleep of pupils of various ages, made clear that sleep needs differ considerably, even among children of the same age, so that it was not possible to specify the exact amount of sleep required at any particular age. The most useful guide we have is 11 hours at 7 years of age, 10 hours at 11 years and 9 hours at 15 years. Half an hour seems a reasonable time between the end of a meal and the resumption of vigorous exercise. (1)

Dental Supervision

The school doctor should be concerned with the provision of good dental care. In maintained schools, the Health Authority is obliged to arrange for all children to be dentally inspected by the Community Dental Service, and the school medical officer may refer pupils to the Community Dental Officer. In independent schools, it is possible for the children to miss this service unless the school doctor takes steps to see that there is a reliable routine by which children see a dentist during the school holidays.

An alternative solution is for boarding schools to arrange for a dentist to carry out regular inspections and treatment in term-time of all pupils except those whose parents wish them to remain under the care of a dental surgeon at home. Such an arrangement is particularly appropriate with increasing numbers of pupils undergoing treatment with orthodontic appliances, and the use of mouthguards in contact sports. It can also be most helpful to have a local dental surgeon to provide immediate care in cases of dental injury. The dental surgeon attending a school may also make a contribution to group and individual health education on the preventive aspects of oral health. This should include the care of teeth and gums, the discouragement of caries-producing diets and the prevention of sports injury by the use of mouthguards. (See 'Sports Injuries').

If there is no visiting dental surgeon problems may arise in the care of pupils from overseas who are away from home for long periods of time and who have no constant or holiday address in the UK. Usually, satisfactory arrangements for the dental care of these pupils can be made locally: hopefully with minimal disruption of their schooling. (See Appendix E for Dental Care in schools.)

Counselling

The school doctor should be in a position to arrange counselling or to co-ordinate the agencies which are available, to act as a link between teaching staff and the school psychological service. Some independent schools have their own counsellor. Other independent schools have found it valuable to retain the services of a psychiatrist with an interest in child and adolescent emotional disorders. (See also, 'School Nursing' for further information about counselling.)

Remuneration

Doctors on the staff of the Consultant Community Paediatrician working in the maintained sector are remunerated according to the National Scale.

Independent Schools

At the beginning of the National Health Service in 1948, it was established that medical officers of independent schools would normally accept pupils attending such schools as patients on their NHS list, and receive, in addition to their NHS remuneration for this, a fee from the school for duties outside the NHS. (See earlier in this Chapter.)

For large schools, say those with in excess of 400 pupils, the doctor may be paid on a sessional basis in accordance with the rates of pay appropriate for a part-time occupational physician. These rates are available from local offices of the BMA and, in accordance with the DDRB, are revised annually.

For smaller schools, MOSA and the BMA recommend a 'per capita' fee and it is common practice in many fee-paying schools for these charges to be passed on to the parents by the school authorities. It must be emphasised that no fee can be claimed for any duty which is covered by the National Health Service Act, 1946. The duties which are covered by the fee are listed earlier in this chapter. Doctors, who are in receipt of the recommended fee for their duties outside the NHS may well waive some of the fees on the list. The exact fee is a matter of negotiation by the medical officer and the school, who are advised to enter into a contract which provides for an annual salary review. (See Appendix K). Guidance on the amount of capitation fee to be negotiated is provided annually by MOSA and the BMA. The MOSA recommended fee is circulated to Members and the BMA recommendation is included in Section VI of the Fees section of the Handbook. Since 1988, the BMA and MOSA have recommended the same fee for medical officers in independent schools. The suggested fee for 1997 was £33.50 per pupil per annum.

In negotiating with the school, the doctor should take into account the other benefits of his office such as use of the school's sporting facilities and (possibly) a discount on school fees, should he choose to have his children educated at the school.

Very recently, changes have taken place in the NHS, with regard to GP on-call duties and school doctors who are in GP partnerships, should be mindful of their contract with the school, if they are contemplating joining deputising organisations and co-operatives. They should make sure that any new arrangements they make with regard to provision of 'out of hours' services have the approval of the head and the school authorities. Most schools readily accept the services of the school doctor's GP partners in providing these services in the school doctor's legitimate absence, since they will be *au fait* with the school and the local medical facilities, but an unknown doctor from another town, without any knowledge of the school or its environs, might not be acceptable to the school.

References

1. Klackenberg, G. (1982) Sleep behaviour studied longitudinally. Acta Pediatr, Scand. 71. 501.

CHAPTER 2

PREVENTIVE MEDICINE IN SCHOOLS

General Hygiene

The school doctor should interest himself in the general hygiene of the school, reports on which, to the School Governing Body may be part of his contract. His colleagues in Public Health Medicine are available for guidance.

School Premises

Standards are laid down in the Education (School Premises) Regulations 1995; a summary of the main provisions are in Chapter 1.

Swimming Pools
Treatment and Quality of Water in Swimming Pools.

There is no obvious alternative to chlorine as a water disinfectant, but chlorine gas has been phased out and an alternative source of chlorine has to be used. Whichever chlorine donor is decided upon, the active constituent is hypochlorous acid, which is measured in a swimming pool as the 'free chlorine residual.' This kills micro-organisms and also reacts with other bather contaminants, mainly urea and creatinine, to produce various irritants to mucous membranes. Some of these are volatile and produce the characteristic swimming pool odour. They also cause irritation of the eyes and the respiratory system, e. g. conjunctivitis and pharyngitis. All these irritant substances are combined in the 'combined chlorine residual.' To minimise irritation, this should not be allowed to rise above one part per million. With a high bathing load and therefore heavy bather contamination, the combined chlorine residual should be kept low by frequent back washing of the filters to dilute the pool water. Additional fresh water may be added to the pool. Chlorine itself does not cause eye and respiratory irritation in the absence of bather contaminants; a free chlorine residual high enough to bleach hair and costumes is comfortable for swimming in the absence of contamination.

A well-maintained pool will be clear and colourless, but the pool and its surrounds may give the water a blue appearance. It should not be obviously cloudy, and it should be possible to see clearly through 40 feet of water, not only for aesthetic reasons but also to minimise the risk of drowning accidents. Green colouration which is thought to be due to algae should be treated with five times the usual level of free chlorine residual; the filters should be kept running 24 hours a day and the high chlorine left to attain normal levels before bathing is resumed.

Eye Irritation

Any liquid which is not isotonic causes some eye irritation, but the main causes are the substances contained in the combined chlorine residual. Other chemicals can aggravate eye irritation, such as algicides, which should preferably be avoided, and other salts which are used to correct pH. Non-physiological pH can also affect the eyes. There is no evidence that eye irritation is any less with non-chlorine based disinfectants, despite advertisements to the contrary.

Swimming Pool Rash and Swimmers' Ear

The pre-disposing and causal factors for these conditions are very similar. They include wetting, wetting/drying cycles, degreasing and dewaxing by the disinfectants, infection (usually with some serotypes of Pseudomonas aeruginosa), chemical irritation and lack of acclimatisation. In subjects who swim less than once a day, otitis externa should affect less than 1% of a large sample at any time, unless a failure of disinfection has allowed bacteria to build up in the pool. If more than 10% are affected by otitis externa, then infection of the pool is almost certain. When infection builds up in a pool, swimmers are first affected by otitis externa. Swimming pool body rash occurs only with heavy bacterial contamination of the pool or, because of an individual's susceptibility to the disinfectant.[1]

Choice of Disinfectant

Technical details of the choice of swimming pool disinfectants and methods of working for pool staff are given in Appendix D.

Swimming Pool Safety

This is dealt with in the Chapter 'Safety at School.'

Water and Food Hygiene
Water Supply

Nearly all schools are supplied with mains water from the local Water Authority which is responsible for the supply. In rare cases where schools have their own water supply the school medical officer will need the assistance of his local Environmental Health Officer to ensure that the water is regularly tested and where essential, chlorinated. Another important check is to ensure that plumbo solvency and pH are satisfactory. In some older school premises a search should be made for lead lined storage tanks and lead pipes.

Milk Supply

All milk supplied to schools should be pasteurised. Domestic methods of heat treatment are unreliable and home produced milk is best disposed of to The Milk Marketing Board, which carries out bulk pasteurisation. Milk borne outbreaks of salmonellosis and campylobacter jejuni enteritis appear to be increasing even though they can be completely prevented by pasteurisation. In Scotland, it has been illegal to supply unpasteurised milk since 1983.

Kitchen Hygiene

School kitchens come within the provision of the Food Hygiene (General) Regulations 1970. The Environmental Health Officer has the responsibility for the inspection and maintenance of satisfactory standards. The school doctor should not only be familiar with these regulations, but he should visit kitchens and dining rooms and be prepared to advise catering staff.

Adequate sanitary facilities, including wash basins with hot water, soap and disposable paper towels or hot air driers must be provided for catering staff. Notices should be displayed near lavatories advising users to wash their hands. First Aid boxes which include waterproof dressings, must be provided. The contents must be frequently inspected and replaced as necessary. Adequate ventilation and lighting are important for the efficient working of kitchen staff. Waste should be removed from the kitchen. Refuse bins, galvanised with lids or disposable plastic sacks should be placed in a dry area outside the kitchen. Some authorities will hire out large refuse containers for institutional use.

Separate stores should be provided for dry goods and for prepared foods. Adequate refrigeration is essential. The time between cooking and eating all moist dishes especially those containing meat, should be as short as possible, unless provision is made for storage at a temperature above 145 degrees F (62. 5 degrees C) or in the cold. The Food Hygiene Regulations require hot food to be kept at a temperature of not less than 145 degrees F (62.5 degrees C) and food can be eaten cold below 50 degrees F (10 degrees C). Masses of food are more difficult to heat and slower to cool, hence cuts of meat should be limited in size to 6lbs (2.73 kg) or less. Meat should be prepared and cooked on the day it is eaten. The reheating of all food must be actively discouraged and it should never be left overnight in a warm kitchen. Meat eaten cold should be cooled rapidly, preferably in a cold room with a fan, and transferred to the refrigerator within one and a half hours of cooking. The temperature of refrigerators should be checked to ensure that a temperature of 34-38 degrees F (1-4 degrees C) is being maintained.

In a review of over 1000 outbreaks of food poisoning and salmonellosis, the Food Hygiene Laboratory at Colindale found that in more than 60% of the outbreaks the food had been prepared for over half a day before it was consumed.[2] The report continued:'This alone would not necessarily cause food poisoning but in combination with inadequate cooking and storage, food prepared earlier becomes an extremely important factor. The main factors were storage at ambient temperature (39%), inadequate cooking (31.9%), inadequate reheating (28.5%) and use of contaminated food (19.1%). Contaminated foods included meats and poultry, pies and 'Take Away 'meals prepared in premises other than those in which the final dish was consumed, but not canned foods.' The report notes that infected food handlers did not play a significant role in causing food poisoning except in Staph. aureus food poisoning.

The school doctor should be available to advise on the health of kitchen staff. Superficial cuts on the fingers or hands should be carefully covered and supervised. In the event of skin sepsis or gastrointestinal infection, those who handle food should be excluded from work until symptomatically recovered and bacteriologically free from infection. The local Environmental Health Officer will advise in cases of difficulty, but a negative swab from a skin lesion and three consecutive negative samples of faeces taken at intervals of two days would be reasonable.

Health of Staff

School doctors are often asked whether an applicant for a teaching, administrative or domestic post is medically fit to be employed. In doing so, he cannot reveal the reasons for his decision without the applicant's permission.

Before an important post is filled it is advisable for the school doctor to examine the applicant and possibly to contact the applicant's general practitioner, before declaring him fit for employment. DFEE regulations no longer require a chest X-ray for entrants to the teaching profession. Female staff should be advised regarding protection against rubella. Vigilance is required in the case of part-time workers as well as full-time domestic staff. Immigrants have a risk of importing tuberculosis and other diseases. Immigrant workers may also be employed by catering contractors whose own standards of surveillance may not be as high as that of the school to which they are contracted. (See Appendix G).

Isolation

Now that dangerous communicable diseases are rare and treated in hospitals, there is much less need for isolation in schools. Single rooms should be used for treating patients with extensive skin sepsis, streptococcal throat infections, gastro intestinal infections and viral hepatitis. Individual towels and eating utensils are helpful but strict barrier nursing is unlikely to be practicable in a school sanatorium.

Scrupulous attention to personal hygiene and hand washing is essential and if any blood is to be taken, then disposable gloves should always be worn and the specimen container put in a sealed plastic bag, clearly labelled, before transmission to the laboratory. If there is a suspected or known hepatitis risk then the specimen bag must be appropriately labelled. The needle should not be resheathed and the used syringe and needle should be placed in the special 'Sharps' container for this purpose. If anyone is pricked by a hypodermic needle after it has been used on a patient the skin should be washed immediately. The incident should then be reported to the school doctor and the appointed accident officer in maintained schools, or to the bursar in independent schools, observing the agreed local procedure.

Spilled blood, faeces, vomit or urine should be covered with a one in ten hypochlorite disinfectant solution, before being mopped up by a member of staff wearing disposable gloves and apron. The mopping up material and gloves and aprons shall be disposed of in a 'dirty dressing' plastic bag for incineration. Used 'sharps' should not be left lying around and the sharps container should not be overfilled.

Disposable urinals and bedpans are preferable to the older variety which required sterilising after use, and of course, hands must be thoroughly washed after using them. School doctors, nurses and all sanatorium staff should be immunised against hepatitis B.

Quarantine

There is no justification for excluding contacts of communicable disease from schools, except in the very rare cases of diphtheria, typhoid and poliomyelitis. Even then, the local Director of Public Health or his Communicable Disease Consultant Colleague should be consulted about the need for, and duration of exclusion. It may be advisable to exclude nursery school children whose siblings have bacillary dysentery.

School Medical Examinations

School medical examinations have been a vital part of preventive medicine ever since their compulsory introduction in 1907.

Since April 1990, there has been a more structured form of child surveillance carried out by most GP practices so that children should have had any defects identified and appropriate treatment instituted long before their examination on school entry.[3]

Repeated routine medical examinations have been abandoned in favour of selective follow-up of children with identified special needs. Court recommended that 'every boy and girl about the age of 13 should have a private interview with the school doctor': in the independent sector, this may conveniently be on entry to school.[3,4] However, regular screening for visual acuity and for colour vision, hearing, height and weight are necessary throughout school life. Recent discussion on the value of blood pressure measurement has indicated that perhaps this is not justified at this stage, yet it is always helpful to have an early base line reading at about 13 years of age, especially for girls, in anticipation of their need for oral contraception in a few years.

The School Medical Examination

This is perhaps the most important medical examination of school life and is, preferably, conducted in the child's second term. However, children already identified as having special needs or handicaps ideally, should be seen as soon as possible after school entry, thus minimising the delay in informing staff who need to know about their condition. Preferably too, the parents and the teacher should be present at the unhurried examination which should take at least 15 minutes. This will allow time for assessment of the child's physical, intellectual and emotional development.

Screening tests, which are usually carried out by nursing staff, take place a day or so before the examination and in maintained schools, the results of the tests and the examination findings are entered, with the social and medical history on Form 10. Independent schools will usually use their own forms.

Screening Tests
Height and Weight

Reference to the Height and Weight charts (see Appendix C) will identify children falling outside the normal range for their age and sex and these will require scrutiny. Obesity is a common finding and the doctor should take the opportunity of advising parents and the child regarding ways of combating this. Rarely, children with growth hormone deficiency or hypothyroidism are detected at such examinations when there still may be time for useful treatment.

Hearing

Even mild, intermittent or selective hearing loss, if undiagnosed will place the child at an educational and social disadvantage. Parents, who are usually very astute at detecting hearing loss in their children, occasionally may fail. Thus, all children on school entry should be screened by pure tone audiometry. The test should be carried out in optimum conditions and any child with impaired hearing should be monitored carefully throughout his school days. The school doctor will arrange appropriate ENT consultant referral and will advise teaching staff.

Vision

The Gardiner-Sheridan Stycar test or the Snellen's test may be used. The Ishihara Colour vision tests are used to detect defective colour vision. The earlier this condition is diagnosed the better, since even toddlers are disadvantaged by it. Teaching staff, especially those in art and craft, design and technology departments shall be required to be advised, as well as parents to whom it must be explained that certain careers are not possible. No treatment is of any avail. (See Appendix F, 'Colour Vision and Eye Care in Sport')

Urine

Each child should have a urine test on school entry. The dip sticks for sugar and albumin in current use are very sensitive and any positive test for albuminuria must be checked by a laboratory examination of a 'clean catch' early morning sample. Any malodorous or cloudy urine should have further laboratory examinations, with follow up and investigations as indicated.

Screening for Haemoglobinopathies

The trait of sickle cell anaemia and other haemoglobinopathies may be carried by African-Caribbean, Mediterranean and some Eastern races. If the children of these races are born in the UK, they are screened soon after birth, Children from these races who are born overseas should have their blood taken for haemoglobinopathy screening preferably as soon as possible after entry into school. (See Chapter 11.).

Parental Attendance

With the results of the screening tests, and a brief medical history regarding the patient, obtained in advance by means of a questionnaire, the examination may commence. Parents have a legal right to be present in maintained schools and should be encouraged to do so. If parents express a wish to be present at a medical examination of their child in an independent school, then they too, must be made welcome.

Education authorities have a duty to examine children unless the parent objects and examinations should proceed in the absence of the parent. When possible, the doctor obtains the obstetric and perinatal history from the parent and also information from the clinical notes. He should enquire about past illnesses and discuss any parental worries or anxieties.

The Physical Examination

During the early stages of each examination, the doctor will note the general appearance of the children, the colour of their mucous membranes, their gait, the presence of any asymmetry and whether their development and behaviour are appropriate to their age and situation. As they draw a picture, observation should be made about their laterality and their pencil grasp. A request to copy a square at the 5-year level or a circle, at the 3-year level, is a quick test to indicate any developmental retardation and other tests can be added if necessary. Children will often explain what they have drawn and so give the doctor an opportunity to hear them speak. If not, then some gentle questioning should elicit a response.

A full physical examination is required, but preferably undressing should not be attempted until the end of the interview when most children are then ready to accept removal of their clothes, including socks and shoes. By this stage, the majority of children will have spoken, but if not, the doctor should assess their speech and articulation by asking them to repeat sentences or to name pictures in a book. Abnormalities of speech in school children are commonly found amongst infants and it is important to be sure that their hearing is normal before they are referred for speech therapy.

Children who, on screening, have been found to have visual defects should be examined promptly for abnormalities such as inequality of pupils or nystagmus and should be tested for squint, using the corneal light reflex and the cover test. Fundoscopy, an assessment of the ocular tension and an estimate of the visual fields on rough confrontation should be undertaken to complete the examination. Squints, especially permanent ones, must be referred promptly for ophthalmological assessment.

The general examination is best started with the child standing as this is convenient for examining the head, eyes, ears, nose, throat and chest. Both radial and femoral pulses should be palpated. If these are present, synchronous and with normal pulsation, then an aortic coarctation will be excluded. In this position many heart murmurs are inaudible and the heart and chest should then be examined with the child supine, before and after exercise. The laterality and the position of the apex beat should be checked and the chest wall palpated there with the flat of the hand in order to detect any thrill. The heart rhythm and sounds should be checked and any murmurs noted. These should be timed and careful note taken of the direction in which the murmurs are propagated. Next, the child should be asked to take a breath and hold it, and then breath normally, before being asked to extend the neck, whilst the heart is again auscultated. These manoeuvres are then repeated after the child has exercised for a short time. Occasionally, this will reveal the presence of murmurs not previously noted at rest. Murmurs which disappear on neck extension or on breath holding, only to reappear when breathing normally and in the usual position of the neck, are most likely to be due to turbulence of blood in the great vessels, the diameters of which are altered on neck extension or downward travel of the diaphragm, and these murmurs are almost certainly benign.

If a murmur persists despite neck extension or deep breathing then any propagation to the axilla or up to the carotid arteries must be carefully noted, bearing in mind the possibilities of a ventricular septal defect and aortic stenosis respectively. If a systolic, or (especially) a diastolic murmur is heard, or a thrill is palpated, then cardiological advice should be sought early. This will permit the timely assessment of any cardiac lesion and indicate the need for prophylactic antibiotics for dental visits. The doctor should also bear in mind that suspicion of any degree of aortic stenosis requires prompt evaluation, with particular reference to the amount of strenuous exercise the child may undertake, since this is one cardiac lesion which can cause sudden death. Pending such cardiological evaluation, the child must avoid severe exertion.

The chest should be percussed and auscultated and even in the absence of adventitious sounds, peak flow readings should be taken and plotted against the height and age curves.

The hernial orifices and the external genitalia should be examined. Checks should be made on the retractability of foreskins and advice given regarding removal of smegma, where necessary. Boys with undescended testicles, varicoceles, epididymal cysts and dense degrees of phimosis should be referred for an early surgical opinion. It is reassuring to note, in girls, the presence of a normal hymenal orifice and the absence of cysts in the breasts.

The child should be asked to bend forward with knees straight, to touch toes, This should reveal the presence of any scoliosis, especially if the scapulae are viewed along the line of the flexed spine and at right angles to it. Any asymmetry of the scapulae, or bunching of the ribs on one side of the chest would strongly suggest a scoliosis. An X-ray of chest, and/or referral would be helpful, if suspected.

If the child is unable to touch toes, then this may indicate an osteochondritic vertebral lesion, especially if there is a complaint of, or history of backache. Then an X-ray of the thoraco lumbo sacral spine or perhaps an orthopaedic opinion should be considered.

Minor degrees of flat feet, especially if they are asymptomatic, do not usually require referral, but cases of knock knee, bowed tibiae or disturbances of gait certainly do require referral, to a podiatrist or orthopaedic surgeon, according to availability and local policy.

Finally, the lymph glands and the abdomen must be examined for the presence of any abnormality.

Subsequent Examination

The school entrance examination provides a medical history of each child. Children showing developmental delay should be reviewed regularly by the school doctor, as should those children in whom there is a physical condition likely to result in a continuing abnormality. The physical conditions which require supervision are visual or hearing defects, asthma, epilepsy, diabetes, congenital abnormality and other physical handicaps.

The adverse effects of any defect on a child's educational progress should be discussed by the doctor with the teachers and other staff who need to know, and ways of minimising these should be considered. Screening of hearing and vision should be repeated at two yearly intervals. Audiometry should be carried out again at about eight years as secretory otitis media may cause undetected hearing impairment and there must be frequent follow-up in cases of doubt.

Visual acuity must be tested on alternate years during school life because of the common onset of myopia in the years around puberty, due to orbital growth and an increase in the axial length of the eye.

Although weighing and measuring of children is no longer routine practice in many schools, there is much to commend it now that obesity and eating disorders are relatively common. The highest incidence of anorexia nervosa is among girls in independent schools, and it may readily be detected if there is a regular routine weighing and measuring of all pupils, say annually. In any case, children falling outside the 3rd and 97th centiles should have their weights and heights regularly measured and charted.

Subsequent medical examinations of first school children are performed on a selective basis. The parents complete questionnaires which are then returned to school and a decision to call up the children for further examination is made after consultation between the school doctor and the teaching staff. Examination after transfer to middle school is advisable, particularly as this may coincide with puberty and a period of rapid growth. The parents and teachers should be encouraged to bring to the school doctor's attention any emotional or behaviour problems which their children may show. If there is insufficient time to deal with a particular child adequately during the medical examination, the doctor should arrange another visit to the school or for an appointment at an appropriate clinic.

Children who are under-achieving should always be considered first of all from the medical point of view, before being referred to an educational psychologist. Apart from defective vision and hearing, other (treatable) conditions like anaemia and undiagnosed epileptic absence seizures require to be considered. If emotional or behavioural disorders are significant, then perhaps referral to a child or to an adolescent psychiatrist may be indicated.

The School Leaver Examination

This should be carried out at some time between 13 years of age and leaving school. The school leaver's fitness for all types of work should be assessed and Form Y9 completed for any pupil whose choice of employment should be restricted for health reasons, including all those with defective colour vision. Copies of the form are sent to Careers Officers and the Employment Medical Adviser. For pupils with severe handicaps, Form Y 10 may be appropriate: it is used for children in special schools and those who may qualify for registration as a disabled person.

School Medical Examination in Independent Schools

All the foregoing principles apply to independent schools as well as maintained schools. Not all independent schools arrange for medical examination and screening of their pupils, and there is no statutory duty for them to do so. It is therefore doubly important for the doctor of an independent school to examine pupils entering the schools, having obtained as full a history as possible. Briscoe has described the advantages in terms of pupil-doctor-parent relationships as well as the purely medical benefit of a thorough medical examination on public school entry.[5] Special examinations are often required for those embarking on hazardous sports or adventure training, and a suitably high standard of physical fitness must be sought.

Most independent schools make use of the following procedures to make up the confidential medical record of each pupil.

(a) A health questionnaire of the family history, previous health and immunisation history. A specimen questionnaire is provided in Appendix L.

(b) Screening tests to assess visual acuity, colour vision, hearing, weight, height, urine tests, tuberculin tests and when necessary, chest and other X-rays.

(c) The physical examination by the school doctor, who should be in possession of the above information.

In addition to these, but not necessarily as part of the medical procedures, schools may request the following which are of value to the doctor in broadening his knowledge of the pupil:

(d) A report from the child's school concerning learning, perceptual difficulties and emotional problems.

(e) Special examinations, such as psychometric testing.

References

1. Rycroft, R. J. G., and Penny, P. T. (1983) Dermatoses associated with brominated swimming pools. *Br. Med. J.,* 284, 462.

2. Roberts, D. (1982) Factors contributing to outbreaks of food poisoning in England and Wales, 1970-79. *J. Hygiene,* 89, 491.

3. Hall, D. M. B., (Ed.) (1989) *Health for all children – A Programme for Child Health Surveillance.* (Oxford Medical Publications.)

4. Court. S. D. M. (1976) Cmnd 6684 Fit for the Future. Vol 1. The report of the Committee on Child Health Services, p. 150. (London). HMSO.

5, Briscoe, J. H. D., (1982) *Evaluation of the routine medical examination of 13-year old 'public school' pupils.* Publ. Hlth. Lond., 96, 231.

Further Reading

Bain, J. (1989) Developmental Screening for all pre-school children; is it worthwhile? *J. R. Coll. Gen. Pract.* 39. 133.

Kennedy, F. D. (1988) Have school medicals had their day? *Arch. Dis. Child.* 63. 1261.

Hart, C. and Bain, J. (1989) *Child Care in General Practice 3rd. Edition. Edinburgh.* Churchill Livingstone.

Buckler, J. M. H. (1997) *A Reference Manual of Growth and Development.* (second edition) Blackwell science Ltd. Oxford and London.

CHAPTER 3

SCHOOL NURSING

Introduction

This is the first time that a chapter on school nursing has been included in the handbook. It is envisaged, with some certainty, in view of today's changing and challenging times, that it will be subjected to much criticism and will require alteration and updating very soon after publication. However, as a first attempt to describe some of the relevant issues, it is hoped that it will be of some value.

School nurses are referred to as 'she'. It was too laborious to 'he/she' every personal pronoun, but this can be altered quite easily if many male nurses become school nurses.

The title of this handbook is the first of many valuable points it has to make. School nurses should be fully integrated into the school community and thereby influence the 'health' status of the school.[1] This can be achieved opportunistically or through planned intervention eg, asthma clinics, but efforts must be made to promote good health and prevent disease, as well as to treat illness. To do this good codes of practice must have been agreed and established between all the relevant parties. This entails a high level of co-operation between the school doctor, the school nurses and the school, which is usually the employer: i.e. the board of governors, the local education authority, headmaster and bursar.

Background

School nursing has recently celebrated its centenary. However over the years many independent schools were slow to adopt change. Consequently, nurses fell behind their colleagues in terms of their professional development. The reasons were complex and in many instances were directly related to poor pay which was not linked to any RCN grading. Long hours on duty and multi-purpose roles which were professionally unsupported were offset by free accommodation. For many bursars their responsibility to the school nurse ended with writing her a cheque for pocket money at the end of the month.

All of this has seen rapid and dramatic change in recent years with an encouraging number of schools employing well qualified nurses on salaries recommended by the RCN, with contracts and conditions of employment which allow them to work and develop professionally.[2] Now, registration with the UKCC and the holding of a PIN number should be prerequisites to employment whether working as a school nurse in the independent sector or for the NHS.

In return the school is surely gaining from this investment by having a sanatorium/surgery which is professionally accountable and which offers the pupils and staff a quality of care equal to or greater than that available in the community. Independent school nurses are responsible for other peoples' children. Their duties are not only delivering medical care but they must fill the void left by parents who may be on the other side of the world.

Parents rightly have very high expectations of the medical and welfare facilities in the school of their choice, especially when they know that a break from the family unit through their decision to send a child to boarding school, may lead to emotional or physical problems. Many people play a part in addressing the needs of the growing child, but the school nurse is often in a unique position to make a valuable contribution.

> 'The practice of nursing... requires the application of knowledge and the simultaneous exercise of judgment and skill. ... Practice must be sensitive, relevant and responsive to the needs of individual patients... and have the capacity to adjust, where and when appropriate, to changing circumstances.'[2]

Role

Has the traditional role of nurses as providers of skill based, tender loving care given way to more academic principles? Is the traditional relationship between doctors and nurses acceptable to all? This is a debate that affects the whole of nursing and one in which all nurses should take part. Nursing in independent schools has been marginalised for so long, that it has been difficult for nurses to be a part of any professional discussion but if their 'house is in order' perhaps now is the right time. The profession has been subjected to accelerated evolution but if it is professionally accountable in its:

scope of practice
training and education
legal responsibilities

and if it is able to justify the trust and confidence of those whom they serve, employers and professional colleagues, they should be ready to enter into this debate. As in other areas of nursing, this rapid change will lead to some very good nurses deciding to change course or to stop practising. Obviously, age and years of service will be important factors in their decision. *But it is vitally important that the lamp is handed on!*

Nurses working in independent schools have an added responsibility to the children placed in their care. Many come from happy and caring homes to which they return for all holidays and exeats. Their medical needs may be restricted to routine medical examinations, health promotion and the occasional paracetamol tablet or plaster. But there is always a small group of children, who, as a result of chronic disease, need more help in achieving a 'normal' lifestyle. For other children, help or intervention in their lives will be needed, short or long term, as a direct result of their displaying inappropriate patterns of behaviour. Occasionally this help will include the support of professional counselling or Social Services. All nurses should be familiar with The Children Act and their local Child Protection Handbook. (See Chapter 8)[3]

'The philosophical basis of nursing is concerned with enabling the individual, whether adult or child, and his or her family to achieve and maintain their optimal physical, psychological and social well-being when that individual or his or her carers cannot achieve this unaided.' The nursing issues which surround this have been identified.[4]

Practitioners should:

work with parents to enable them to care for their children to the best of their ability;

ensure that when working with children they listen to each child, provide appropriate information and take account of the child's wishes and feelings;

identify children in need and, where appropriate, refer to Social Services;

co-operate with Social Services departments to meet the health needs of children.

Child Protection:

Health visitors and school nurses in particular may identify children in need of protection.

Practitioners may need to attend child protection conferences;

Practitioners may have to attend or write a report for the court.[4]

To all these groups of children, whose needs may range from plasters to child protection, nurses must continue to show that they care. The mutual trust and professional support of school staff particularly house parents, can only enhance this care. Nurses must not 'drop the lamp' in their efforts to keep up with innovation and change.

The relationship of school nurses with school doctors is crucial to the service which is provided and a high level of collaboration is essential. 'There are many cases where who provides the help – nurses or doctors – is less important than ensuring that the help is provided promptly'.[5]

It is dangerous to put on permanent record any conclusive statements on subjects of much current debate. However it is not possible to define the nurse's role without reference to important documents which relate to these issues.[3,4,6]

There were 586,965 pupils attending 2,431 independent schools in England, Scotland and Wales in 1994/5. This represented 7.2% of the total school population.[7] Nurses in independent schools carry a burden of responsibility daily for the welfare of these children. At the same time their personal and professional responsibility must remain at the highest level of skill based care. There is no instant solution to finding a model for the future but perhaps, within the varied and unique service which is provided in boarding schools, these debates are not so relevant. Has a good practical base on which to build been found already?

Accountability

It is most important that the school nurse is adequately trained and professionally accountable in all areas of her work.

The code of Professional Conduct states that each registered nurse, midwife and health visitor shall act at all times, in such a manner as to:

safeguard and promote the interests of individual patients and clients.

serve the interests of society.

justify public trust and confidence and

uphold and enhance the good standing and reputation of the professions.

It is important to ask to whom nurses are accountable when working in unusual settings,

in the workplace?

the patients?

ourselves?

and apply this on a daily basis.

'As a registered nurse... you are personally accountable for your practice.' The principles against which to exercise that accountability are detailed in a UKCC Advisory Document which all nurses and their employers should read frequently.[8,9]

Responsibilities

The school nurse must consider each case separately and decide where her professional and legal responsibilities lie.

The International Code of Nursing Ethics (1973) states:

The fundamental responsibility of the nurse is fourfold:

to promote health

to prevent illness

to restore health

to alleviate suffering.

The need for nursing is universal. Inherent in nursing is respect for life, dignity and the rights of human-kind. It is unrestricted by consideration of nationality, race, creed, colour, age, sex, politics or social status. Nurses render health services to the individual, the family and the community and coordinate their services with those of related specialities. The nurse's primary responsibility is to those people who require nursing care. 'The nurse holds in confidence personal information and uses judgment in sharing this information'.[8]

This is particularly important with sensitive issues such as child protection, abuse, HIV positive students, contraception and termination of pregnancy. There should be clear guidelines and agreed procedures within the school in order to protect students from further harm and to promote a return to health.[9] These and other sensitive issues such as bullying and eating disorders are discussed in the relevant chapters of this book but they do require specialist training and the skills to deal with these increasingly common problems must be acquired by the nurse if she is to be a fully active member of the pastoral and professional care team within the school.

Record keeping in a school

'The important activity of making and keeping records is an essential and integral part of care and not a distraction from its provision.'[10] The principles underpinning record keeping by nurses are set out in Standards for Records and Record Keeping and cover:

purpose
importance
standards
ethical features
essential elements
legal status
patient and client held records
computer held records
shared records.

Decisions on resuscitation and individualised care recording are discussed separately.[10]

Where NHS notes are stored on school premises, the Health Authority guidelines must be adhered to and many Health Authorities reserve the right to carry out checks on premises which are not the designated health centre or surgery of the GP practice.

The Data Protection Act has been in force since 1987. Nurses who process information on to a computer should be aware of:

the eight data protection principles
security of systems access
patient access to records
the required UKCC standards
the potential effects of inadequately kept records.[11]

'There is, however, substantial evidence that inadequate and inappropriate record keeping concerning the care of patients and clients neglects their interests through:

impairing continuity of care
introducing discontinuity of communication between staff thus creating the risk of medication or other treatment being duplicated or even omitted.
failing to focus attention on early signs of deviation from the norm, and failing to place on record significant observations and conclusions'[10].

A day book, Cardex system, computer and Heath Authority notes can all be used to record patient care and, where several people might be responsible for the administration of medicines eg. house matrons in a school boarding house, a register of signatures should be kept.

Training and Professional Development

Good basic training is essential for any nurse. However, it is what she does after that training and how she uses that knowledge that should enable her to understand more about the human condition and to use appropriate nursing models to minimise the interruption of a patient's usual way of life. She should continue to develop within the setting of her own practice and now, for the first time, all RGNs must maintain an effective registration. The transition from student to practitioner is no longer a once-only and permanent step.

Post Registration and Practice (PREP) came into force on April 1st 1995.
It is a legal requirement.

There are many articles in the professional papers defining the implications in detail and all members of the RCN will have received advice and information.

The structure of PREP is defined by UKCC's Position Statement on Policy and Implementation:[12]

> a period of support for newly registered practitioners under the guidance of a preceptor
> maintenance of an effective registration
> standards for post registration education in both institutional and community settings.

All nurses must:

> submit a Notification to Practice form
> undertake at least five days study every 3 years
> complete personal and professional profiles
> undertake return to practice programmes (where appropriate).[13]

Study

Study is flexible and varied and there are many options. A school nurse like all other nurses must define her own specific programme. It is important that she identifies needs rather than wants and she must negotiate with the school bursar for the funding and time to complete these statutory requirements. This will require collaboration.

The Department of Health is not at present providing extra funding for the implementation of PREP for any nurses. Therefore it is the responsibility of the individual to persuade her employer to identify areas for investment in staff training.[13]

All employers are likely to be selective about who studies what and when and this strengthens the case for the increasing provision of a range of good cost effective study options. This may include organised private study, formal study days and distance learning.

Five categories are identified for study:

> reducing risk
> care enhancement
> patient, client, family, and colleague support
> practice development
> education development.

It is important for study to be accredited and course participants should receive appropriate certification as proof of their attendance.

Guidance will be given on:

self assessment
identifying learning needs
evaluating outcomes of study
self verification.

The process of how clinical support and personal reviews take place is still uncertain but is being addressed.[14] Personal and professional profile folders can be bought from a number of sources including the ENB, nursing journals and some commercial companies. They are expensive and care needs to be exercised over choice.

Study days on all of these changes are being held in most areas and help is available for those on their own who find this a minefield. However, ignoring it is not an option. Contact the local colleges of nursing and identify your needs to them. Use their research facilities to obtain information from their libraries. This all provides the school nurse working in the private sector with the opportunity to bring her education into line with other areas of nursing and through this, to gain some formal recognition of her job and skills.

School Profile

Each school is unique, just as each child is unique. In order to identify and undertake specific training and then to offer a service to the community, the nurse must understand what is required of her and that necessitates a thorough understanding of her surroundings.

A school profile will provide some surprising and useful insights into the client group she is serving as well as defining more clearly areas of need both in the school population and in the service provided. A number of aspects of school life should be examined as well as the more obvious nature of the practice population, for example:

ethos of the school
environmental characteristics
other support services
morbidity rates e.g. asthma, diabetes, epilepsy.
accident rates (accident forms and Health and Safety reports).

The school population can be analysed in a number of ways, for example:

geographical location of the child's home
racial and religious origins
age
gender
numbers in each year
skills and I.Q.
physical ability
single parent families
prevalence of extended families.
social class distribution.

This information should identify the health and social needs of the practice population, the current service provision and the particular skills, expertise, knowledge and interest required to meet those needs. It should enable the primary health care team to:

> set shared team objectives
> target services
> audit and evaluate services in order to set future objectives.

Although this exercise can be time consuming it is very valuable and without it one cannot offer a service which is relevant to the differing needs of the whole school. Finally it is perhaps important to look at the profile in the setting of the GP practice to which it belongs and recently, the RCN issued a framework document which should be very helpful.[15]

Setting protocols which lead to standards of care, measurement, evaluation and audit

Some results are measurable and an outcome easy to define. The setting of standards through protocols provides a structure for nursing care which even in its simplest form demonstrates and promotes a need for discipline. This is sometimes hard to achieve as a school nurse working alone.

Simple protocols can be set and adhered to in such areas as:

> immunisation
> asthma
> diabetes
> wound management
> measurement of growth
> eating disorders
> severe allergy, e.g. peanut
> drug administration
> anaphylactic shock
> counselling

As Richard Asher says in his book, 'Talking Sense', 'Kipling gives us an admirable summary of the way we get most of our knowledge:

> 'I keep six honest serving men
> (They taught me all I knew);
> Their names are What and Why and When
> And How and Where and Who.'[16]

This provides an invaluable checklist when working on protocols and profiles.

Protocols should be specific to your own practice
A protocol:

> is an agreed strategy for carrying out a procedure or an activity

> is useful when there is a need for health professionals to have clarification with complex issues

> offers the opportunity for teamwork (not something inflicted by one on others).

It should be dated, signed and a review date agreed by all health professionals involved

They are commonly used;

to assist diagnosis
to improve medical care of a disease, once diagnosed
to manage or reduce costs
for legal protection.

However, the disadvantages of protocols have been identified as:

making it difficult to meet the individual needs of patients
restricting the desirable use of clinical discretion.[17]

The structure of writing any protocol can be divided into:

What   Aim – to carry out any procedure according to the guidelines
Objectives – to provide information and consistent advice
– to target specific groups.

Why   Rationale.

Where   Surgery/Private space.

When   Protected time/Opportunistically.
Time of year.
Schedule.
Circumstances.

Who   Areas of responsibility—Doctor/Nurse/Lay.
Training/Teaching responsibilities.
Target group.
Exclusions.

Which   – Range of Treatment – e. g. drugs, dressings.
Clinical information.
Measurement/audit.

How   – Permission.
Indication for referral to GP.
Communication.
Equipment and Storage.
Site (of treatment).
Prescription.
Emergency procedures.
Record keeping.
Disposal.
Evaluation.
Assessment.

A good protocol which is observed by all allows evaluation, audit and measurement of outcomes to take place easily and at any time.

Asthma

It would be easy to discuss nearly every topic in the handbook from the nurse's perspective and to select one may invite criticism. However, it would be wrong to omit an area where nurse expertise in understanding the disease, clinical judgement, teaching and management can have such a dramatic effect on the health of the school child.

'It is an accepted fact that in any large sample of school aged children, 10-15% will have suffered asthma symptoms in the last year. This means that:

– there are 4 or 5 children per class,

– about half of these remain undiagnosed.

There are about 2, 000 deaths per year in the UK from asthma.[17]

If a protocol is completed in collaboration with the school doctor and the nurse has undertaken asthma training to agreed levels of competence, the children with asthma in their care should gain immediate benefit.

The protocol should contain:

strategy for carrying out procedures
height and peak exploratory flow measurement chart
instructions for use of the PFM (peak flow meter)[18]
PEFR (peak expiratory flow rate) chart
PF action level calculator chart (70%, 50% and 30% of potential normal PF)
self management plans for boarding house and home.
teacher's strategy.

Equipment should include charts, instruction leaflets, video recordings, placebo inhalers in all the methods of delivery and, most important of all, a peak flow meter. The drug companies who make inhalers and other medications for the treatment of asthma produce excellent teaching aids as well. They will usually visit a school and in some areas there is a specialist representative. These drug companies are also involved in educational sponsorship.

Check List.

Do all the children with asthma have easy access to their inhalers at all times?

Do you:

have a management plan worked out for every child with severe asthma?

hold a nurse run asthma clinic (NRAC) regularly in which you monitor height, PEFR, technique and discuss trigger factors?

check maintenance therapy, technique and control opportunistically?

alter systems of delivery and increase medication if control is poor or in order to pre-empt an asthma attack? (i. e. a management plan.)

nebulise when necessary using PF action level calculator chart?

add prednisolone as appropriate?

alert GP at agreed time (protocol)?

refer for alteration in medication if PEFR fails to improve sufficiently?

reduce medication to maintenance levels when symptom free?

continue to monitor child in NRAC and opportunistically?

teach all staff about the condition?

Peak flow meter:

'For a patient with asthma, recording peak flow can be just as important as measuring blood sugar is for a patient with diabetes and they should be given every encouragement'.[17,18]

Is the PFM your main tool?

do all children with asthma have instant access to one, at school, in the boarding house and at home?

do all children with asthma, know how to measure their peak flow correctly, chart it and what action to take at given levels?

Children may feel stigmatised because of their asthma and having to use inhalers and peak flow meters in front of their peers. As a school nurse, one of the primary tasks is in educating everyone, not just children with asthma, to understand the importance of his/her preventative medication for this variable condition, even when they are symptom free.

For some children with a severe pre-existing medical condition it is worth considering the use of a Medic-Alert bracelet or necklace (older children only). Many different staff can be responsible for these children and will they always remember a severe drug allergy or other hidden condition? Parents often welcome the opportunity to discuss safeguards.

Assessment

The school nurse in the independent sector frequently works alone and without any opportunity for objective assessment. Clinical support and supervision should become available as the effects of PREP are seen in the community. Discussions are being held at every level about the development of clinical support systems for all nurses, whatever their field of practice'. Nurses and health visitors require support in the development of their practice.'[4] Even among practice nurses and other community based health professionals, an external assessment programme such as the mentor scheme is not always in place and therefore some kind of honest self assessment is required.

A form can be devised to complement the protocols in which:

knowledge
skills
attitudes

can be examined and rated 1 to 5, hence:

1=little or no competence
5=competent enough to accept accountability.

In low scoring areas the nurse needs to consider how she can improve her competence by:

reading journals and articles
using a nurse mentor, clinical supervisor
discussion with the GP or other nurse colleagues.

NB. A specimen self-assessment form is reproduced in Appendix J.

Communication skills and teaching

Learning some teaching skills from your staffroom colleagues can greatly enhance your practice. They come to us for medical expertise: go to them for teaching expertise.

As school nurses we are constantly imparting knowledge to children, parents (sometimes on the other side of the world), teaching staff and other professionals. Good communication skills are essential. How we pass on information can often make the difference between compliance and failure of treatment. Do we make sure that the parent understands the importance of finishing a course of antibiotics, even when the child has arrived home seemingly fit?

Do we describe the need for immunisation accurately and fully so that the parents give their **informed** consent? This does not have to be in writing but where a parent is not present it is desirable. Even when faced with a request for immunisations which should begin immediately, a facsimile transmission or a letter will back up that verbal permission. The initial telephone call gives you the opportunity to discuss the request, assess its suitability and inform parents of the timing. (See remarks on 'Consent' at the commencement of the next Chapter:' Immunisation').

The responsibility for a child's health is often in the hands of a number of people over a period of 24 hours: the child, parent, house parent and teaching staff, all need to be given appropriate, accurate and consistent advice which has been sympathetically presented. How often does a child, parent or member of staff leave your surgery without information or instruction?

Remember: What – Why – When – How – Where – Who.

Who is the child and have they understood?

Does the child have learning difficulties, has the child impaired hearing or is he/she just scared? It has been suggested that most people will retain only five consecutive instructions. Where the topic is medicine, the 'teachers' are the doctors or nurses and the setting is clinical, there is a great danger of a total memory shutdown as soon as the patient leaves the room.

Listening and counselling

Whilst all the academic and intellectual aspects of any profession can at times overwhelm the task in hand, they do only provide the bedrock of one's experience. We should never forget that the ability to listen sympathetically and thus to demonstrate that we care about the child is often enough to help them to mature and develop. This is particularly important during adolescence when their needs can be greatest and are combined with an emotional state which is lacking in self-confidence, limited in understanding and dominated by overwhelming feelings. Our skills in early problem solving can sometimes make the need for long term and more serious help unnecessary. However, recognising when that help is necessary is equally vital.

The following can help a nurse to be more concise and focussed when dealing with emotional adolescents:

establishing rapport
clarifying issues and intentions

gathering and giving information
help with problem solving on mutually identified issues.

It is possible to use complex and multiple-model approaches in setting priorities but Maslow's Hierarchy of Needs is the role model for many of them and is shown here in simplified form.[18]

Self-activation	Self-fulfilment
Status	Approval, respect, dignity
Belonging	Love, affection, kindness, friendship, feeling part of a group.
Safety	Physical safety and comfort, security
Physiological	Food, water, oxygen, elimination, shelter, exercise, rest, sex, pain—free

Networking

Keeping up to date on the many aspects of a school nurse's job is a hard task when much of her working life is spent in isolation from other health professionals.

The primary healthcare team, especially the school doctor and his practice nurse, is a vital source of information. They are providing a similar service out in the community and have easier access to other professionals, a whole range of services, information and medical technology. Their professional papers eg. *Practice Nurse* and magazines such as *Pulse*, publish articles on up-to-date clinical issues.

The Royal College of Nursing School Nurses' Forum has an independent School Nurse Representative. Also, there are regional groups, some of which play a very active role in the education and support of their members. Isolation can also mean that nurses do not always have an easy time within their own practice setting and are often near the bottom of the Bursar's or the Headmaster's lists. Salary, contract, insurance (professional and life), capital expenditure budgets, equipment replacement funds, investment in staff training are all potentially contentious issues unless there is already good dialogue between the relevant parties.

Conclusion

It is important not to confuse the weakness and at times the unsuitability of individuals with the institution. We are all imperfect. The strength of any institution is the way it creates rules, adopts standards of behaviour and strives as far as possible to overcome its own imperfections.'[19] This quotation is as true for the school child trying to adopt and adhere to the standards of the institution in which they find themselves as it is for doctors and nurses working together to provide a service within that setting.

Frequently it will be the school nurse who is confronted with a problem first and she may well be on duty alone. While she works in a team, she is also an independent practitioner, so that 'who provides the care-nurses or doctors is less important than ensuring that help is provided promptly.'[5]

However, it is the confidence of the school doctor in her ability to create rules for good nursing practice, to adopt and adhere to professional standards and in her judgment in any situation, that is paramount to the service she provides.

References

1. MOSA (1992) *The Handbook of School Health17th Edn,*. Appendix H. p. 225. Trentham Books Ltd.

2. UKCC, *The Scope of Professional Practice.*

3. Department of Health, Welsh Office (1989) *Child Protection: Clarification of Arrangements Between the NHS and Other Agencies. Addendum to Working Together Under the Children Act.* HMSO. London.

4. NHS Management Executive, (1993) *A Vision for the Future,*. (HMSO.)

5. *Br. MedJ.* (1995) Vol. 311. p271 See also Pp. 273, 274, 287, 303, 309, 325, 338, 339. (29. Jul 95)

6. DOH Community Guide (1994) *Health Needs of School Age Children*, paras 7.18 and 7.19 The Royal College of Paediatrics and Child Health, formerly The British Paediatric Association.

7. ISIS, Independent Schools Information Service.

8. International Council of Nurses, (1973) *International Code of Nursing Ethics.*

9. UKCC (1992) *Code of Professional Conduct for the Nurse, Midwife and Health Visitor.*

10. UKCC, Standards for Records and Record Keeping.

11. Office of the Data Protection Registrar 1989. DOH 1984, *Report from the Confidentiality Working Group.*

12. UKCC (1994). *The Future of Professional Practice: The Council's Standards for Education and Practice Following registration.*

13. Melville, E., (April 1995) 'The Implications of PREP for Practitioners'. *Professional Nurse.*

14. Faugier and Butterworth. (1994) 'Clinical Supervision: A Position Paper' School of Nursing Studies, University of Manchester.

15. Dukes and Stewart, (January 23 1993) 'Be Prepared.' *Health Service Journal.*

16. Asher, R. (1972) 'Talking Sense' Pitman Press.

17. The Asthma Training Centre. (1992) *'Asthma Who Cares? A Recipe Book to Help with the Management of Asthma in Schools.'*

18. Jeffree, P. (1995) *'The Practice Nurse',* second edition, Chapman and Hall.

19. *The Times.* (1992.) An article on the monarchy.

Addresses

UKCC, 23 Portland Place, London W1N 3AF. Tel: 0171-637-7181.

The Royal College of Nursing, 20, Cavendish Square, London W1M OAB. Tel: 0171-872-0840/0171-409-3333.

National Asthma Campaign, Providence House, Providence Place, London. N1 ONT. Tel: 0171-226-2260.

The Asthma Training Centre, Winton House, Church Street, Stratford-upon-Avon CV37 6HB. Tel:: 01789-296974.

ISIS, 56, Buckingham Gate, London SW1E. Tel: 0171-630-8793/4.

Medic Alert Foundation, Brit. Isles and Ireland, 12, Bridge Wharf 156, Caledonian Road, London N1 9UU. Tel: 0171-833-3034.

CHAPTER 4

IMMUNISATION

Immunisation plays a vital part in the prevention of infectious diseases in children. Carers who are concerned with the health and welfare of children have a responsibility which embraces health education, administration, treatment and communication with the pupils and their parents. They should be satisfied with nothing less than complete efficiency in the compilation of immunisation histories and schedules so that appropriate procedures are undertaken. There is an additional responsibility towards children who travel abroad or live overseas.

Most areas have computerised immunisation schedules which notify parents when their children's immunisations are due. Records of immunisation status may therefore be centrally held and in a day school the responsibility shall be shared with the general practitioner and the school health service, which may, in particular, be involved with BCG vaccination. In most boarding schools, the school doctor has an undivided responsibility, although in some areas the Consultant Community Paediatrician undertakes responsibility for BCG vaccination. A full record of immunisations should be kept and the parents informed of the child's protective state. Parents should be requested to inform the school doctor of any immunisation procedure carried out on their child during school holidays.

Consent

The matter of consent before any medical or surgical treatment, including immunisation procedures, can be undertaken, has been revised recently. The earlier, rather 'blanket' forms of consent have been abandoned in favour of rather more specific consent for individual procedures.

First of all, the consent requires to be informed and care should be taken at all times to ensure that children and parents are fully informed about proposed procedures. Adequate time must be devoted to explanation and to answering any questions, taking extra specialist advice where necessary. This advice may be obtained from a Consultant Paediatrician, a Communicable Diseases Consultant or Immunisation Co-ordinator of a District Health Board.

Details of consent specifically for immunisation procedures are given on page 7 of 'Immunisation against Infectious Disease'(1996), and are reproduced, below by kind permission of HMSO.

Written consent provides a permanent record, but consent either written or verbal is required at the time of each immunisation after the child's fitness and suitability have been established.

Consent obtained **before** the occasion upon which a child is brought for immunisation is only an agreement for the child to be included in the immunisation programme.

Bringing a child for immunisation after an invitation to attend for this purpose may be viewed as acceptance that the child may be immunised. When a child is brought for this purpose, and fitness and suitability have been established, consent to that immunisation may be implied in the absence of any expressed reservation to the immunisation proceeding at that stage.

Similarly, the attendance of a child at school on the day that the parent/ guardian has been advised that the child will be immunised may also be viewed as acceptance that the child may be immunised, in the absence of any reservation expressed to the contrary. However, because of the parent/ guardian's legal responsibilities in respect of the child's attendance at school, the possibility that immunisation will be offered should be made clear to the parent/guardian.

A child under 16 years of age may give consent for immunisation, provided he or she understands fully the benefits and risks involved. However, the child should be encouraged to involve a parent or guardian in the decision if at all possible.

Where a child under 16 who fully understands the benefits and risks of the proposed immunisation wishes to refuse the immunisation, that wish should be respected.

If a child's fitness and suitability cannot be established, immunisation should be deferred. Specialist advice may need to be obtained, as in the case of the provision of extra information before consent is given, as discussed above.

Vaccine Induced Immunity

Immunity induced against a variety of bacterial and viral infecting agents or their products may be passive or active.

Passive Immunity

Passive immunity results from injecting antiserum containing antibodies, which are usually human in origin. This protection is immediate, but short-lived, lasting only until the anti-serum has been eliminated from the body. The two main types are:

(1) Human normal immunoglobulin (HNIG) derived from the pooled plasma donors containing antibodies to infectious agents which are currently prevalent in the general population. Examples are the use of human normal immunoglobulin in protecting immunocompromised children against measles and protection of patients against hepatitis A.

(2) Specific immunoglobulins for tetanus, hepatitis B, rabies and varicella -zoster, which are obtained from the pooled blood of convalescent patients, donors recently immunised with the relevant vaccine or those who, on screening, are found to have sufficiently high antibody titres.

Active Immunity

Active immunity provides protection for months or years, and can be induced by the administration of vaccines containing an attenuated living organism of the disease concerned, as in oral poliomyelitis and measles vaccines, or by giving a vaccine in which the organism has been inactivated during manufacture, as in whooping cough and typhoid vaccines. Other examples are vaccines inactivated by treatment with formaldehyde, which inactivates the vaccine, thus rendering it harmless, but the resultant product, the toxoid, still retains its immunising properties. Diphtheria and tetanus are two vaccines treated in this way.

These vaccines confer protection by inducing cell mediated immunity and the production of antibodies, whose presence can be detected in the serum. BCG vaccine, (the Bacillus of Calmette and Guerin, which is an attenuated strain of bovine tuberculosis) produces active immunity against tuberculosis by a cell mediated immunity mechanism, following intradermal injection, which is demonstrated by a positive tuberculin skin test.

The first dose of an inactivated vaccine or of a toxoid preparation, in a subject not previously exposed to the disease, produces only a slow antibody response, predominantly of IgM antibody, – the 'primary response'. When, after a suitable interval, a second dose is given, the response is quicker and to a higher level of antibody or antitoxin titre (IgG) – the' secondary response'. After a full course, (usually two or three injections) the antibody or the antitoxin levels remain high for months or years. If the immune mechanism has been set up, and later, serum levels are noted to fall, then immunity can be reinforced and reinstated by a further dose of the vaccine.

Some of the inactivated vaccines are combined with substances, like aluminium phosphate and aluminium hydroxide which enhance their antibody response, e. g. adsorbed diphtheria/tetanus/pertussis vaccine (DTP) and the adsorbed diphtheria/tetanus vaccine (DT).

In most individuals, one dose of a live attenuated virus vaccine, such as measles, mumps and rubella will produce a full and long-lasting protective antibody response. Live oral poliomyelitis vaccine requires three doses for a similar response. An important additional effect of oral poliomyelitis vaccine is the establishment of local immunity in the intestine.

Viruses which are used in the production of vaccines are grown in a variety of cells. For example, measles, mumps, influenza and yellow fever viruses are grown in chick cells, some polio viruses in monkey kidney cells and rubella, hepatitis A and other polio viruses are grown in human diploid cells.

Immunisation Procedures

After the necessary consent has been obtained and suitability for immunisation has been established, the school doctor should ensure that the necessary trained personnel, drugs and equipment are in place in order to deal with any anaphylactic reactions or other emergencies. It is assumed of course, that all personnel (doctors and nurses) will have had the requisite training so that they are competent in vaccination techniques.

Vaccines must have been properly transported and stored and their identity and expiry date must be verified before use. Of course, time expired vaccines should on no account be administered. With such important procedures as immunisation and vaccination, it is important that the description and the batch number of the product and the date of the procedure should be recorded on the child's medical record. When two vaccines are administered simultaneously, then the relevant sites must be recorded, so that in the event of untoward reactions the responsible product can be identified. Contra-indications to immunisation must always be borne in mind. No vaccine should be given during an acute febrile illness. Live vaccines should not normally be given in pregnancy or to immunocompromised patients, those on steroids or those receiving radiotherapy.

The recommendations set out in 'Immunisation Against Infectious Disease 1996' ('The Green Book') are based on the expert advice, currently available to the Joint Committee on Vaccination and Immunisation and reflect the present national policy on immunisation, which of course, is very closely followed by MOSA. The above work contains detailed information on the distribution, storage and disposal of vaccines and details of immunisation techniques and vaccine damage payments. The chapters in 'The Green Book' on 'Indications and Contraindications', 'Adverse Reactions' and 'Anaphylaxis' are quoted here, by kind permission of HMSO., because of their immediate importance to the school doctor.

Indications and Contraindications
Special risk groups
Some conditions increase the risk of complications from infectious diseases and children and adults with such conditions should be immunised as a **matter of priority**. These conditions include the following: asthma, chronic lung and congenital heart diseases, Down's syndrome, Human Immuno-deficiency Virus (HIV) infection, small for dates babies and those born prematurely.

When children are immunised opportunistically in Accident and Emergency Units or whilst hospital in-patients, it is most important that a record is sent to the school medical officer, general practitioner or to the Health Authority or Trust Board by way of an 'unscheduled immunisation' form.

Unimmunised children and others with unknown immunisation histories
Some children, for a variety of reasons, may not have been immunised or their immunisation history may be unknown. If children coming to the UK, to attend school, for example, are not known to have been completely immunised, they should be assumed to be unimmunised and a full course of immunisations planned. For children under 10 years of age, this should be the full UK primary immunisation schedule of three doses of diphtheria, tetanus, pertussis and oral polio vaccine (Hib only up to four years, three doses for children under one year, only one dose for children aged one to four years) with boosting for diphtheria, tetanus and polio five and ten years thereafter. Children of all ages above 12 months should receive two doses of MMR, separated by at least 3 months. For children over 10 years of age, Td should be used along with MMR and OPV. Boosting with Td and OPV should be

given five and ten years later. In the event of a severe adverse reaction, blood should be taken for tetanus antibody titres as these may provide a marker for previous immunisation. No further diphtheria, tetanus and pertussis immunisations are needed in children where there is evidence of previous immunisation including booster doses; immunisation should be completed with OPV and Hib if appropriate.

Children coming to the UK, part way through their immunisation schedule, should be transferred on to the standard UK schedule, as appropriate for their age.

Children and adults with no spleen, or who have functional hyposplenism, are at increased risk of bacterial infections, most commonly caused by encapsulated organisms. Such infection is most common in the first two years after splenectomy; the risk is greatest amongst children but persists into adult life. The following vaccines are recommended in addition to those in the routine schedule: pneumococcal vaccine (over two years of age, see later), Hib vaccine (irrespective of age, see later), influenza, (see later) and meningococcal A and C vaccine (see later) Where possible, immunisation should be given two weeks before splenectomy together with advice about the increased risk of infection.

Adults and children who receive dialysis are at increased risk of hepatitis B and hepatitis C although these risks have declined. Haemodialysis patients should be screened for serological evidence of hepatitis B immunity and antibody negative individuals should have three doses of hepatitis B vaccine, ideally before dialysis commences or as soon as possible thereafter. In haemodialysis patients, protection only lasts as long as anti-HBs antibodies remain over 10 miu/ml. Patients on haemodialysis should be monitored annually for anti-HBs antibodies and re-immunised if antibodies fall below this level. Recipients of renal transplants and individuals with chronic renal disease are at increased risk of infection and should be considered for annual influenza immunisation, Hib and pneumococcal immunisation.

General considerations

If an individual is suffering from an acute illness, immunisation should be postponed until recovery has occurred. Minor infections without systemic upset are not reasons to postpone immunisation. Antibody responses and the incidence of adverse reactions were the same in children with or without acute mild illness, when given MMR vaccine. The acute illnesses were respiratory tract infection, diarrhoea and otitis media.

Immunisation should not be carried out in individuals who have a definite history of a severe local or general reaction to a preceding dose. Detailed enquiry may reveal that the reported reaction may not match the specifications below and immunisation can proceed. Appropriate specialist advice should be sought if there is doubt. The following reactions should be regarded as severe.

Local: an extensive area of redness and swelling which becomes indurated and involves most of the antero-lateral surface of the thigh or a major part of the circumference of the upper arm.

General: fever equal to or more than 39.5 degrees Centigrade within 48 hours of the vaccine; anaphylaxis; bronchospasm; laryngeal oedema; generalised collapse. Prolonged unresponsiveness;prolonged inconsolable or high pitched screaming for more than four hours;convulsions or encephalopathy occurring within 72 hours.

Although there is evidence to suggest that rubella and polio vaccines are not teratogenic (See later), live vaccines should not be administered to pregnant women because of the theoretical possibility of harm to the foetus. When there is a significant risk of exposure to the disease, for example to poliomyelitis or yellow fever, the need for immunisation outweighs any possible risk to the foetus.

Live Vaccines – special risk groups

There are some individuals for whom there may be risks if they are given live vaccines. Inactivated vaccines are not dangerous to these recipients but may be ineffective. These individuals may not be able to make a normal immune response to live vaccines and could suffer from severe manifestations such as disseminated infection with BCG, or paralytic poliomyelitis from vaccine virus. These individuals include:

(a) All patients currently being treated for malignant disease with chemotherapy or generalised radiotherapy, or within six months of terminating such treatment.

(b) All patients who have received an organ transplant and are currently on immunosuppressive treatment.

Patients who within the previous six months have received a bone marrow transplant. Such individuals, irrespective of age, should have their immunity to diphtheria, tetanus, poliomyelitis, measles, mumps, rubella and Hib checked six months after transplant and be immunised appropriately. Such tests are difficult to interpret if performed within three months after the receipt of any blood product, including HNIG.

Children who receive prednisolone, orally or rectally, at a daily dose (or its equivalent) of 2 mg/kg/day for at least one week, or 1mg /kg /day for a month. For adults, an equivalent dose is harder to define, but immunosuppression should be considered in those who receive 40 mg prednisolone per day for more than a week. Corticosteroids administered by other routes, such as aerosols, topically or intra-articularly, are not immunosuppressive. Administration of live vaccines should be postponed for at least three months after immunosuppressive treatment has stopped, or three months after levels have been reached that are not associated with immunosuppression.

Lower doses of steroids, given in combination with cytotoxic drugs (including anti thymocyte globulin or other immunosuppressants) should be considered to cause immunosuppression. The advice of the physician in charge or immunologist should be sought.

Occasionally, there may be individuals on lower doses of steroids or other immunosuppressants for prolonged periods, or who, because of their underlying disease, may be immunosuppressed, and are at increased risk of infection. The clinician should ideally discuss their management with a consultant in infectious disease, microbiology, paediatrics or relevant specialist physician.

Patients with evidence of impaired **cell-mediated immunity**, for example HIV infection with current symptoms, severe combined immunodeficiency syndrome, Di George Syndrome and other combined immunodeficiency syndromes. Patients with minor **deficiencies of antibodies** are not at risk; those with major antibody deficiencies will be receiving antibodies in their immunoglobulin treatment preparations and hence are not at risk from live vaccines. Because the patient is receiving immunoglobulin preparations, live vaccines are likely to be ineffective, apart from yellow fever vaccine as it is most unlikely that there are significant amounts of anti-yellow fever antibodies in immunoglobulin.

After exposure to measles or chickenpox (See later), individuals who fulfil the above criteria, and are susceptible to measles or chickenpox on the grounds of history or antibody titres, should be given an injection of the appropriate preparation of immunoglobulin as soon as possible.

Immunisation of individuals with antibody to the Human Immunodeficiency Virus (HIV positive)

HIV positive individuals **with or without symptoms** should receive the following as appropriate:

Live vaccines: **measles;mumps;rubella; and polio.**

Inactivated vaccines: **pertussis; diphtheria; tetanus; poliomyelitis; typhoid; cholera; hepatitisB; and Hib.**

For HIV positive symptomatic individuals, inactivated polio vaccine (IPV) may be used instead of OPV, at the discretion of the clinician.

HIV positive individuals should **not** receive **BCG** vaccine; there have been reports of dissemination of BCG in HIV positive individuals.

Yellow fever vaccine should not be given to either symptomatic or asymptomatic HIV positive individuals since there is, as yet, insufficient evidence as to the safety of its use. Travellers should be told of this uncertainty and advised not to be immunised unless there are compelling reasons. If such travellers still intend to visit countries where a yellow fever certificate is required for entry, then they should obtain a letter of exemption from a medical practitioner.

No harmful effects have been reported following live attenuated vaccines for **measles, mumps, poliomyelitis** and **rubella** in HIV positive individuals who are at increased risk from these diseases. Immunisation of known measles seronegative HIV positive individuals is advised;a measurable antibody response may occur in only some vaccinees. It should be noted that in HIV positive individuals, poliomyelitis virus may be excreted for longer periods than in other people. Contacts of a recently immunised HIV positive individual should be warned of this, and of the need for washing their hands after changing an immunised infant's nappies. For HIV positive contacts of an immunised individual (whether that individual is HIV positive or not) the potential risk is greater than that in non-HIV individuals.

Vaccine efficacy may be reduced in HIV positive individuals. Consideration should be given to the use of normal immunoglobulin for HIV positive individuals after exposure to measles.

For symptomatic HIV positive individuals exposed to **chicken pox or zoster**, Human Varicella-Zoster Immunoglobulin (VZIG) should be given . VZIG is not indicated for asymptomatic HIV positive patients with normal CD4 counts as there is no evidence of increased risk of severe varicella in these individuals.

HIV positive individuals may also receive; pneumococcal, rabies, hepatitis A and meningococcal A&C vaccines.

NB. Some of the above advice differs from that for other immuno-compromised patients

Note Specific contraindications to individual vaccines must be observed.

Immunisation intervals

Live virus vaccines, with the exception of yellow fever vaccine, should not be given during the three months following injection of immunoglobulin because the immune response may be inhibited. Human normal immunoglobulin obtained from UK residents is unlikely to contain antibody to yellow fever virus which would inactivate the vaccine. In travellers, when time is short and there is a significant risk of exposure to poliomyelitis, vaccine **should** be given even if immunoglobulin has been given at any time in the previous three months.

If it is necessary to administer more than one live vaccine at the same time, they should either be given simultaneously in different sites (unless a combined preparation is used) or in theory be separated by a period of at least three weeks. There are no current data using presently available vaccines to support this recommendation which came from earlier observations about 'take rates' of smallpox vaccination; these may have been reduced if other live vaccines had been given shortly before smallpox vaccination. It probably has little relevance for intervals between oral polio vaccine and other presently used live virus vaccines. It is recommended that a three week interval should be allowed between the administration of live virus vaccines especially measles vaccine, and tuberculin testing; there is experience that shows that measles infection or immunisation can give false negative results in tuberculin positive individuals. No interval needs to be observed between the administration of live and inactivated vaccines.

The following conditions are NOT contraindications to immunisation:

    a.   Family history of any adverse reactions following immunisation.

    b.   Previous history of pertussis, measles, rubella or mumps infection.

    c.   Prematurity: immunisation should not be postponed.

    d.   Stable neurological conditions such as cerebral palsy and Down's syndrome.

    e.   Contact with an infectious disease.

f. Asthma, eczema, hay fever or 'snuffles'.

g. Treatment with antibiotics or locally -acting (e.g. topical or inhaled) steroids.

h. Child's mother is pregnant.

i. Child being breast fed.

j. History of jaundice after birth.

k. Under a certain weight.

l. Over the age recommended on the immunisation schedule.

m. 'Replacement' corticosteroids.

Other contraindication issues

A history of allergy is **not** a contraindication. Hypersensitivity to egg contra-indicates influenza vaccine; previous **anaphylactic** reaction to egg contra-indicates influenza and yellow fever vaccines.

There is increasing evidence that MMR vaccine can safely be given even to children with a history of previous anaphylaxis after egg ingestion.

A personal or family history of inflammatory bowel disease (Crohn's or ulcerative colitis) does not contraindicate measles or MMR immunisation. Evidence for an association between measles vaccine and inflammatory bowel disease is not convincing.

Where there is a close family history (parents or sibling) of febrile convulsions, there is an increased chance that a febrile convulsion could follow a fever in a vaccine recipient. Immunisation should be carried out after advice on the prevention of pyrexia has been given.

Siblings and close contacts of immunosuppressed children **should** be immunised against measles, mumps and rubella. There is no risk of transmission of virus following immunisation.

Oral poliomyelitis vaccine (OPV) should **not** be given to immunosuppressed children, their siblings or other household contacts. Inactivated poliomyelitis vaccine (IPV), should be given instead; this should also be given to immunosuppressed adults and their contacts. (See pages 96 and 97).

Recently immunised children may be taken swimming, even if they have been given OPV. Similarly, there is no risk of an unimmunised child contracting vaccine associated poliomyelitis from a recently immunised child if they are taken swimming. In such public places, care must be taken to dispose of soiled napkins without contaminating facilities that others might use.

Surgery is not a contraindication to immunisation, nor is recent immunisation a contraindication to anaesthesia or surgery. Recent receipt of OPV does not contraindicate tonsillectomy. In the United States, where recent OPV administration has never been considered a contraindication to tonsillectomy, there has been no recorded case of vaccine associated poliomyelitis following this procedure.

Homoeopathy: the Council of the Faculty of Homoeopathy strongly supports the immunisation programme and has stated that immunisation should be carried out in the normal way using the conventional tested and approved vaccines, in the absence of medical contra-indications.

Adverse Reactions

The success of the spontaneous reporting system for vaccines depends on early, complete and accurate reporting of suspected adverse drug reactions (ADRs) through the Yellow Cards, which are supplied to general practitioners and pharmacists and are available through the CSM Freefone, or by writing to 1 Nine Elms Lane, London SW8 5NQ.

For currently marketed vaccines, **serious** suspected reactions, including those which are fatal, life-threatening, disabling, incapacitating or those which result in hospitalisation should be reported; this applies to all serious reactions whether or not such reactions have been previously recognised. For new vaccine formulations, which have a black triangle, all suspected reactions should be reported. When submitting a Yellow Card for an adverse reaction, it is most important that the vaccine is correctly identified, so that it is clear which formulation has been used;for example, combined Tetanus and low-dose diphtheria vaccine (Td) should be distinguished from Diphtheria/Tetanus vaccine (DT). Wherever possible, the batch number should be provided.

It is important to give as much information as possible about the nature, timing and severity of the observed reaction, if the patient was hospitalised, what treatment was given and the final outcome. Information about other factors such as concomitant medication, underlying disease, allergies or family history should be provided wherever possible. The provision of additional information such as test results or relevant hospital correspondence is always helpful. If further information becomes available after reporting a reaction, this should be sent to the MCA to help in the assessment of a suspected reaction.

Most of the reports submitted on Yellow Cards are of self-limiting illness, such as fever, rashes or injection site reactions which are associated with a complete recovery. More serious reactions are reported less frequently. Although a reaction might occur in close temporal association with an immunisation, often it can be very difficult to assess whether or not there is a causal link. Most reported reactions can occur independently of immunisation and there are few specific tests that can establish or exclude whether a vaccine caused a reported reaction. The probability that a vaccine has played a causal role in an event is increased if the event has occurred at a time interval after the immunisation which is in accordance with the known incubation periods of live organisms. For example, pyrexial illness occurring five to ten days after measles immunisation or parotid swelling three weeks after mumps immunisation, would be consistent with the incubation periods for these particular viruses. Pyrexia occurring less than three days after measles vaccine is unlikely to be caused by the immunisation and an intercurrent infection is more likely.

Assessing the probability of whether a reaction is caused by a vaccine is particularly difficult in young children. Illness such as fever or convulsions occur frequently in the first year of life and almost every child is immunised on three separate occasions during this period. Interpretation of the significance of clinical events occurring after immunisation depends on the biological plausibility, an identified excess of events in a specified post-immunisation period compared against background rates, and laboratory evidence that support the association. Generally, the risk of serious illness following natural infection far outweighs any possible risk from the relevant vaccine.

In 1995, there were 648 Yellow Card reports of suspected adverse reactions relating to routinely administered childhood vaccines for the whole UK., 152 of which were classified as 'serious'. Since 14 million doses of these vaccines were distributed in the UK in 1995, this means that the reported 'serious' suspected reactions were one per hundred thousand distributed doses of vaccine.

Immunisation can rarely increase the risk of a specific disease. Also, the evidence of harm from immunisation is not supported. Whilst natural rubella infection is often associated with arthropathy, especially in adult women, one recent retrospective case control study showed no increase in risk of arthropathy in under immune women immunised post-partum, compared with unimmunised controls.[1] A US study of re-immunisation of college students with MMR vaccine showed no increase in fever or rash in immunised students, compared with unimmunised controls.[2]

Acceptance and Establishment of Evidence of Causal Relationships of Adverse Reactions for Vaccines Currently on Offer

	Evidence favours acceptance of a causal relationship.	Evidence establishes a causal relationship.
DTP	Acute encephalopathy, shock and unusual shock-like state.	Anaphylaxis, Protracted inconsolable crying.
OPV/IPV	Guillain Barré Syndrome Syndrome (OPV) ***	Poliomyelitis in vaccine recipient or contact (OPV). Death from polio vaccine strain viral infection.*
Hib	–	–
Measles	Anaphylaxis	Thrombocytopenia (MMR) Anaphylaxis (MMR). Death from measles vaccine strain viral infection.*
Mumps	–	–
Rubella**	Chronic arthritis	Acute arthritis
T/DT/Td	Guillain Barré Syndrome Brachial neuritis	Anaphylaxis
Hepatitis B	–	Anaphylaxis

* These data come primarily from individuals proven to be immunocompromised.

** for counter view, see current 'Green Book, ' page 31 et seq.

***Subsequently retracted.

NB. See 'Green Book'pages 35 and 36 for information regarding the Vaccine Damage Payments Scheme.

Serious neurological reactions such as encephalitis may occur very rarely after vaccines. All such cases should be investigated and referred to hospital in the normal way and a final diagnosis of a suspected reaction to a vaccine should be made only after all other causes have been excluded. A suspected serious adverse reaction can be reported on a Yellow Card pending the availability of other results and further information can always be submitted at a later date.

The National Childhood Encephalopathy study concluded, after three years of case finding and follow up that if there was an increased risk of encephalopathy and permanent cerebral damage or death after pertussis vaccine, it was too small to be demonstrated statistically. Also, American studies have concluded that whole-cell pertussis vaccine has not been proven to be a cause of brain damage.

Anaphylaxis

Recipients of any vaccine should be observed for an immediate adverse reaction and should remain under observation until they have been seen to be in good health and not to be experiencing an immediate adverse reaction. As vaccines are administered subcutaneously or intramuscularly, the time of onset of anaphylaxis is variable and onset may be delayed for up to72 hours. Patients should be advised to seek medical attention if they develop early symptoms such as breathlessness, swelling and rash. Parents should be advised to seek medical advice should unexpected symptoms develop after immunisation. All cases of anaphylaxis should be reported using the Yellow Cards.

Clinical Characteristics of Anaphylaxis

Anaphylaxis is typically rapid and unpredictable with variable severity and clinical features. The most serious features include cardiovascular collapse, bronchospasm, angio-edema, pulmonary oedema, loss of consciousness and urticaria. Asthmatic patients often develop bronchospasm during anaphylaxis. Anaphylaxis generally responds promptly to adrenaline.

Anaphylactic reactions to vaccines are therefore probably very rare, (see page 37 of the 'Green Book' for recent studies), but they are unpredictable and have the potential to be fatal. Most anaphylactic reactions occur in individuals who have no known risk factors, making it difficult to advise on special precautions. It is uncertain whether a history of hypersensitivity significantly increases the risk of anaphylaxis.

Management of anaphylaxis
Differential diagnosis

It is most important to be able correctly to diagnose anaphylactic reactions, convulsions and fainting. Most convulsions reported after measles and rubella vaccine occurred within an hour of immunisation and had features suggesting syncope rather than epileptic fits. Syncope occurs commonly after any injection such as an immunisation in adults and adolescents. Very young children rarely faint and sudden loss of consciousness at this age should be presumed to be anaphylaxis if a central pulse (such as the carotid) cannot be felt. **A central pulse is maintained during a faint or convulsion.**

Anaphylaxis can occur without warning. Therefore, adrenaline and an appropriate sized oral airway must always be immediately available whenever immunisation is given. All health professionals responsible for immunisation must be familiar with techniques for resuscitation of a patient with anaphylaxis to prevent disability and loss of life.

Identification of Anaphylaxis, Syncope and Panic Attack

0-72 hours after vaccine

Symptoms suggestive of *anaphylaxis*

General signs:	*pallor, limpness, apnoea*
Cardiovascular:	*profound hypotension in association with tachycardia;sinus tachycardia*
Upper airway obstruction:	*angioedema – swelling of lips, face, neck and tongue;difficulty in breathing, speaking, swallowing;hoarseness and stridor.*
Lower airway obstruction:	*subjective feelings of retrosternal tightness and dyspnoea, bronchospasm-audible expiratory wheeze.*
Skin:	*diffuse erythema* *urticaria—itchy weals with erythematous edges and pale blanched centres.* *peripheral oedema.*

Treatment

1   Lie the patient in the left lateral position. If unconscious insert airway.

2   Send for professional assistance. Never leave the patient alone.

Mild anaphylaxis/allergic reactions (slowly progressing peripheral oedema changes restricted to the skin eg. urticaria)
oral antihistamines or subcutaneous *adrenaline* with observation and reassurance. Nebulised salbutamol oral or parenteral steroids, parenteral antihistamine, if necessary and/or available.

Severe anaphylaxis (with cardiovascular collapse)
Administer intramuscular adrenaline immediately. If appropriate, begin cardio-pulmonary resuscitation. If there is no improvement in the patient's condition in 5/10 minutes, repeat the dose of adrenaline to a maximum of three doses.

Chlorpheniramine maleate (piriton) may be given intravenously by appropriately trained individuals. Intravenous hydrocortisone may also be given to prevent further deterioration in severely affected cases.

If available, volume replacement with colloid solutions should be considered.

Bronchospasm
Administer nebulised adrenaline or adrenaline by intramuscular injection immediately.

Steroids may also be administered. Other nebulised bronchodilators, such as Beta 2 agonists (e.g. salbutamol) or parenteral aminophylline should be considered.

Angio—oedema/laryngeal oedema
Administer nebulised adrenaline or adrenaline by intramuscular injection.

Antihistamines should be given and intubation may be necessary.

Patients with anaphylaxis should be referred to hospital for assessment and further treatment may be necessary, such as provision of bronchodilators, adrenaline by infusion, colloids and assisted ventilation. NB. patients should be monitored after IV administration of adrenaline as adverse effects may be more common when the drug is given this way.

All cases of anaphylaxis should be observed for at least 6 hours, in case of any delayed reactions, and the Yellow Card should be used to report the reaction to the Medicines Control Agency.

Adrenaline Dosage: Adrenaline 1/1, 000 (1mg/ml) by intramuscular or subcutaneous injection.

Adults: 0.5 to 1. 0 ml repeated as necessary up to a maximum of three doses. The lower dose should be used for the elderly or those of slight build.

Infants and children:

Age	Dose of adrenaline
less than 1 year	0.05 ml
1 year	0.1 ml
2 years	0.2 ml
3-4 years	0.3 ml
5 years	0.4 ml
6-10 years	0.5 ml

Slow intravenous injection may be considered only in extreme emergency. Dilute adrenaline (1/10,000) should be used for the intravenous route. Where intramuscular injection might succeed, time should not be wasted seeking intravenous access. Patients should be monitored after intravenous administration as adverse effects may be more common when the drug is administered in this way.

Chlorpheniramine maleate	Age	Dose of chlorpheniramine maleate
	up to 1 year	200 µg/kg body weight
	1-5 years	2.5-5 mg
	6-12 years	5-10 mg
	over 12 years	10-20 mg

By slow intravenous injection over 1 minute.

Hydrocortisone

Age	Dose of hydrocortisone
up to 1 year	25 mg
1-5 years	50 mg
6-12 years	100 mg
adult	100-500 mg

By slow intravenous injection

This table is based on the Alder Hey book of childrens' doses, which provides guidelines on suitable doses of chlorpheniramine maleate for children. Chlorpheniramine maleate is not licensed for injection in children and clinicians take responsibility for its use in this group.

0-1 hour after vaccine
Symptoms suggestive of syncope or panic attacks

General signs:	*sweating, nausea, dizziness, ringing in the ears, dimmed vision, weakness, may precede the event. Choking and difficulty breathing may lead to hyperventilation, paraesthesiae and spasms of the hands.*
Cardiovascular:	*hypotension* *bradycardia*
Neurological:	*transient jerking movements and eye rolling can occur rarely.*

There should be rapid recovery . Although symptoms of malaise may persist, the patient should regain consciousness in 1-2 minutes. Any abnormal cardiovascular signs usually revert within a few minutes.

VERY YOUNG CHILDREN RARELY FAINT AND SUDDEN LOSS OF CONSCIOUSNESS AT THIS AGE SHOULD BE PRESUMED TO BE ANAPHYLAXIS IN THE ABSENCE OF A STRONG CENTRAL (CAROTID) PULSE, WHICH PERSISTS DURING A FAINT OR CONVULSION.

TREATMENT: The patient should remain lying down for 10—15 minutes with their feet raised. At any age, if in doubt, treat the patient for anaphylaxis

NB For further information consult the references detailed at the end of this chapter.

Immunisation Schedules

The schedule for primary immunisation with DTP and Hib and polio starts at two months, with an interval of one month between each dose, except in some parts of Scotland, where the schedule is started at two months and completed at six months with intervals between injections of not less than one month. This is summarised as follows:

Vaccine	Age		Notes
D /T /P and Hib	First dose	2 months)	
Polio	Second dose	3 months)	Primary Course
	Third dose	4 months)	
Measles/mumps rubella (MMR)	12-15 months		Can be given at any age over 12 months.
Booster DT and polio MMR second dose	3-5 years		Three years after completion of primary course
BCG	10-14 years or infancy		
Booster tetanus diphtheria and polio.	13-18 years		

Children should, therefore have received the following vaccines:

By 6 months:	3 doses of DTP, Hib and polio
By 15 months:	measles/mumps/rubella
By school entry:	4th DT and polio; second dose measles/mumps/rubella
Between 10 and 14 years:	BCG.
Before leaving school	5th polio and tetanus diphtheria (Td).

Diphtheria (See Chapter on Communicable Diseases)

The recommended vaccines for immunisation are:Adsorbed diphtheria/ tetanus/pertussis (DTP), adsorbed diphtheria/tetanus (DT), Adsorbed diphtheria (D), Adsorbed low dose diphtheria for adults (d), Adsorbed tetanus/ low dose diphtheria for adults (Td). Plain vaccines are less immunogenic, have no advantage in terms of reaction rates and are no longer available. The dose is 0.5ml given by intra muscular cutaneous injection.

Consult the 'Green Book'with regard to the storage and disposal of diphtheria vaccine and remember that vaccine which has been frozen must never be used.

Recommendations
For primary immunisation of infants and children up to ten years of age

a. Primary immunisation

Diphtheria vaccine as a component of triple vaccine (diphtheria toxoid, tetanus toxoid and Bordetella Pertussis toxoid) is recommended for infants from two months of age. Adsorbed vaccine should be used as it has been shown to cause fewer reactions than the plain vaccine which is no longer available. If the pertussis component is contraindicated, adsorbed diphtheria/tetanus vaccine should be used. A course of primary immunisation consists of three doses starting at two months with an interval of one month between each dose. If a course is interrupted it may be resumed; there is no need to start again.

b. Reinforcing immunisation

Booster doses of vaccine containing diphtheria and tetanus toxoids are recommended for: (i) children before school entry – DT, preferably at least three years after the last dose of the primary course, and (ii) before leaving school at 13 to 18 years of age – Td, both at the same time as OPV.

In approximately 25% of children, a fifth tetanus vaccine dose is said to have been given by the time the school leaving booster (Td) is due. If a child requires a tetanus booster after a tetanus prone wound, **after the fourth dose** has been given (at around 4 years of age) and ten years has elapsed, then Td should be given. The school leaving Td dose is then unnecessary.

If there is a documented history of a fifth dose of tetanus vaccine having already been given when the school leaving booster is due, **and** supplies of a low dose diphtheria vaccine product are readily available, (either low dose diphtheria vaccine (d) or 0.1ml of paediatric strength diphtheria vaccine (D)), then one of these latter two products should be used. If neither is available, then Td should be given with an interval of at least one month since the last dose of tetanus vaccine. Recent experience has shown that when Td is given to children who have already had 5 doses of tetanus vaccine, there is some increase in the number who have local reactions and low grade pyrexias, but no increase in the numbers with pyrexias over 38. 5 degrees C.

Immunisation of persons aged ten years or over
a. Primary immunisation

Low dose diphtheria vaccine for adults (d) must be used because of the possibility of a reaction in an individual who is already immune.

Past experience has shown that when full strength vaccine preparations (D) were given to adults, there were considerably more localised and generalised reactions, such as high fever. Three doses (0.5ml) of low dose vaccine for adults (d) should be given by deep subcutaneous or intramuscular injections at intervals of one month. When this product is not available, then a 0.1ml injection of the standard paediatric diphtheria vaccine (D) may be given as an alternative. For adults who have never received either diphtheria or tetanus vaccine previously, three doses of Td should be used, each given one month apart.

b. Reinforcing immunisation

A single dose of low-dose diphtheria vaccine (d) must be used for all persons aged ten years and over.

When this product is not available, then a 0.1 ml injection of the standard paediatric diphtheria vaccine (D) may be given as an alternative. When a reinforcing dose of tetanus vaccine is also required, then Td should be used. Prior Schick testing is not necessary and the material is no longer available.

Children given DTP at monthly intervals without a booster dose at 18 months have been shown to have adequate levels of diphtheria and tetanus antibody. A booster dose at 18 months for such children is therefore unnecessary.

Travel
Primary or reinforcing doses are recommended for travellers to epidemic or endemic areas.

Contacts of a diphtheria case, or carriers of a toxogenic strain
Individuals exposed to such a risk should be given a complete course or a reinforcing dose according to their age and immunisation history as follows:

a. **Immunised** children up to ten years.
   One injection of diphtheria vaccine (D).

b. **Immunised** children ten years and over, and adults.
   One injection of low dose diphtheria vaccine for adults (d orTd).

c. **Unimmunised** children under ten years.
   Three injections of diphtheria (D) vaccine (or DTP and polio vaccines if appropriate) at monthly intervals.

d. **Unimmunised** children ten years and over, and adults.
   Three injections of low dose diphtheria vaccine for adults (d) or (Td) at monthly intervals.

Unimmunised contacts of a case of diphtheria should in addition be given a prophylactic course of erythromycin or penicillin. Symptomatic contacts (including close contacts)of cases of sore throat associated with non-toxogenic C *diphtheriae* should be swabbed and treated accordingly; asymptomatic contacts do not require swabbing or antibiotic prophylaxis. Contacts of cases of C. *ulcerans* do not require prophylaxis as human to human transmission does not occur.

HIV positive individuals may be immunised against diphtheria in the absence of any contraindications.

Adverse reactions
Swelling and redness at the injection site are common. Malaise, transient fever and headache may also occur. A small painless nodule may form at the injection site but usually disappears without sequelae. Severe anaphylactic reactions are rare. Neurological reactions have been reported occasionally.

Severe reactions should be reported to the Committee on Safety of Medicines using the Yellow Card.

Contraindications
a. If a child is suffering from any acute illness, immunisation should be postponed until the child has fully recovered. Minor infections without fever or systemic upset are not reasons to postpone immunisation.

b. Immunisation should not proceed in children who have had a severe local or general reaction to a preceding dose, if it is thought that the diphtheria component has caused the preceding reaction. Reactions to the pertussis component of the DTP are the most likely and immunisation should proceed with DT; acellular pertussis vaccine can be used if the previous reaction was a local one.

When there is a need to control an outbreak, diphtheria vaccine may have to be given to individuals suffering from acute febrile illness. Low-dose diphtheria vaccine for adults (d or TD) must be used for persons aged ten years and over.

Diphtheria Antitoxin

Diphtheria antitoxin is now only used in suspected cases of diphtheria. Tests with a trial dose to exclude hypersensitivity should precede its use. It should be given without waiting for bacteriological confirmation since its action is specific for diphtheria. It may be given intramuscularly or intravenously, the dosage depending on the clinical condition of the patient. This is shown in the following table. It is no longer used for diphtheria prophylaxis because of the risk of provoking a hypersensitivity reaction to the horse serum from which it is derived. Unimmunised contacts of a case of diphtheria should be promptly investigated, kept under surveillance and given antibiotic prophylaxis and antibiotics as described on the previous page.

Dosage of antitoxin recommended for various types of diphtheria.

Type of Diphtheria	Dosage (units)	Route
Nasal	10,000 – 20,000	Intramuscular
Tonsillar	15,000 – 25,000	Intramuscular or Intravenous
Pharyngeal or laryngeal	20,000 – 40,000	Intramuscular or Intravenous
Combined types or delayed diagnosis	40, 000 – 60, 000	Intravenous
Severe diphtheria e. g. with extensive membrane and/or severe oedema (bull-neck diphtheria)	40,000 – 1000,000	Intravenous or part intravenous and part intramuscular

If acute anaphylaxis develops, intravenous adrenaline (0.2 to 0.5 ml of 1:1000 solution) should be administered immediately by intravenous injection. Antitoxin is probably of no value for cutaneous disease, although some authorities use 20,000 to 40,000 units of antitoxin because toxic sequelae have been reported.

Pertussis

Pertussis vaccine is a suspension of killed *Bordetella pertussis* organisms and is usually given as a triple vaccine combined with diphtheria and tetanus vaccine (DTP), with an adjuvant, usually aluminium hydroxide. The plain vaccine is no longer supplied as it is less immunogenic and causes more in the way of systemic reactions, especially fever.

At the present time there is no monovalent whole cell pertussis vaccine, but as an alternative, an acellular monovalent preparation (Acellular Pertussis Vaccine (APV)) is available on a named patient basis, and, as with the dose of DTP, it is given by deep subcutaneous or intramuscular injection. The DTP vaccine is given as in the schedule described earlier and the monovalent pertussis vaccine can be given when the pertussis component has been omitted from earlier immunisations. Children who have received a full course of immunisation against diphtheria and tetanus should be given three doses of monovalent pertussis vaccine at monthly intervals. APV has been made available solely for this purpose and should not be used in place of the existing DTP vaccine for routine primary immunisation.

For further details regarding pertussis vaccine and vaccination, together with information about pertussis vaccination and children with problem histories, the reader is referred to the 'Green Book', pages 158-163.

Haemophilus influenzae Type b (Hib)

The dose of Hib vaccine is 0.5ml., which should be given by deep sub-cutaneous or intramuscular injection, in a different limb from other con-currently administered vaccines. The recording of these sites allows any local actions to be attributed to the appropriate antigen(s). However, there is now sufficient evidence of preservation of immunogenicity and no increase in reactogenicity to allow recommendations for Hib vaccines to be mixed with DTP vaccines for simultaneous administration.[3]

The conjugate Hib vaccines are not live, and at the present time, there is no evidence of its safety or lack of safety in pregnancy. No reinforcing booster doses are recommended for children who have received three injections at the appropriate times (See Injection Schedule) and because the incidence of invasive H *influenzae* disease diminishes rapidly after the age of four years, routine immunisation of older children and adults is not recommended. Hib Vaccine can be given at the same time as any other vaccine. Also, HIV positive individuals may receive Hib vaccine.

Children under the age of thirteen months are at high risk of disease and should receive 3 doses of Hib vaccine, even if they have already commenced or completed their immunisations against Diphtheria, Tetanus, Pertussis and Poliomyelitis. Hib vaccine can be given at the same time as any other vaccines and any outstanding Hib doses should be given after the completion of the other antigens separated by one month from the last Hib dose.

Unimmunised children between 13 and 48 months should be given a single dose of Hib vaccine, either simultaneously with MMR vaccine, or singly if the MMR has already been given. Children in this age group are at a lower risk of disease and the vaccine is effective after a single dose.

Recent studies undertaken by the PHLS have shown that there is no loss of immunogenicity or increase in reactogenicity when children are immunised with different sequences of Hib vaccines from different manufacturers. Thus, children who start a course of Hib vaccine with one product can have the course completed with another product should the need arise.

Asplenic children and adults, irrespective of age and interval since splenectomy, should receive a single dose of Hib vaccine. Data are available suggesting that a single dose of Hib vaccine is immunogenic in splenectomised adults. Those under one year should be given three doses. At present, there are no data to indicate a need for further booster doses. In the case of an elective splenectomy, the vaccine should be given preferably at least two weeks earlier.

Adverse reactions

Swelling and redness at the injection site have been reported at a rate of up to 10%, following the first dose, but the size of these reactions was rarely sufficient to contraindicate further doses. These reported effects usually appear within 3 to 4 hours and resolve completely within 24 hours. The incidence of these reactions declines with subsequent doses, supporting the recommendation that courses of immunisation should be completed despite the occurrence of such reactions.

When a severe local reaction follows the administration of combined DTP/Hib vaccines, the course should be continued with the products given separately (DTP at one site, Hib at another site). Should a severe generalised reaction follow the administration of combined DTP Hib vaccine, the Hib vaccine should be given at one site and DT vaccine at another. Incidentally, the addition of Hib vaccine to routine immunisation does not lead to an increased incidence in the number of febrile convulsions that occur in the 72 hours after immunisation, compared to control periods. Surveillance in the UK of adverse events following Hib immunisation has not revealed any severe reactions that are not routinely reported after either DTP or MMR, which have most often been administered at the same time.

Contraindications

If a child is suffering from any acute illness, immunisation should be postponed until the child has recovered. Minor infections without fever or systemic upset, are not reasons to postpone immunisation.

However, immunisation should not proceed in children who have had a severe local reaction or a general reaction which can be confidently related to a preceding Hib immunisation. When Hib vaccine has been given with DTP, generalised reactions are more likely to have been caused by the pertussis component of the DTP vaccine.

Immunisation of cases and contacts of Hib disease

Household contacts of a case of invasive Hib disease have an increased risk of contracting the disease themselves. Any unimmunised household contact, under four years of age, should receive Hib vaccine (three doses if under 13 months, one dose if over 13 months and under four years). Independently of immunisation, rifampicin prophylaxis should be given to household contacts. The recommended dose is 28mg/kg/day (up to a maximum of 600 mg daily) once daily for four days. Chemoprophylaxis is not indicated for those contacts under **four** years who have been fully immunised against Hib disease. The index case should also be immunised, irrespective of age.

When a case occurs in a playgroup, nursery or creche, the opportunity should be taken to identify any unimmunised children under four years of age. Chemoprophylaxis should be offered to all room contacts – teachers and children – when **two or more** cases of Hib disease have occurred in a playgroup, nursery or creche within 120 days. There is little evidence, however, that children in such settings are at significantly higher risk of Hib disease than the general population of the same age.

NB Regarding rifampicin prophylaxis, where applicable, warn contact lens wearers of irritation and staining and advise extra contraception, where necessary, because of liver enzyme induction reducing the efficacy of oral contraception and indicating the temporary need for additional contraceptive measures.

For Supplies of all the above vaccines and anti-toxins. See the 'Green Book' Pages 75 and 83.

Hepatitis A
Vaccine
Hepatitis A vaccine is a formaldehyde – inactivated vaccine of a strain of hepatitis A virus (HAV) grown in human diploid cells. It is supplied as a suspension in pre-filled syringes. The vaccine should not be frozen, should be protected from light, stored at temperatures between 2 and 8 degrees C and not diluted or mixed with any other vaccines in the same syringe. Immunogenicity studies show that levels of antibody produced after a primary course of vaccine administered by intramuscular injection, are well in excess of those found after administration of HNIG. The primary course produces anti – HAV antibodies which persist for at least one year and antibody persistence can be prolonged by administration of a booster dose of vaccine six to 12 months after the initial course. Human normal immunoglobulin (HNIG) may be administered at the same time as the vaccine if protection is required less than 10 days after the first dose of hepatitis A vaccine.

Recommendations
1. Travellers
Protection against hepatitis is recommended for travellers to areas of moderate or high HAV endemicity particularly if sanitation and food hygiene are likely to be poor. Active immunisation with hepatitis A vaccine is the preferred method of protection particularly for frequent travellers to such areas or for stays longer than three months. Immunisation is **not** considered necessary for those travelling to Western Europe (including Spain, Portugal and Italy), or to North America, Australia or New Zealand.

When practicable, testing for antibodies to hepatitis A virus prior to immunisation may be worthwhile in those aged 50 and over, those born in areas of moderate or high hepatitis A endemicity and those who have a history of jaundice. Similar conditions will apply to military and diplomatic personnel being posted or likely to be posted to hepatitis A virus endemic countries. Also, this could well apply to school leavers contemplating a career in one of the armed forces of the crown.

Patients with chronic liver disease
Although patients with chronic liver disease are at no greater risk of acquiring hepatitis A infection, it can produce a much more serious illness in these patients who should therefore be considered for immunisation with hepatitis A vaccine. This will include intravenous drug misusers with chronic liver disease.

Haemophiliacs

Transmission of hepatitis A has been associated with the use of Factor VIII and Factor IX concentrates where viral inactivation procedures do not destroy hepatitis A and it is especially important that haemophiliacs receiving such products should be immunised against hepatitis A. Because of the high incidence of previous infections with hepatitis B and hepatitis C and of pre-existing liver disease in haemophiliacs, infection with hepatitis A can be particularly severe and these haemophiliacs should be immunised against hepatitis A. Those who are immunosuppressed may respond less well to the vaccine, and post-immunisation antibody testing should be considered. Haemophiliacs should be immunised subcutaneously and haemophiliacs and patients with chronic liver disease should be checked for previous exposure before immunisation.

Occupational exposure

Immunisation is recommended for laboratory workers who are working directly with the virus. There is no evidence that most health care workers are at increased risk of hepatitis A and routine immunisation is not indicated.

Outbreaks of hepatitis A have been associated with residential institutions for the mentally handicapped. Transmission does occur more readily in such institutions and immunisation of staff and residents may be appropriate in the light of local risk assessment. Similar considerations apply in other institutions where standards of personal hygiene are poor.

Infection in young children is likely to be sub-clinical and those working in day-care centres and other settings with children who are not yet toilet-trained may be at increased risk of infection. Under normal circumstances, the risk of transmission to staff and children can be minimised by careful attention to personal hygiene but, for example, in the case of local community outbreaks the need for the immunisation of children and staff should be discussed with the local Consultant in Communicable Disease Control or in Scotland the CPHM (CD and EH).

Food packers or food handlers in the UK have not been associated with HAV transmission sufficiently often to justify their immunisation as a routine measure.

Homosexuals

Cases of hepatitis A in homosexual males have been reported in the UK. Immunisation should be offered to those whose behaviour is likely to put them at risk.

Outbreaks

There is evidence that the use of hepatitis A vaccine can interrupt ongoing community outbreaks of hepatitis A when given to a defined population. Further guidance on the management of outbreaks should be sought from the Consultant in Communicable Disease Control or from the PHLS Communicable Disease Surveillance Centre. In Scotland this should be from the CPHM (CD/and/EH); or from the Scottish Centre for Infection and Environmental Health. Post exposure prophylaxis for contacts of cases will be dealt with later.

Route of administration and dosage.

The immunisation regimen for adults consists of a single dose of vaccine. Antibodies produced in response to this persist for at least a year. A booster at six to twelve months after the initial dose results in more persistent antibodies, a substantial increase in antibody titre and will give immunity for up to10 years.

The immunisation regimen for children and adolescents up to 15 years consists of a single dose of vaccine (720 ELISA units of the HM 175 strain) administered intramuscularly and produces antibodies for at least a year. In order to obtain more persistent immunity for up to ten years a booster dose (720 ELISA units) is recommended between six and twelve months after the primary course.

The former regimen for children and adolescents up to15 years consisted of two doses of vaccine (360 ELISA units) administered intramuscularly, two weeks to one month apart with a booster dose (360 ELISA units) recommended between six to twelve months after the primary course for prolonged immunity. Where initiated, the manufacturer recommends this regimen should be completed at this dosage.

The vaccine should be given intramuscularly in the deltoid region. It should not be given in the gluteal region because the vaccine efficiency may be reduced; nor should it be administered intravenously, or intradermally and should not be routinely given subcutaneously, although the subcutaneous route should be used in haemophiliacs.

Dosage

The dose in adults (16 years and over) is 1440 ELISA units (1ml) of the HM 175 strain or 160 Antigen units (0.5ml) of the GBM strain. The dose in children/adolescents (1-15 years), in a separate presentation is 720 ELISA units (0.5 ml) of the HM 175 strain. This will replace the earlier formulation where the dose was 360 ELISA units (0.5ml) (See 'Route of administration and dosage' immediately above.)

Adverse reactions

Adverse reactions are usually mild and confined to the first few days after immunisation. The most common reactions are mild transient soreness, erythema and induration at the injection site. General symptoms such as fever, malaise, fatigue, headache, nausea and loss of appetite are reported less frequently. It is important that all serious adverse reactions are reported to the Committee on Safety of Medicines by the Yellow Card.

Contraindications

Immunisation should be postponed in individuals suffering from severe febrile Illness.

Immunoglobulin

Human normal immunoglobulin (HNIG) offers short-term protection (up to about four months) against infection with hepatitis A to those in close contact with cases and to those travelling to areas where infection is more prevalent, particularly if sanitation and food handling are poor. Although infection is commonly subclinical in young children and severe infection uncommon, the decision to use HNIG may be influenced by the wish to protect parents and other adult contacts. Evidence suggests that, even if HNIG modifies disease rather than prevents infection, it is effective in preventing secondary cases.

There is no evidence associating the administration of intramuscular immunoglobulin with transmission of HIV. Not only does the processing of the plasma from which it is prepared render it safe, but the blood is derived from donors screened for HIV, and hepatitis B and C.

Recommendations

Use of HNIG should be considered in the following circumstances:

a. Contacts of cases of hepatitis A infection.

Prophylaxis restricted to household and close contacts may be relatively ineffective in controlling further spread. If given to a wider social group of recent household visitors (kissing contacts and those who have eaten food prepared by the index case) spread may be more effectively prevented.

b. Outbreaks

The appropriate approach to prophylaxis and the use of HNIG, with or without hepatitis A vaccine, should be discussed with the Consultant in Communicable Disease Control or CPHM (CD and EH) in Scotland.

In schools, particularly nursery and primary schools, HNIG may be used to protect teachers, adult helpers, including those responsible for cleaning the toilets, and the children and parents of the affected classes.

In closed communities where personal hygiene may be poor, widespread use of HNIG should be considered.

c. Travellers

HNIG is an alternative to vaccine for those travelling occasionally and for short periods outside Northern and Western Europe, North America, Australia and New Zealand. Hepatitis A vaccine is preferable for those visiting such countries frequently or staying for longer than three months. (See earlier notes on travel).

Where practicable, testing for antibodies to hepatitis A virus prior to immunisation may be worthwhile in those aged fifty years and over, those born in areas of high or moderate endemicity and those who have a history of jaundice.

HNIG may interfere with the development of active immunity from live virus vaccines. It is therefore wise to administer live virus vaccines at least three weeks before the administration of immunoglobulin. If immunoglobulin has been administered first, then an interval of three months should be observed before administering a live virus vaccine. This does not apply to yellow fever vaccine since HNIG does not contain antibody to this virus. For travellers, if there is insufficient time, the recommended intervals may have to be ignored, especially where polio vaccine is concerned. Alternatively, hepatitis A vaccine may be used in these circumstances.

Dosage

At present, the dosage of HNIG is expressed either by weight (mg) or by volume (ml). 1 ml of a 16% solution contains 160 mg. There are two dosage levels. The higher dose is recommended for those at greater risk (i. e. contacts) and for extended protection (i. e. those travelling abroad for 3-5 months).

Age	Low dose For travel lasting 2 months or less	High dose For travel lasting 3-5 months and for contacts.
Under 10 years	125mg	250 mg
10 years and over	250 mg	500 mg
or		
All ages	0.02-0.04 ml/kg	0.06-0.12 ml/kg

NB. For Contacts and the control of outbreaks only:

PHLS Communicable Disease Surveillance Centre,

Public Health Laboratories, England and Wales. Tel. 0181 200 6868

Scottish Centre for Infection and Environmental Health, Glasgow. (Tel: 0141 946 7120).

For Supplies of Hepatitis A immunoglobulin: See the 'Green Book' Page 93

Hepatitis B

Hepatitis B is the only sexually transmitted infection which may be prevented by immunisation.

There are two types of immunisation product; a **vaccine** which produces an immune response, and a **specific immunoglobulin** (HBIG) which provides passive immunity and can give immediate but temporary protection after accidental inoculation or contamination with antigen positive blood. Passive immunisation with specific immunoglobulin does not affect the development of active immunity in response to vaccine and combined active/passive immunisation is recommended in certain circumstances. (See later).

ACTIVE IMMUNISATION

Vaccine

Hepatitis B vaccine contains hepatitis B surface antigen (HBsAg) adsorbed on aluminium hydroxide adjuvant. It is currently prepared from yeast cells using recombinant DNA technology. The plasma derived vaccine is no longer marketed in the UK. The vaccine should be stored at 2-8 degrees C but not frozen, because **freezing destroys the potency of the vaccine**.

The vaccine is specific in preventing infection in individuals who produce specific antibodies to the hepatitis B surface antigen (anti-HBs). Overall, about 80-90% of individuals mount a response to the vaccine with anti-HBs levels greater than 10 miu/ml. Those over the age of 40 are less likely to respond. Patients who are immunodeficient or on immunosuppressive therapy may respond less well than healthy individuals and may require larger doses of vaccine or an additional dose.

An antibody level below 10 miu/ml is classified as a non-response to the vaccine whilst an antibody level of 100 miu/ml is considered to be protective. Those with antibody levels below 10miu/ml two to four months after completing a primary course of immunisation will require HBIG for protection if exposed to infection. (See later). Poor responders (anti-HBs 10-100 miu/ml) should receive a booster dose and in non-responders (anti-HBs less than 10miu/ml) a repeat course of vaccine should be considered.

Immunisation may take up to six months to confer adequate protection when the usual dose schedule is followed. (See Later.) Antibody titres should be checked in health care workers and babies born to hepatitis B carrier mothers two to four months after completion of the course. Post immunisation testing may also be indicated for other groups.

The duration of antibody persistence is not known precisely and there is no consensus of opinion on the need for booster doses. On present evidence it is felt that a single booster dose five years after the completion of a primary course is sufficient to retain immunity in those who continue to be at risk of infection unless they have already received a booster dose following possible exposure to the virus. (See later.)

Antibody levels greater than 100 miu/ml persist in some individuals for much longer than five years and there is some evidence that protective immunity is still present when antibody levels have fallen below 100 miu/ml.

Recommendations

Immunisation is recommended in individuals who are at increased risk of hepatitis B because of their lifestyle, occupation or other factors, such as close contact with a case or carrier (See later). In some groups the risk is similar for all, but in other cases it will be necessary for an individual assessment of risk to be made. This is particularly the case for those who may be at risk because of their occupation. The Control of Substances Hazardous to Health (COSHH) Regulations 1994 require employers to undertake their own risk assessment and to bring into effect measures necessary to protect workers and others who may be exposed, as far as is reasonably practicable against these risks.

NB. It is important that immunisation against hepatitis B does not encourage relaxation of good infection control procedures.

The vaccine should **not** be given to individuals known to be hepatitis B surface antigen positive, or to patients with acute hepatitis B, since in the former it would be unnecessary and in the latter, ineffective.

Hepatitis B vaccine **may** be given to HIV positive individuals and should be considered in those not already known to be infected or immune. Response rates are of the order of 70%.

Risk Groups

Immunisation is recommended for the following groups, – **excluding mothers and babies**: (for whom, see Green Book, page 99 for details)

Parenteral drug misusers

Individuals who change sexual partners frequently

Particularly homo and bi sexual men, and men and women who are prostitutes. Hepatitis B is the only sexually transmitted infection which can be prevented by immunisation.

Close family contacts of a case or carrier

Sexual partners are most at risk but close household contacts may also be at increased risk.

Contacts should have their hepatitis B markers checked to see if they have already become infected. Contacts who are HBsAg, anti-HBs or anti-HBc positive do not require immunisation but, in the case of sexual partners, it may be unwise to delay the administration of the first dose of the vaccine whilst awaiting test results. Advice should be given regarding the use of condoms until immunity is established. Sexual contacts of patients with acute hepatitis B should also receive HBIG (See later).

Families adopting children from countries with a high prevalence of hepatitis

(Particularly some in Eastern Europe, SE Asia and S America) may be at risk as some of these children could be chronic carriers. When the status of the child to be adopted is not known, families adopting children from any high prevalence country should be counselled as to the risks and offered immunistion against hepatitis B. There are grounds to consider testing such children because there could be benefits from referring an infected child for further management.

NB Although this paragraph may be considered not immediately relevant to schools medicine, it is retained for information, since the adopted children will be required to attend school.

Haemophiliacs

Those receiving regular blood transfusions or blood products, or those carers responsible for the administration of such products.

Patients with chronic renal failure

The response to hepatitis B vaccine is poor in those who are immunocompromised. Only 60% of patients on haemodialysis develop anti-HBs and therefore, in addition to those already on haemodialysis, the immunisation of all patients with chronic renal failure is recommended, as soon as it is anticipated that they may require dialysis or transplantation. A better response among patients with chronic renal failure may be obtained if higher doses (e. g. 40 mcg) are used.

Health care workers including students and trainees

Those who have direct contact with patients' blood or blood-stained body fluids or with patients' tissues. This group will include doctors, surgeons, dentists, nurses, midwives, laboratory workers, mortuary technicians, police and prison officers, but immunisation should be considered for any other staff who are at risk of injury from blood stained sharp instruments, contamination of surface lesions by patients' blood or blood stained body fluids, or of being deliberately injured or bitten by patients. Advice should be obtained from the appropriate Occupational Health Department.

Staff and residents of residential accommodation for those with severe learning disabilities (mental handicap)

A higher prevalence of hepatitis B carriage has been found among certain groups of those with learning difficulties (mental handicap) in residential accommodation than in the general population. Close daily living contact, and the possibility of behaviour problems, may lead to staff and other clients being at increased risk of infection. Similar considerations may apply to children and staff in day care settings and special schools for those with severe learning disabilities. Decisions on immunisation should be made on the basis of local risk assessments.

Those travelling to areas of high prevalence

Those who intend to seek employment as health care workers or those who plan to remain there for lengthy periods and who may therefore be at increased risk of acquiring infection as the result of medical and dental treatment carried out in those countries. Short term tourists or business travellers are not generally at increased risk of infection unless they place themselves at risk by their sexual behaviour when abroad.

Route of administration and dosage

The basic immunisation regimen consists of three doses of vaccine, with the first dose at the elected date, the second dose one month later and the third dose at six months after the first dose. An accelerated schedule has also been used where more rapid immunisation is required, for example for travellers or following exposure to the virus, when the third dose may be given at two months after the initial dose with a booster at 12 months. This dosage schedule for the rapid acquisition of immunity can be used to prevent perinatal transmission if given to neonates born to hepatitis B carrier mothers.

The vaccine should normally be given intramuscularly. The injection should be given in the deltoid region, though the anterolateral thigh is the preferred site in infants. **The buttock must not be used because vaccine efficiency may be reduced.**

In patients with haemophilia, the subcutaneous or intradermal route may be used. The likelihood of an effective antibody response is, however, reduced following use of the intradermal route and doctors are advised that until such times as the manufacturers apply for and are granted variations to their product licences for the intradermal route of administration, the use of this route is on their own personal responsibility. (See under). The response may be poor in those who are immunosuppressed and further doses of vaccine may be required.

Dosage

Currently licensed products contain different concentrations of antigen per ml. The particular manufacturers dosage schedules should be strictly observed.

Engerix B (Smith Kline Beecham)
　　Age 0-12 years　　10 mcg (0.5 ml)　　**Adults** 20 mcg (1.0 ml)

The intradermal dose (**but see above, regarding responsibility**) of Engerix B is 2 mcg (0.1 ml).

H-B-Vax II (Pasteur Merieux MSD)
　　Age 0-10 years　　5 mcg (0.5 ml)　　**Adults** 10 mcg (1. 0ml)

Adverse reactions

Hepatitis B vaccine is generally well tolerated and the most common adverse reactions are soreness and redness at the injection site. Injection intradermally may well produce a persisting nodule at the site of the injection, sometimes with local pigment changes. Other reactions which have been reported include fever, rash, malaise, an influenza like syndrome, arthritis, arthralgia and myalgia. Serious neurological reactions such as Guillain Barré syndrome and demyelinating disease have very rarely been reported although a causal relationship with hepatitis B vaccine has not been established. (NB. Yellow Cards!)

Contraindications

Immunisation should be postponed in individuals suffering from severe febrile illness.

Pregnancy

Hepatitis B infection in pregnant women may result in serious disease for the mother and chronic infection of the newborn. Immunisation should not be withheld from a pregnant woman if she is in the high risk category.

Information available on the outcome in those immunised during pregnancy does not reveal any cause for concern.

Supplies of Hepatitis B vaccine: Consult the 'Green Book'
Post-exposure prophylaxis

Specific hepatitis B immunoglobulin (HBIG) is available for passive protection and is normally used in combination with hepatitis B vaccine to confer passive/active immunity after exposure. Guidance is given in 'Exposure to hepatitis B virus;guidance on post exposure prophylaxis'. PHLS Hepatitis Sub-committee. *CDR Review* 1992: 2; R97-R101. A summary of this guidance is given below:

Whenever immediate protection is required, immunisation with the vaccine should be combined with simultaneous administration of hepatitis B immunoglobulin (HBIG) at a different site. It has been shown that passive immunisation with HBIG does not suppress an active immune response. A single dose of HBIG (usually 500 iu for adults;200 iu for the newborn) is sufficient for healthy individuals. If infection has already occurred at the time of immunisation, virus multiplication may not be inhibited completely, but severe illness, and, most importantly, the development of the carrier state may be prevented.

Immunoglobulin should be administered as soon as possible after exposure. In babies born to hepatitis B carrier mothers it should be given not later than 48 hours after birth (but see below) and in other types of exposure it should preferably be given within 48 hours and certainly no later than a week after exposure.

There is no evidence associating the administration of HBIG with acquisition of HIV infection. Not only does the processing of the plasma from which it is prepared render it safe, but the screening of blood donations is now routine practice.

Groups requiring post-exposure prophylaxis

Babies born to mothers who are HBeAg positive carriers, who are HBsAg positive without e markers (or where the marker status has not been determined), or who have had acute hepatitis during pregnancy. See 'Green Book' page 105.

Persons who are accidentally inoculated, or who contaminate the eye or mouth or fresh cuts or abrasions of the skin, with blood from a known HBsAg positive person. Individuals who sustain such accidents should wash the affected area well with soap and warm water and seek medical advice. Advice about prophylaxis after such accidents should be obtained by telephone from the nearest Public Health Laboratory or from the CPHM on call for the local Health Board in Scotland. Advice following accidental exposure may also be obtained from the Hospital Control of Infection Officer or the Occupational Health Services.

Health care workers who have already been successfully immunised should be given a booster dose of vaccine unless they are known to have adequate protective levels of antibody.

Sexual partners and in some circumstances, family contacts judged to be at high risk of individuals suffering from acute hepatitis B, and who are seen within one week of onset of jaundice in the contact.

Dosage

Hepatitis B immunoglobulin is available in 2ml ampoules containing 200 iu and 5 ml ampoules containing 500 iu.

Newborn	200 iu as soon as possible after birth

If administration of HBIG is delayed for more than 48 hours see above.

Children

Age 0-4 years	200 iu
Age 5-9 years	300 iu

Adults and children aged 10 years or more 500 iu

For adults and children not exposed at birth, HBIG should be given preferably within 48 hours and not later than a week after exposure.

For Supplies of Hepatitis B Immunoglobulin See the 'Green Book' Page 108

Note: Supplies of this product are limited and demands should be restricted to patients in whom there is a clear indication for its use.

HBV Prophylaxis for reported exposure incidents

HBV status of person	Significant exposure			Non-significant exposure	
	HBsAg +ve	Unknown	HBs Ag negative	Continued risk	No further risk
≤1 dose HB vaccine pre-exposure	Accelerated course of HB vaccine* HBIG x 1	Accelerated course of HB vaccine*	Initiate course of HB vaccine	Initiate course of HB vaccine	No HBV prophylaxis Reassure
≥ 2 doses HB vaccine pre-exposure (Anti-HBs not known)	One dose of HB vaccine followed by second dose 1/12 later	One dose of HB vaccine	Finish course of HB vaccine	Finish course of HB vaccine	No HBV Prophylaxis Reassure
Known responder to HB vaccine (anti-HBs>10miU /ml	Consider booster dose of HB vaccine	Consider booster dose of HB vaccine	Consider booster dose of HB vaccine	Consider booster dose of HB vaccine	No HBVprophylaxis Reassure
Known non-responder to HB vaccine (anti-HBs<10 miU/ml 2 – 4 months post-immunisation	HBIG x 1 Consider booster dose of HB vaccine	HBIG x 1 Consider booster dose of HB vaccine	No HBIG Consider booster dose of HB vaccine	No HBIG Consider booster dose of HB vaccine	No prophylaxis Reassure

*An accelerated course of vaccine consists of doses spaced at 0, 1 and 2 months.
A booster dose may be given at 12 months to those at continuing risk of exposure to HBV.
Source:PHLS Hepatitis Subcommittee. CDR Review1992;2; R 97 – R101. (further details and explanation of definitions are contained in this article.

Immunoglobulin

Information on specific immunoglobulins is provided in the chapters on particular vaccines. All immunoglobulins are prepared from the blood of donors who are negative for hepatitis B surface antigen (HBsAg) and for antibody to human immunodeficiency viruses types 1 and 2 (HIV), and to Hepatitis C virus (HCV). The materials are treated to inactivate viruses.

Human Normal Immunoglobulin (HNIG)

This is prepared from pooled plasma of blood donors and contains antibody to measles, varicella, hepatitis A and other viruses which are currently prevalent in the population. Immunoglobulin prepared by Bio Products Laboratory, and supplied as below, is available in 1.7 ml ampoules containing 250 mg, and 5ml vials containing 750 mg. It is given by intramuscular injection. It must be stored at 0-4 degrees C and the expiry date on the packet must be observed. It has a shelf life of three years when correctly stored. Unused portions of the vial must be discarded.

Recommendations for the use of HNIG for prophylaxis of measles and hepatitis A are given on the appropriate pages. It is not recommended for the protection of rubella and mumps.

HNIG may interfere with the immune response to live virus vaccines which should therefore be given at least three weeks before or three months after an injection of HNIG. This does not apply to yellow fever vaccine since HNIG obtained from donors in the UK is unlikely to contain antibody to this virus. For travellers going abroad this interval may not be possible. In the case of live polio vaccine, this is likely to be a booster dose for which the possible inhibiting effect is less important.

For Supplies of Human Normal immunoglobulin and Specific Immunoglobulins for anti-tetanus, anti-hepatitis B, anti-rabies and anti-varicella-zoster. See 'Green Book' p110-111.

Influenza vaccine

This is prepared each year using virus strains or genetic reassortants similar to those considered to be most likely to be circulating in the forthcoming winter. The highly purified viruses are grown in embryonated hens' eggs, chemically inactivated, and then further treated and purified. Current vaccines are trivalent containing two type A and one type B sub-types and in recent years have given a good match with subsequently circulating viruses. A monovalent vaccine containing the antigens of only one strain of virus might be more appropriately produced if a new virus with epidemic or pandemic potential emerged.

Two types of vaccine are available; 'split virus' vaccines contain virus components prepared by treating whole viruses with organic solvents or detergents and then centrifuging; 'surface antigen' vaccines contain highly purified haemagglutinin and neuraminidase antigens prepared from disrupted virus particles. The vaccines are equivalent in efficiency and adverse reactions.

Currently available influenza vaccines give 70-80% protection against influenza virus strains related to those in the vaccine. In the elderly, protection against infection may be less, but immunisation has been shown to reduce the incidence of bronchopneumonia, hospital admissions and mortality. Protection lasts for about one year. To provide continuing protection, annual immunisation is necessary with vaccine containing the most recent strains. The vaccines should be stored at 1-8 degrees C and protected from light. They must not be frozen, should be allowed to reach room temperature and shaken well before they are given.

For many years MOSA has been involved in studies of influenza and its vaccination, because this disease is capable of causing widespread disruption to school life, especially in boarding schools. Although the immunisation of fit children and adults against influenza is not normally recommended by the Department of Health, such vaccination is recommended for those living in residential homes and the like, and boarding schools will fit into this category, yet the final decision regarding whether or not to immunise against influenza must rest with the school doctor.

Annual influenza immunisation is strongly recommended by the Department of Health for adults and children with any of the following conditions: chronic respiratory disease, including asthma, chronic heart disease or renal failure, diabetes mellitus and immunosuppression due to disease or treatment, including asplenia or splenic dysfunction.

The departments of Health in the UK, by means of the annual letters from their Chief Medical Officers, advise doctors of details of the composition and doses of each year's vaccines and of any changes in recommendations for vaccination.

Route of Administration and dosage
Adults and children aged 13 and over:
a single injection of 0.5 ml im or deep sc

Children aged 4-12 years:
0.5ml im or deep sc, repeated 4-6 weeks later if receiving influenza vaccination for the first time

Children aged 6 months – 3 years:
0.25 ml im or deep sc, repeated 4-6 weeks later if receiving influenza vaccine for the first time

The deltoid muscle is the recommended site for adults and older children. For infants and young children, the preferred site is the antero-lateral aspect of the thigh.

Antibody levels may take up to 10-14 days to rise. Influenza activity is not usually significant before the middle of November, and therefore the ideal time for immunisation is October/early November. Patients and their parents, should be warned that many organisms cause respiratory infections similar to influenza during the influenza season, and influenza vaccine will not prevent these other infections. The 'common cold' is completely uninfluenced by the influenza vaccine, contrary to popular belief. Also, influenza vaccine contains inactivated virus and therefore cannot cause influenza.

Adverse reactions

Influenza vaccine is usually well tolerated apart from occasional soreness at the immunisation site. In rare instances it can, however, cause:

a.) Fever, malaise, myalgia and /or arthralgia beginning 6 to12 hours after immunisation and lasting up to 48 hours.

b) Immediate reactions such as urticaria, angio-oedema, bronchospasm and anaphylaxis, most likely due to hypersensitivity to residual egg protein.

Guillain-Barré syndrome has been reported very rarely after immunisation with influenza vaccine, although a causal relationship has not been established.

Contraindications

The vaccines are prepared in hens' eggs and should not be given to individuals with known anaphylactic hypersensitivity to egg products.

There is no evidence that influenza virus prepared from inactivated virus causes damage to the foetus. However, it should not be given during pregnancy unless there is a specific indication.

Amantadine in the prevention of influenza A

Amantadine hydrochloride is an effective antiviral agent against influenza A and may be used prophylactically to control an outbreak proven to be due to, or occurring during an epidemic of, influenza A, for unimmunised patients suffering from a condition likely to be made worse by influenza, for a fort – night, pending the vaccine taking effect. Similarly, it can be used for such patients for whom immunisation is contraindicated or unavailable. Healthcare workers, eg, house care and temporary sanatorium staff, could also benefit from the drug. (See Influenza in the Chapter on Communicable Diseases).

The recommended dose is 100 mg daily. Higher doses are associated with a greater incidence of adverse reactions, which include insomnia, restlessness and anxiety, nausea and anorexia. (In the elderly taking doses higher than 100mg daily, epileptic fits have been reported.) The use of amantadine should not be used for influenza prophylaxis outside the above recommendations because of the risk of inducing drug resistance in the virus.

For Supplies of Influenza vaccine: Consult the 'Green Book' Page 118.

Measles, Mumps and Rubella (MMR)
Measles

Following the introduction of MMR vaccine in October 1988 and the achievement of coverage levels in excess of 90%, notifications of measles fell progressively to the lowest levels since records began in 1940. The high coverage of MMR vaccine and the ensuing reduction in the transmission of the measles virus, meant that after 1988, children who had not been immunised no longer had the opportunity to be exposed to measles infection and remained susceptible until early teenage. Age stratified seroepidemiology confirmed that a rising proportion of school children were susceptible to measles and the high probability of a major resurgence of measles affecting the greater part of the school age population was predicted. (Similar epidemics of measles had been observed in many other countries following periods of low incidence of the disease achieved by high immunisation coverage.)

After further outbreaks in 1993, including a significant one in the West of Scotland, a national immunisation campaign throughout the UK was implemented the following year, in which over eight million children between the ages of five and 16 years were immunised with measles/rubella vaccine.

Consequently, susceptibility to measles in the target population fell by about 85% and only very few confirmed cases of measles have occurred in school children. Sometimes the disease is imported from abroad and adults can be affected. Reports of serious adverse reactions to the vaccine were very rare(0.007%) (See under 'Communicable Diseases'.)

Mumps

This is an acute viral illness which is described in greater detail under Communicable Diseases. It can affect all ages and is characterised by salivary gland swellings, with the potential for neurological and other complications. It was made a notifiable disease in 1988 and there has been a marked reduction in notifications of late. Accurate diagnosis is available by the discovery of mumps immunoglobulin in saliva.

Rubella

This mild infectious disease is capable of causing severe damage to the developing foetus in the early months of pregnancy. See under Communicable Diseases.

MMR Vaccine

This is a freeze dried preparation containing live attenuated measles mumps and rubella viruses. It must be stored in a dry state, between 2-8 degrees C, not frozen and protected from light. It should be reconstituted with the diluent supplied by the manufacturer and used within the hour. Immunisation provides protection for approximately 90% of recipients for measles and mumps and over 95% for rubella. Vaccine-induced antibody has been shown to persist for at least 18 years in the absence of endemic disease. Since the vaccine viruses are not transmitted, there is no risk of infection from vaccinees.

One vaccine is currently available, viz.

MMR II (Merk); Enders' Edmonston strain measles, RA 27/3 rubella, Jeryl Lynn mumps.

Single antigen measles, mumps and rubella vaccines are available.

For details of supplies: See 'Green Book' Pages 141 for vaccine and 143 for immunoglobulin.

Route of administration and dosage

0.5ml is given by deep intramuscular injection.

Recommendations

Observations over the last few years have indicated that the potential for the re-emergence of epidemics of measles can be prevented with a two dose programme. Thus, since1st October1996, all children except those with a valid contraindication should receive two doses of MMR vaccine: one shortly before the age of one and the other before school entry, irrespective of a history of measles, mumps or rubella.

MMR vaccine may be given to children of **any age** on request from the parents. If the primary immunisations of DTP, polio and Hib have not been completed by the time that MMR vaccine is due, they can be given at the same time using separate syringes and different sites. For maximum effect, MMR vaccine must be given soon after the first birthday. If the parents do not wish MMR vaccine to be given at the same time as other injected vaccines, the OPV should be given with MMR and the child recalled for the other vaccines as soon as possible; in these circumstances no three week interval between immunisations is necessary.

When children who have not received their first dose of MMR attend for their pre-school boosters (DT and polio vaccines), they should be offered their first MMR and arrangements made for a second dose to be given three months after the first dose.

There is a group of children who were too young to be included in the measles rubella immunisation campaign of 1994 and who have already been given their pre-school boosters. These children should be recalled and given their MMR vaccine. Similarly, any children known not to have received measles and rubella vaccine, should be offered MMR vaccine.

When children attend for their school leaving immunisations, there is an opportunity to check that all recommended immunisations have been completed. Boys and girls who have not had measles and rubella vaccine, should be offered MMR vaccine. There is no contraindication to the simultaneous administration of MMR, Td and OPV.

MMR vaccine can be given to non-immune adults and should be considered for those in long-term institutional care who might not have developed immunity. Entry into college, university or other centres for further education provides an opportunity to check the immunisation history. Students who have not received MR or MMR vaccine should be offered MMR immunisation.

Children with a personal or close family history of convulsions should be given MMR vaccine, provided that the parents understand that there may be a febrile response. As for all children, advice for reducing fever should be given. Doctors should seek specialist paediatric advice rather than refuse immunisation. Dilute immunoglobulin, as formerly used with measles vaccine for such children is no longer used since it may inhibit the immune response to the rubella and mumps components.

Unimmunised children in the following groups are at particular risk from measles infection and should be immunised with MMR vaccine:

a). Children with chronic conditions such as cystic fibrosis, congenital heart or kidney disease, failure to thrive and Down's syndrome.

b). Children from one year upwards in residential or day care, including play groups and nursery schools.

As vaccine induced **measles** antibody develops more rapidly than that following natural infection, MMR vaccine can be used to protect susceptible contacts during a **measles** outbreak. To be effective the vaccine must be administered within three days of exposure. If there is doubt about a child's immunity, vaccine should be given since there are no ill effects from vaccinating children who are already immune. Immunoglobulin is available for individuals for whom vaccination is contraindicated. (See later).

NB: Antibody responses to the rubella and mumps components of MMR vaccine are too slow for effective prophylaxis after exposure to these infections.

Re-immunisation is necessary when vaccine has been given before 12 months of age.

Measles virus inhibits the response to tuberculin, so that a false negative tuberculin test may be found for up to a month following MMR vaccine.

HIV positive individuals may be given MMR vaccine in the absence of contraindications.

Adverse reactions

Following the first dose of MMR vaccine

Malaise, fever and/or a rash may occur, most commonly about a week after immunisation and last about two to three days. In a study of over 6,000 children aged one to two years, the symptoms reported were similar in nature, frequency, time of onset and duration to those commonly reported after measles vaccination. During the sixth to the eleventh days after the vaccine, febrile convulsions occurred in 1/1000 children, the rate previously reported in the same period after the measles vaccine. Parotid swelling occurred in about 1% of children of all ages up to four years, usually in the third week and occasionally later.

Up until September 1992, MMR vaccines containing the Urabe strain of mumps virus were in routine use. These vaccines were found to be rarely associated with mumps meningitis, most often occurring around three weeks after immunisation. **No cases have been confirmed with the presently used Jeryl Lynn mumps vaccine.** When mumps virus is isolated from the cerebrospinal fluid, laboratory tests can distinguish between wild and vaccine strains. Advice should be sought from the National Institute for Biological Standards and Control. (Tel: 01707 654753).

Thrombocytopenia, which usually resolves spontaneously, occurs in about 1 in 24,000 children given a first dose of MMR at 12-15 months. Arthropathy (arthralgia and arthritis) has been reported to occur rarely after MMR immunisation. If it occurs other than 14-21 days after immunisation, it is most unlikely to have been caused by the vaccine.

Because MMR vaccine contains live attenuated viruses, it is biologically plausible for it to cause cases of encephalitis. However, a recent review of the published evidence on encephalitis, and measles or MMR immunisation, concluded that the evidence is inadequate to accept or reject a causal relationship between measles or mumps vaccine and encephalitis or encephalopathy. This suggests that if there is a risk of encephalitis or encephalopathy, induced by the vaccine, it is exceptionally small.

23 cases of neurological disease following measles immunisation were investigated in the USA between 1965 and 1967. 18 cases were characterised as 'encephalitis'. The interval from immunisation to the onset of symptoms ranged from 3 to 24 days. The estimated rate of encephalitis within a four week period of measles immunisation was 1.5 cases per million distributed doses of vaccine. The background rate of encephalitis (unrelated to immunisation) was 2.8 cases per 1 million children for any 4 week period. The authors of the study concluded that 'no single clinical or epidemiological characteristic appears consistently in the reports of cases of possible neurological sequelae of measles immunisation'.

After the second dose of MMR vaccine.

Adverse reactions are consistently less common than after the first dose. One study showed no increase in fever or rash after re-immunisation of college students compared to unimmunised controls. Only three cases of thrombocytopenia were reported in association with the immunisation of over eight million children in the November 1994 measles/rubella campaign. This suggests that the risk (of an adverse reaction) in children receiving a second dose is considerably less than in children receiving a first dose. An analysis of adverse reactions reported through the US Vaccine Adverse Events Reporting System in1991-93 showed fewer reactions among children aged 6 to 19 years, considered to be second dose recipients, than among those aged 1 – 4 years, considered first dose recipients.

Three cases of Guillain Barré syndrome (GBS) were reported following the November 1994 MR immunisation campaign. Between one and eight cases would have been expected in this population over this period in time in the absence of an immunisation campaign. Analysis of reporting rates of GBS from acute flaccid paralysis surveillance undertaken in the region of the Americas has shown no increase in rates of GBS following measles immunisation campaigns when over 70 million children were immunised. It was concluded from this evidence that measles immunisation does not cause GBS.

Parents should be told about possible symptoms after immunisation and given advice for reducing fever, including the use of paracetamol in the period five to ten days after immunisation. They should also be reassured that post immunisation symptoms are **not** infectious.

Serious reactions should be reported to the Committee on Safety of Medicines using the yellow card system.

Contraindications

i. If a child is suffering from an acute illness, immunisation should be postponed until recovery has occurred. Minor infections without fever or systemic upset are not reasons to postpone immunisation. Antibody responses and incidence of adverse reactions were the same in children with or without acute mild illness, when given MMR vaccine. The acute illnesses were upper respiratory tract infection, diarrhoea, or otitis media.

ii Children with untreated malignant disease or altered immunity;those receiving immuno-suppressive or X-ray therapy or high-dose steroids. (See earlier) iii Children who have received another live vaccine – including BCG – within three weeks. As explained earlier, in the section on poliomyelitis vaccination, (immunisation intervals), it is recommended that a three-week interval should be allowed between the administration of live virus vaccines, especially measles vaccine and tuberculin testing. There is experience to show that measles infection or immunisation can give false negative results in tuberculin positive individuals.

iv Children with allergies to neomycin or kanamycin.

v If MMR vaccine is given to women of child-bearing age, pregnancy should be avoided for one month, as for rubella.

vi MMR vaccine should not be given within three months of an injection of immunoglobulin.

Allergy to egg

There is increasing evidence that MMR vaccine can be safely given to children even when they have had an anaphylactic reaction (generalised urticaria, swelling of the mouth and throat, difficulty in breathing, hypo-tension and shock) following food containing egg. MMR was administered safely to 1209 patients with positive skin tests for egg. There were only two reports suggestive of anaphylaxis (0.16%). The combined data indicate that over 99% of children who are allergic to eggs can safely receive MMR vaccine. Dislike of egg, or refusal to eat it is **not** a contraindication. If there is concern, paediatric advice should be sought with a view to immunisation under controlled conditions such as admission to hospital as a day case.[4,5]

Measles

Children and adults with compromised immunity who come into contact with measles should be given human normal immunoglobulin (HNIG) as soon as possible after exposure. Testing for measles antibody may delay the administration of HNIG and neither immunisation nor low level antibody guarantees immunity to measles in the immunocompromised.

Children under 12 months in whom there is a particular reason to avoid measles, (such as recent severe illness), can also be given immunoglobulin; MMR vaccine should then be given after an interval of at least three months, at around the usual age.

Dose:

To prevent an attack:	Age	Dose
	Under 1 year	250 mg
	1-2 years	500 mg
	3 and over	750 mg
To allow an attenuated attack:		
	Under 1 year	100 mg
	1 year or over	200 mg.

An interval of at least three months must be allowed before subsequent MMR vaccination.

Dilute immunoglobulin as previously used with measles vaccine for children with a history of convulsions is no longer used since it may inhibit the immune response to rubella and mumps.

Mumps

HNIG is no longer effective for post exposure protection since there is no evidence that it is effective. Mumps -specific immunoglobulin is no longer available.

Rubella

Post-exposure prophylaxis does **not** prevent infection in non-immune contacts and is therefore **not** recommended for the protection of pregnant women exposed to rubella. It may however, reduce the likelihood of clinical symptoms which may possibly reduce the risk to the foetus. It should only be used when termination of pregnancy for proved rubella infection is unacceptable to the pregnant woman, when it should be given as soon as possible after exposure; serological follow-up of recipients is essential.

Dose: 750mg.

See the 'Green Book' pages 141 and 143 for details of supplies of vaccine and immunoglobulin.

Tetanus

Effective protection against tetanus is provided by active immunisation and in1970, it was recommended in the UK that active immunisation should be routinely provided in the treatment of wounds, when immunisation against tetanus should be initiated if appropriate, and subsequently completed.

Tetanus vaccine and adsorbed tetanus vaccine

The recommended vaccines for immunisation are, Adsorbed tetanus (T), Adsorbed diphtheria/tetanus (DT), Adsorbed tetanus/low-dose diphtheria vaccine for adults (Td) and Adsorbed diphtheria/tetanus/pertussis (DTP).

Plain vaccines are no longer supplied as they are less immunogenic and have no advantage in terms of reaction rates. Vaccines should be stored at 2-8 degrees C, not frozen and protected from light. Disposal should be by incineration at not less than 1100 degrees C at a registered waste disposal contractor.

The dose is 0.5ml given by intramuscular or deep subcutaneous injection.

Recommendations

a. Primary immunisation

Triple vaccine, i. e., vaccine containing diphtheria toxoid, tetanus toxoid, and Bordetella pertussis, is recommended for infants from two months of age. Adsorbed DTP vaccine is used as it has been shown to cause fewer reactions than plain vaccine. If the pertussis component is contraindicated, adsorbed diphtheria/tetanus vaccine should be given. **A primary course of immunisation consists of three doses starting at two months with an interval of one month between each dose**. If a course is interrupted it may be resumed; there is no need to start again, whatever the interval. The dose is 0.5ml given by intramuscular or deep subcutaneous injection.

b. Reinforcing doses in children

A booster dose of adsorbed diphtheria/tetanus (DT) should be given at least three years after the final dose of the primary course. If the primary course is only completed at school entry, then the booster dose should be given three years later. A further reinforcing dose of tetanus and low dose diphtheria vaccine (Td) is recommended for those aged 13-18 years or before leaving school. **Teenagers being treated for tetanus prone wounds and who had earlier received their fourth dose of tetanus vaccine approximately ten years earlier, should be given Td vaccine and the school leaving dose omitted.**

Children given DTP at monthly intervals for primary immunisation, without a booster dose at 18 months, have been shown to have adequate antibody levels at school entry. A booster dose at 18 months is therefore not recommended.

For immunisation of adults and children over ten years

Adults most likely to be susceptible to tetanus are the elderly, especially women and men who have not served in the Armed Forces.

a. For primary immunisation the course consists of three doses of 0.5ml of adsorbed tetanus vaccine (T) by intramuscular injection or deep sub-cutaneous injection, with intervals of one month between each dose. If there is no record of diphtheria immunisation either, then three doses of Td vaccine should be given.

b. A reinforcing dose (T or Td) ten years later after the primary course and again ten years later maintains satisfactory levels of protection which will probably be life-long.

c. For immunised adults who have received five doses, either in childhood, or as above, booster doses are not recommended, other than at the time of tetanus prone injury, since they have been shown to be unnecessary and can cause considerable local reactions. There are data that show that tetanus has occurred only exceptionally rarely in fully immunised individuals despite the passage of many years since the completing dose of a standard course of immunisation, and without subsequent boosting. Cases that have occurred were not fatal. **There is little justification for boosting with tetanus vaccine beyond the recommended five dose regime.**

Treatment of patients with tetanus-prone wounds

The following are considered tetanus-prone wounds:

a. Any wound or burn sustained more than six hours before surgical treatment of the wound or burn.

b   Any wound or burn at any interval after injury that shows one or more of the following characteristics:

   (i)   A significant degree of devitalised tissue.

   (ii) Puncture-type wound.

   (iii) Contact with soil or manure likely to harbour tetanus organisms.

   (iv) Clinical evidence of sepsis.

Thorough surgical toilet of the wound is essential whatever the tetanus history of the patient.

Specific anti-tetanus prophylaxis is as follows:

Immunisation status	Type of Wound Clean	Type of Wound Tetanus Prone
Last of 3 dose course, or reinforcing dose within last 10 years	Nil	(A dose of human tetanus immunoglobulin may be given if risk of infection is considered high, e. g. contamination with stable manure).
Last of 3 dose course or reinforcing dose more than 10 years previously.	A reinforcing dose of adsorbed vaccine.	A reinforcing dose of adsorbed vaccine plus a dose of human tetanus immunoglobulin.
Not immunised or immunisation status not known with certainty.	A full 3 dose course adsorbed vaccine	A full 3 dose course of vaccine, plus a dose of tetanus immunoglobulin in a different site.

Dosage human tetanus immunoglobulin

Prevention	Treatment
250 iu by intramuscular injection, or 500 iu, if more than 24 hours have elapsed since injury, or there is risk of heavy contamination or following burns.	150 iu/kg given in multiple sites.

Available in 1ml ampoules containing 250iu.

Routine tetanus immunisation began in 1961, thus individuals born before that year will not have been immunised in infancy. After a tetanus-prone injury such individuals will therefore require a full course of immunisation unless it has been previously given, as for instance in the armed services.

Immunised individuals respond quickly to a subsequent single injection of adsorbed tetanus vaccine, even after an interval of years.

For wounds not in the above categories, such as clean cuts, antitetanus immunoglobulin should **not** be given.

Patients with impaired immunity who suffer a tetanus-prone wound may not respond to vaccine and may therefore require antitetanus immunoglobulin in addition.

HIV positive individuals **should** be immunised against tetanus in the absence of contra indications.

Adverse reactions

Local reactions, such as pain, redness and swelling round the injection site may occur and persist for several days. General reactions, which are uncommon, include headache, lethargy, malaise, myalgia and pyrexia. Acute anaphylactic reactions and urticaria may occasionally occur and, rarely, peripheral neuropathy. Persistent nodules may arise at the injection site if the injection is not given deeply enough. Severe or unusual reactions should be reported to the Committee on Safety of Medicines using the Yellow Card.

Contraindications

(a) Tetanus vaccine should not be given to an individual suffering from acute febrile illness except in the presence of a tetanus prone wound. Minor infections without fever or systemic upset are not reasons to postpone immunisation.

(b) Immunisation should not proceed in individuals who have had an anaphylactic reaction to a previous dose. A large study of individuals (740) with case histories of reactions after tetanus immunisation showed that tetanus immunisation could be completed and none of the patients when challenged, suffered an adverse reaction. The authors conclude that an adverse reaction to tetanus toxoid does not preclude further immunisation with this same material. If this is to be done in patients with an adverse reaction to a previous dose, then it is best performed in a setting where there are facilities to deal with any acute allergic reactions.[4]

For details of suppliers of tetanus vaccines and anti tetanus immunoglobulin, including human anti tetanus immunoglobulin for intravenous use, see the 'Green Book' p. 212.

Tuberculosis and BCG Vaccination

BCG vaccine, containing a live attenuated strain, derived from M. bovis, has been shown to have an efficiency of between 70 and 80% in conferring protection against tuberculosis for 10-15 years to UK schoolchildren. Adverse reactions to BCG vaccine are rare, if proper attention is paid to the selection of subjects and the techniques for tuberculin testing and actual BCG vaccination. A Department of Health video, demonstrating the techniques, 'Heaf Testing and BCG Vaccination' is available to Nursing and Medical Professionals on 5 day's free loan (in England only) from Immunisation Coordinators in England. Alternatively, it may be bought, for £19.90 incl. VAT, from CFL Vision, PO Box 35, Wetherby, Yorkshire. LS23 7EX. Tel: 01937 541010 (cheques payable to CFL Vision)

Recommendations for immunisation

The following groups are recommended for immunisation with BCG provided:

a. BCG immunisation, as evidenced by the presence of a characteristic pale, flat, circular scar, on the upper arm or lateral aspect of the thigh, has not previously been carried out.

b. The tuberculin skin test is negative, as defined below:

For the Heaf Test. The reaction is graded 0-4 according to the degree of induration produced (NB erythema alone should be ignored). The results should be recorded as a number and not merely as positive or negative.

Grade 0 – no induration at the puncture sites.

Grade 1 – discrete induration at 4 or more needle sites.

Grade 2 – induration around each needle site merging with the next, forming a ring of induration but with a clear centre.

Grade 3 – the centre of the reaction becomes filled with induration to form one uniform disc of induration 5-10 mm wide.

Grade 4 – solid induration over 10mm wide. Vesiculation or ulceration may occur.

NB (Coloured illustrations of Heaf test responses are shown on the inside rear cover of the 'Green Book')

Heaf grades 0 and 1 or a Mantoux response of 0-4mm induration are regarded as negative. Individuals who have not previously received BCG immunisation may be offered immunisation in the absence of contraindications. However, those who give a history of previous BCG should only be re-immunised if there is no evidence of a characteristic scar and they are tuberculin negative.

Those with a grade 2 reaction (or a Mantoux response of induration of diameter 5-14 mm following injection of 0.1ml of Purified Protein Derivative (PPD) 100 units/ml) are positive. They are hypersensitive to tuberculin protein and should not be given BCG vaccination. When the immunisation is performed as part of a routine health promotion programme such as the schools programme, no further action is required. In other circumstances (e.g. new immigrants under 16 years, contacts of tuberculosis), subjects with a grade 2 reaction who have not previously had a BCG immunisation should be referred to a chest clinic.

Contacts of tuberculosis, children in the schools immunisation programme and new immigrants who show a strongly positive reaction to tuberculin (grade 3 or 4 or a Mantoux response with induration of at least 15mm diameter following 0.1 ml PPD 100 units/ml) should be referred for further investigation and supervision (which may include prophylactic chemotherapy).

Factors affecting the tuberculin test
The reaction to tuberculin protein may be suppressed by the following:
a. infectious mononucleosis.

b. viral infections in general, including those of the upper respiratory tract.

c. live viral vaccines. Tuberculin testing should not be carried out within three weeks of receiving a live viral vaccine: immunisation programmes should be arranged so that tuberculin testing is carried out before live viral vaccines are given.

d. Hodgkin's disease

e. sarcoidosis

f. corticosteroid therapy

g. immunosuppressant therapy or diseases, including HIV

Subjects who have a negative test but who may have had an upper respiratory tract or other viral infection at the time of testing or at the time of reading should be re-tested two to three weeks after clinical recovery before being given BCG. If a second tuberculin test is necessary it should be carried out on the other arm: repeat testing at one site may alter the reactivity either by hypo- or more often hyper sensitising the skin and a changed response may reflect local changes in sensitivity only.

NB For details of the preparation, supply and storage of BCG vaccine, the details of the BCG standard immunisation technique and details of the per- cutaneous BCG immunisation of infants and very young children, the reader is referred to the: 'Green Book', pages 233-236.

Immunisation reaction and care of the BCG immunisation site

Following intradermal administration of BCG, normally a local reaction develops at the immunisation site within two to three weeks, beginning with a small papule which increases in size for a few weeks widening into a circular area up to 7 mm in diameter with scaling, crusting and occasional bruising. Occasionally, a shallow ulcer 10mm in diameter develops. It is not necessary to protect the site from becoming wet during washing and bathing, but should any oozing occur, a temporary dry dressing may be used until a scab forms. It is essential that air is not excluded. If absolutely essential an impervious dressing may be applied but only for a short period (for example, to permit swimming) as it may delay healing and cause a larger scar. The lesion slowly subsides over several months and eventually heals leaving only a small, flat scar.

After immunisation with BCG vaccine there is a high tuberculin con- version rate and routine further observation of those at normal risk is not necessary, nor is further tuberculin testing recommended. However, in large immunisation programmes, some check should be made of the severity of the reactions six weeks or so later, possibly on a sample basis, as part of monitor- ing the programme.

In health care staff and others who are at occupational risk, the site of immunisation should be inspected six weeks later to confirm that a satis- factory reaction has occurred. Reactions should be recorded by measuring the transverse diameter in mm. Only those who show no reaction to BCG require a post-BCG tuberculin test, after which anyone who is at occupational risk who is still tuberculin negative should be re-immunised. If after re-immunisa- tion there is still no evidence of a satisfactory reaction or of conversion to a positive tuberculin test, the individual should be told the result and considera- tion given to work not involving exposure to patients with tuberculosis or with tuberculous material.

Adverse reactions to BCG

Vertigo and dizziness have occasionally been reported following BCG vaccination, and, rarely, immediate allergic type or anaphylactic reactions.

Severe injection site reactions, large ulcers and abscesses, are most com- monly caused by faulty injection technique where all or part of the dose is administered too deeply (subcutaneously, instead of intradermally). The immunisation of individuals who are tuberculin positive may also give rise to such reactions. To avoid these, doctors and nurses who carry out tuberculin skin tests and administer BCG vaccine must be trained in the interpretation of the results of the tuberculin tests as well as in the technique of intradermal injection with a syringe and needle.

Keloid formation at the injection site is an uncommon and largely avoidable, complication of BCG immunisation. Some sites are more prone to keloid formation than others and those immunising should adhere to the two recommended sites (the lateral aspect of the mid-upper arm or the lateral aspect of the mid-upper thigh). Most experience has been gained in the use of the upper arm and it is known that the risk of keloid formation is increased manyfold when the injection is given at a site higher than the **insertion of the deltoid muscle near the upper middle of the upper arm.**

Apart from these injection site reactions, other complications following BCG immunisation are rare and mostly consist of adenitis with or without suppuration and discharge. A minor degree of adenitis may occur in the weeks following immunisation and should not be regarded as a complication. Very rarely, a lupoid type of local lesion has been reported. A few cases of widespread dissemination of the injected organisms have been reported.

It is important that all complications are recorded and reported to a chest physician. Serious or unusual complications (including abscess and keloid scarring) should be reported to the Committee on Safety of Medicines using the Yellow Card and techniques reviewed. Every effort should be made to recover and identify the causative organism from any lesion constituting a serious complication.

Record keeping and monitoring

It is important that records are maintained to show the result of tuberculin skin testing, whether the subject had previously received BCG, and whether or not BCG was subsequently given. These records should show who administered the skin test or vaccine, the batch number of the vaccine, and who recorded the result or lesion. Particular attention should be paid to unusual or severe reactions. Such records should be kept for at least 10 years.

The results of tuberculin skin tests and of BCG immunisation of hospital staff (including students) should be recorded on appropriate records. If staff or students move to another hospital or training school the record cards should be transferred to the occupational health unit. Individual record cards may be carried by members of staff.

For monitoring selective neonatal and schools BCG programmes, records will need to be kept of numbers in the target groups, the number skin tested and the number found to be negative (for the schools programme), and the number given BCG.

NB: For details of supplies of BCG vaccine, PPD, and devices for Heaf testing, consult the 'Green Book', page 239

Typhoid
Vaccines

Three typhoid vaccines are available.

Monovalent whole cell typhoid vaccine contains not less than 1000 million heat-killed, phenol preserved S. typhi organisms per ml. One 0.5ml injection confers around 70-80% protection which fades after one year. Two doses, four to six weeks apart, give protection for three years or more.

Typhoid Vi polysaccharide antigen vaccine is a parenteral vaccine containing Vi antigen from the capsule of the organism, preserved with phenol. Each 0.5ml dose contains 25mcg of antigen, A single dose gives 70-80% protection for at least three years.

Oral typhoid vaccine contains a live attenuated *Salmonella* typhi strain (Ty 21a) in an enteric coated capsule. One capsule taken on alternate days for three doses appears to produce similar efficacy to parenteral vaccines, although the length of protection may be less: in those not repeatedly or constantly exposed to S. typhi it is recommended the full course is repeated after one year. The vaccine is unstable at normal room temperatures.

The efficacy of typhoid vaccines is partly related to the size of the infecting dose encountered after immunisation. The vaccines are not 100% effective and the importance in preventing infection of scrupulous attention to personal, food and water hygiene must still be emphasised for those travelling to endemic areas.

Typhoid vaccines for injection should be stored at 2-8 degrees C and not frozen.

Any partly used multidose containers should be discarded at the end of an immunisation session.

Oral typhoid vaccine is not stable at normal room temperature. It is essential to replace unused vaccine in the refrigerator between doses. The package should be kept dry and out of the light.

Recommendations

Typhoid immunisation is advised for;

(a) Laboratory workers handling specimens which may contain typhoid organisms.

(b) Travellers to countries in Africa, Asia, Central and South America and the Caribbean where sanitation and hygiene may be poor and for some countries in Eastern Europe, although immunisation against typhoid may be less important for short stays in good accommodation (See 'Health Information for Overseas Travel' for more details.)

Typhoid immunisation is not recommended for contacts of a known typhoid carrier or for controlling common-source outbreaks.

Route of administration and dosage.
Adults

Whole cell vaccine: a primary course of two doses four to six weeks apart. A reinforcing dose every three years for those at continued or repeated risk. (A single primary injection will give short-term immunity;a reinforcing dose will be needed after one year).

The first dose of the primary course must be given by intramuscular or deep subcutaneous injection for a reliable antigenic response. Subsequent doses may be given by intradermal injection, which may reduce the severity of adverse reactions.

Vi polysaccharide vaccine: a single dose by intramuscular or deep subcutaneous injection. Re-immunisation with a single dose every three years for those who remain at risk of infection.

Oral Ty 21a vaccine: one capsule on alternate days for three doses. It should be taken on an empty stomach with a cool drink. Those taking the vaccine home must be instructed to keep it in the refrigerator between doses.

Children

Immunisation against typhoid is not recommended for children under one year of age: the risk of infection is low and none of the vaccines is suitable for use in this age group. Children under 18 months may show a suboptimal response to polysaccharide antigen vaccines;use of vaccines in this age group should be governed by the likely risk of exposure to infection.

Oral typhoid vaccine is not suitable for children under six years of age.

Parenteral typhoid vaccines do not contain live organisms and may therefore be given to HIV positive individuals in the absence of contraindications. The oral vaccine contains live organisms and is contraindicated.

Dose

Vaccine	Primary Course	Boosters
Whole cell vaccine **Adults**	0.5 ml im or deep sc then 0.5ml im or deep sc or 0.1ml id four to six weeks later.	0.5ml im or sc or 0.1ml id every three years.
Children aged 1-10 years	0.25 ml im or deep sc then 0.25 ml im or deep sc or 0.1ml id four to six weeks later	0.25 ml im or deep sc or 0.1ml id every three years.
under one year	not recommended	
Vi polysaccharide antigen vaccine Adults and children above 18 months	0.5ml im or deep sc	0.5 ml or deep sc every 3 years.
Children less than 18 months.	Not recommended. See above.	
Oral Ty 21a vaccine Adults and children over 6 years	1 capsule on alternate days x 3 doses	for residents of non-endemic areas, 3 dose course annually.
under 6 years	not recommended	

Adverse reactions

Whole cell typhoid vaccine commonly produces local reactions such as redness, swelling, pain and tenderness which may persist for a few days. Systemic reactions include malaise, nausea, headache and pyrexia. They usually resolve within 36 hours. Neurological complications have been described but are rare. Reactions are especially common after repeated injections and are often more marked in people over 35 years. They may be reduced by giving the second and subsequent injections intradermally.

Local reactions to Vi polysaccharide vaccine are mild and transient and systemic reactions less common than with whole cell vaccine.

Oral Ty 21a vaccine may cause transient mild nausea, vomiting, abdominal cramps, diarrhoea and urticarial rash.

All severe reactions should be reported to the Committee on Safety of Medicines using the yellow card system.

Contraindications

The following contraindications should be observed:

(a) Acute febrile illness

(b) Severe reaction to a previous dose of the same vaccine.

(c) Pregnancy: as with other vaccines, typhoid vaccine should only be given if a clear indication exists

(d) Oral Ty 21a vaccine should not be given to those taking an antimicrobial agent, and if mefloquine is being taken for malaria chemoprophylaxis the vaccine should be taken at least 12 hours before or after the mefloquine.

(e) Oral Ty 21a vaccine should not be taken during persistent diarrhoea or vomiting.

(f) Oral typhoid vaccine is contra-indicated in those with immuno-suppression due to disease or treatment.

Oral typhoid vaccine and oral polio vaccine should be given at least three weeks apart on the theoretical grounds of possible interference of the immune response in the gut.

Typhoid vaccine is not recommended during an outbreak of typhoid fever in the UK. It affords no immediate protection, it may temporarily increase susceptibility to infection and, by stimulating antibody production, it makes interpretation of diagnostic serological tests more difficult.

Management of outbreaks

The Consultant in Communicable Disease Control (CCDC) or in Scotland, the Chief Administrative Medial Officer (CAMO) should be informed immediately whenever a patient is suspected of having typhoid fever without waiting for laboratory confirmation. Early identification of the source of the infection is vital in containing this disease.

Household or other close contacts of cases should be excluded from work if they are involved in food handling, until at least two, and in some cases three, negative faecal cultures have been obtained.

The need for strict personal hygiene should be stressed.

For details of Suppliers of parenteral and oral typhoid vaccines. See 'Green Book' p. 248

Varicella (Chickenpox)

Varicella vaccine

Live attenuated vaccine has recently been licensed in some countries but as yet, no vaccine is licensed for use in the UK. It is available on a named patient basis from Smith Kline Beecham and Pasteur Merieux MSD Ltd for immuno-compromised individuals, particularly children with leukaemia or solid organ transplants.

Human Varicella-Zoster Immunoglobulin (VZIG)

Two licensed VZIG preparations are available in the UK. See Page 252 'Green Book' for details of suppliers and advice with regard to storage etc. All immunoglobulins are prepared from HIV, hepatitis B and hepatitis C negative donors.

Recommendations

VZIG prophylaxis is recommended for individuals who fulfil all of the following three criteria:

(a) a clinical condition which increases the risk of severe varicella;this includes immunosuppressed patients, neonates and pregnant women.

(b) no antibodies to varicella-zoster virus.

(c) significant exposure to chickenpox or herpes zoster.

Categories of immunosuppressed patients have already been defined. (See 'Communicable Diseases.')

Antiviral chemotherapy may be used for patients with other clinical conditions in whom attenuation of an attack of chickenpox would be desirable.

Note that severe or fatal varicella can occur despite VZIG prophylaxis; varicella immunisation should therefore be considered for susceptible immunosuppressed patients at long term risk. About half of the susceptible immunosuppressed home contacts will develop clinical chickenpox despite VZIG prophylaxis and a further 15% will be infected subclinically. There is no difference in outcome whether VZIG is given within 3 days or 4-7 days after exposure. For management of **pregnant women** and neonates, consult the 'Green Book', page 256

Determination of VZ immune status

The majority of adults and a substantial portion of children without a definite history of chickenpox will be VZ antibody positive. In order to conserve supplies of valuable VZIG, all individuals being considered for VZIG should have a sample of serum tested for VZ antibody; **only those without antibody require VZIG.** Advice on VZ antibody testing may be obtained from the local Public Health or Hospital Laboratory.

VZ antibody detected in patients who have been transfused or who have received intravenous immunoglobulin in the previous three months may have been passively acquired. Although VZIG is not indicated if antibody from any other blood products is detectable, re-testing in the event of a subsequent exposure will be required as the patient may have become antibody negative.

About 15% of patients given VZIG who remain symptom free after a home contact will have had a subclinical infection. Patients who have received VZIG in the past, following a close exposure, should therefore be retested in the event of another exposure, to identify those who have seroconverted asymptomatically and are antibody positive.

The value of a clinical history of chickenpox in determining immune status varies with the patient group:

(a) **Immunosuppressed contacts**: Whenever possible, contacts with a positive history of chickenpox should be tested to confirm the presence of VZ antibody. Those with a positive history in whom antibody is not detected by a sensitive assay should be given VZIG.

VZIG is not indicated in immunosuppressed contacts with detectable antibody as the amount of antibody provided by VZIG will not significantly increase VZ antibody titres in those who are already positive. Second attacks of chickenpox can occasionally occur in immunosuppressed VZ antibody positive patients, but these appear to be related to defects in cell-mediated immunity.

While it is recommended that immunosuppressed patients without a history of chickenpox should be tested for VZ antibody, VZIG administration should not be delayed past seven days after initial contact while an antibody test is done. Under these circumstances VZIG should be given on the basis of a negative history of chickenpox.

(b) **Neonates**: Infants whose mothers develop chickenpox less than eight days before delivery, or after birth, can be presumed to be VZ antibody negative. The VZ antibody status of infants whose mothers have a negative history should be determined by testing a maternal blood sample before VZIG is given.

A small proportion of premature infants who are born before 28 weeks of gestation or with a birth weight less than 1000 gms may not possess maternal antibody despite a positive history in the mother.

(c) **Pregnant women**: Those with a history of chicken pox do not require VZIG. Those with a negative history must be tested for VZ antibody before VZIG is given. The outcome in pregnant women is not adversely affected if administration of VZIG is delayed up to 10 days after initial contact while a VZ antibody test is done.

Definition of a significant exposure to varicella-zoster virus

Three aspects of the exposure are relevant:

(a) **Type of varicella-zoster infection in index case**: The risk of acquiring infection from an immunocompetent individual with non-exposed zoster lesions (e. g. thoraco-lumbar) is remote.

The issue of VZIG should therefore be restricted to those in contact with chickenpox, or the following: disseminated zoster, immunocompetent individuals with exposed lesions (e. g. ophthalmic zoster) or immuno-suppressed patients with localised zoster on any part of the body (in whom viral shedding may be greater).

(b) **The timing of the exposure in relation to onset of rash in index case**: VZIG should normally be restricted to patients exposed to a case of chickenpox or disseminated zoster between 48 hours before the onset of the rash until cropping has ceased and crusting of all lesions, or day of onset of rash until crusting for those exposed to localised zoster.

(c) **Closeness and duration of contact**: The following should be used as a guide to the type of exposure, other than maternal/neonatal and continuous home contact, that requires VZIG prophylaxis:

Contact in the same room (e. g. in a house or classroom or a 2-4 bed hospital bay) for a significant period of time (15 minutes or more).

Face-to-face contact, for example while having a conversation.

In the case of large open wards, where air-borne transmission has occasionally been reported, the necessity of giving VZIG to all susceptible high risk contacts should be considered, particularly in paediatric wards where the degree of contact may be difficult to define.

Dose of VZIG for prophylaxis
The dosage for both the BPL and PFC products are as follows:

0-5 years	250 mg (1 vial)
6-10 years	500 mg (2 vials).
11-14 years	750 mg (3 vials)
15 years and over	1000 mg (4 vials)

VZIG is given by **intramuscular** injection as soon as possible and **not** later than ten days after exposure.

It must **not** be given intravenously.

If a second exposure occurs after three weeks, a further dose is required.

Contacts with bleeding disorders who cannot be given an intramuscular injection should be given intravenous normal immunoglobulin at a dose of 0.2g per kg body weight (ie. 4 mls/kg for a 5% solution) instead. This will produce serum VZ antibody levels equivalent to those achieved with VZIG.

Treatment
There is no evidence that VZIG is effective in the treatment of severe disease. Since antibody production can be delayed in immunosuppressed individuals, intravenous commercial preparations of normal human immunoglobulin may be used to provide an immediate source of antibody.

Safety
VZIG is well tolerated. Very rarely anaphylactoid reactions occur in individuals with hypogamma-globulinaemia who have IgA antibodies, or those who have had an atypical reaction to blood transfusion.

No cases of blood borne infection acquired through immunoglobulin preparations designed for intramuscular use have been documented in any country. Report severe reactions on Yellow Cards.

Management of hospital outbreaks

Susceptible staff with a significant exposure to VZ virus, as described earlier, including those dressing zoster lesions on non-exposed areas of the body, should whenever possible be excluded from contact with high risk patients from eight to 21 days after exposure.

To simplify procedures after the admission or recognition of a case, it is recommended that hospital staff without a definite history of chickenpox should be routinely screened for VZ antibody so that those susceptible are already identified. This is particularly important for staff in contact with high risk groups such as pregnant women and immunosuppressed patients.

Poliomyelitis

Inactivated poliomyelitis vaccine (Salk) was introduced in 1956 for routine immunisation, and was replaced by attenuated live oral vaccine (Sabin) in 1962. **Individuals born before 1958 may not have been immunised and no opportunity should be missed to immunise them in adult life.** Since the introduction of vaccine, notifications of paralytic poliomyelitis (in England and Wales) have dropped from nearly 4,000 in 1955 to a total of 35 cases between 1974-1978. This included 25 cases during 1976 and 1977, in which infection with wild virus occurred in unimmunised persons, demonstrating the continuing need to maintain high levels of immunisation uptake. From 1985-1995, 28 cases were reported. 19 were vaccine associated (14 recipients, 5 contacts), 6 were imported; the source of infection could not be found in 3 cases, but in none of whom could wild virus be detected. By March 1996, coverage for poliomyelitis immunisation was 96% by the second birthday.

The World Health Organisation has included the UK among the countries which are likely to have eliminated indigenous poliomyelitis due to wild virus. **In any case of childhood acute flaccid paralysis (AFP), including Guillain Barré syndrome, it is essential to obtain two faecal samples 24 to 48 hours apart, as soon as possible after the onset of paralysis for viral examination. Ideally, faecal samples should also be obtained from household and other contacts.** In the region of the Americas, where there has been no case of wild virus poliomyelitis since 1991, it was recommended that faecal samples should be obtained from at least 5 close contacts of each AFP case.

In September 1994, after three years with no single case of wild virus poliomyelitis, an international commission certified that polio virus transmission had been interrupted in the region of the Americas and polio could be considered to have been eliminated from that region.

Poliomyelitis vaccine (Live and Inactivated)

Live oral polio vaccine (OPV) is routinely used for immunisation in the UK, always by mouth. It contains live attenuated strains of poliomyelitis virus types 1, 2 and 3 grown in cultures of monkey kidney cells or in human diploid cells. The attenuated viruses become established in the intestine and promote antibody formation both in the blood and in the gut epithelium, providing local resistance to subsequent infection with wild poliomyelitis viruses. This reduces the frequency of symptomless excretion of wild poliomyelitis virus in the community. OPV inhibits simultaneous infection by wild polio viruses and is thus of value in the control of epidemics. Vaccine strain poliomyelitis virus may persist in the faeces for up to six weeks after OPV. This provides an additional community benefit as contacts of recently immunised children may be protected through acquisition of vaccine virus.

Whilst a single dose of polio vaccine may give protection, a course of three doses produces long-lasting immunity to all three polio virus types.

Enhanced potency inactivated polio vaccine (eIPV) contains polio viruses of all three types inactivated by formaldehyde. It should be stored at 2-8 degrees C but not frozen. 0.5ml is given by subcutaneous injection. A course of three injections at monthly intervals produces long-lasting immunity to all three polio virus types. IPV can be given from two months of age.

When IPV has been given previously, subsequent immunisation can be carried out using OPV if appropriate. Similarly, when OPV has been used initially, immunisation can be completed with IPV if needed.

Recommendations

Primary immunisation of infants and children

Oral polio vaccine is recommended for infants from two months of age. **The primary course consists of three separate doses with intervals of one month between each dose given at the same time as diphtheria/tetanus/ pertussis and Hib vaccine.** The dose of vaccine should be repeated if it is regurgitated. Breast feeding does not interfere with the antibody response to OPV and immunisation should not be delayed on this account. Faecal excretion of vaccine virus can last up to six weeks and may lead to infection of unimmunised contacts; such infection may provide protection of previously susceptible individuals, but bear in mind previous details of immuno – compromised individuals, etc.

The contacts of a recently immunised baby should be advised of the need for strict personal hygiene, particularly for washing their hands after changing the baby's napkins.

Unimmunised adults can be immunised at the same time as their children. There is no need to boost previously immunised individuals.

Recently immunised children may be taken swimming, even if they have been given OPV. Similarly, there is no risk of an unimmunised child contracting vaccine associated poliomyelitis from a recently immunised child if they are taken swimming. In such public places, care must be taken to dispose of soiled napkins without contaminating facilities that others might use.

Reinforcing immunisation in children

A reinforcing dose of oral poliomyelitis vaccine (OPV) should be given before school entry at the same time as a reinforcing dose of diphtheria and tetanus vaccine; a further dose of OPV should be given at 15-19 years of age before leaving school.

Immunisation of adults

A course of three doses of OPV at intervals of four weeks is recommended for the primary immunisation of adults. **No adult should remain unimmunised against poliomyelitis**. Reinforcing doses for adults are **not** necessary unless they are at special risk, such as:

a.　Travellers to areas or countries where poliomyelitis is epidemic or endemic (See 'Health information for Overseas Travel' 1995 Edition).

b.　Health care workers in possible contact with poliomyelitis cases.

Health care workers requiring polio vaccine, either for primary immunisation or for boosting prior to travel to a polio infected country, may be given OPV. They must be reminded of the need for strict personal hygiene, especially if their work brings them into contact with immunosuppressed individuals.

There is no known case of nosocomial vaccine related contact poliomyelitis involving a health care worker and an immunosuppressed patient.

For those exposed to a continuing risk of infection, a single reinforcing dose is desirable every ten years.

Polio vaccines and immunocompromised individuals

Inactivated polio vaccine (IPV) is available for the immunisation of individuals for whom a live vaccine is contraindicated. (See earlier). It should be used for siblings and other household contacts of immunosuppressed individuals. A primary course of three doses of 0.5ml with intervals of one month should be given by subcutaneous injection and can be given from two months of age. A course started with OPV can be completed or reinforced with IPV and vice versa. Reinforcing doses should be given as for OPV.

HIV positive asymptomatic individuals **may** receive live polio vaccine but excretion of the vaccine virus in the faeces may continue for longer than in normal individuals. Household contacts should be warned of this and reminded of the need for strict personal hygiene, including hand washing after nappy changes for an HIV positive infant.

For HIV positive symptomatic individuals, IPV may be used instead of OPV at the discretion of the clinician.

Adverse reactions

Cases of vaccine-associated poliomyelitis have been reported in recipients of OPV and in contacts of recipients. In England and Wales there is an annual average of one recipient and one contact case in relation to over two million doses of oral vaccine. Contact cases would be eliminated if all children and adults were immunised. The possibility of a small risk of poliomyelitis induced by OPV cannot be ignored but it is insufficient to warrant a change in immunisation policy. **The need for strict personal hygiene for contacts of recent vaccinees must be stressed**.

Any such cases following immunisation with poliomyelitis vaccine should be reported to the Committee on Safety of Medicines using the Yellow Card system.

Contraindications – OPV

(i) Acute or febrile illness

(ii) Vomiting or diarrhoea: immunisation must be postponed.

(iii) Treatment involving high-dose corticosteroids or immunosuppression including general radiation.

(iv) Malignant conditions of the reticulo-endothelial system such as lymphoma, leukaemia, and Hodgkin's disease, and where the normal immunological mechanism may be impaired as for example, in hypogammaglobulinaemia.

(v) Although adverse effects on the foetus have not been reported, oral polio vaccine should not be given to women during the first four months of pregnancy unless there are compelling reasons, such as travel to an endemic poliomyelitis area.

OPV **may** be given at the same time as the inactivated vaccines and with other live vaccines except oral typhoid. When BCG is given to infants, there is no need to delay the primary immunisations which include polio vaccine, because the latter viruses replicate in the intestine to induce local immunity and serum antibodies, and three doses are given.

OPV may contain trace amounts of penicillin, neomycin, polymixin and streptomycin but these do not contraindicate its use except in cases of extreme hypersensitivity.

OPV should **not** be used for the siblings and other household contacts of immunosuppressed children; such contacts should be given IPV.

OPV should be given for either three weeks before or three weeks after an injection of normal immunoglobulin. This may not always be possible in the case of travellers going abroad, but as in such cases the OPV is likely to be a booster dose, the possible inhibiting effect of the immunoglobulin is less important.

Contraindications to IPV

(i) Acute or febrile illnesses; immunisation should be postponed.

(ii) IPV may contain trace amounts of polymixin B and neomycin but these do not contraindicate its use except in rare cases of extreme hypersensitivity. It does not contain penicillin.

Management of Outbreaks

After a single case of paralytic poliomyelitis from wild virus, a dose of OPV should be given immediately to all persons in the neighbourhood of the case (with the exception of individuals with genuine contraindications such as immunodeficiency, to whom IPV should be given) regardless of a previous history of immunisation against poliomyelitis. In previously unimmunised individuals, the three month course should be completed. If there is laboratory confirmation that a vaccine-derived polio virus is responsible for the case, immunisation of possible contacts is unnecessary since no outbreaks associated with the virus have ever been documented. If the source of the outbreak is uncertain, it should be assumed to be a 'wild' virus and appropriate control measures instituted.

Rabies
Vaccine

Rabies human diploid cell vaccine (HDCV) is a freeze dried suspension of Wistar rabies virus strain PM/WI 38 1503-3M cultured in human diploid cells and inactivated by beta-propiolactone. The potency of the reconstituted vaccine is not less than 2.5 International Units per 1 ml dose. It contains traces of neomycin.

The freeze-dried vaccine should be stored at 2-8 degrees C and not frozen. It should be used immediately and reconstituted with the diluent supplied, and any unused vaccine discarded after one hour. It may be given by deep subcutaneous, intramuscular or intradermal injection, usually into the deltoid region.

Rabies-specific immunoglobulin

Human rabies immunoglobulin (HRIG) is obtained from the plasma of immunised human donors. It is used after exposure to rabies to give rapid protection until rabies vaccine, which should be given at the same time, becomes effective.

Recommendations
Pre-exposure (prophylactic) immunisation

Pre-exposure immunisation with human diploid cell rabies vaccine should be offered, and is available free from the NHS, to:

a. Laboratory workers handling the virus.

b. Those, who in the course of their work, regularly handle imported animals e. g.

- at animal quarantine centres

- at zoos

- at research and acclimatisation centres where primates and other imported animals are housed.

- at ports e. g. certain Customs and Excise officers

- carrying agents authorised to carry imported animals

- veterinary and technical staff at the Ministry of Agriculture, Fisheries and Food (MAFF), the Scottish Office, Agriculture, Environment and Fisheries Department, (SOAEFD) and the depart ment of Agriculture for Northern Ireland (DANI).

- inspectors appointed by local authorities under the Diseases of Animals Act. (This does not include all local authority dog wardens for whom the risk of exposure is low and for whom post exposure prophylaxis in the event of an incident is likely to be more appropriate.)

c. Licensed bat handlers

d. Workers in enzootic areas abroad who by the nature of their work are at special risk of contact with rabid animals (e.g. veterinary staff or zoologists).

e.   Health workers who are likely to come into close contact with a patient with rabies.

Pre-exposure immunisation is also recommended for those living or travelling in enzootic areas who may be exposed to unusual risk of being infected or are undertaking especially long journeys in remote parts where medical treatment may not be immediately available. (More detailed country by country advice is contained in the UK Health Department's book 'Health Information for Overseas Travel'). For these individuals, the vaccine is not supplied free from the NHS

Route of administration and dosage.

For primary exposure protection, three doses of 1.0ml of HDCV should be given, on days 0, 7 and 28, by deep subcutaneous or intramuscular injection in the deltoid region. (The antibody response may be reduced if the gluteal region is used.)

For travellers who are not animal handlers, two doses of 1.0ml by deep subcutaneous or intramuscular injection four weeks apart can be expected to give immunity in 98% of recipients and may be acceptable if post-exposure treatment is likely to be readily available. For those at continued exposure a further dose should be given 6-12 months later.

Use of the intradermal route: When more than one person is to be immunised, the vaccine may be administered in smaller doses (0.1 ml) by the intradermal route in either of the above schedules. The intradermal route may also be used for rapid immunisation of, for example, staff caring for a patient with rabies, giving 0.1ml intradermally into each limb (0.4 ml in all) on the first day of exposure to the patient. **Intradermal immunisation is reliable only if the whole of the 0.1 ml dose is properly given into the dermis and should only be given by those experienced in the intradermal technique. It should not be used in those taking chloroquine for malaria prophylaxis as this suppresses the antibody response. The use of the intradermal route is on the doctor's own responsibility as this is not covered by the manufacturer's Product Licence.**

Reinforcing doses: Where post-exposure treatment is readily available, as in the UK, reinforcing doses are not normally required for the individuals who have received three doses of vaccine unless exposure occurs (when post-exposure treatment should be given) or unless exposure is regular and continuous (e. g. laboratory workers handling the virus, licensed bat handlers).

For those at regular and continuous risk in the UK, and where post-exposure treatment is not readily available and there is continued risk, single reinforcing doses of vaccine should be given at two to three year intervals, the interval to be reviewed after 2-3 reinforcing doses. (But see later.)

The three dose primary post-exposure course produces protective antibody in virtually 100% of recipients and makes routine post-immunisation serological testing unnecessary. Serological testing is advised for those who work with live virus. They should have their antibodies tested every six months, and be given reinforcing doses of vaccine as necessary to maintain protective levels. Serological testing is only advised for those who have had a severe reaction to a previous dose of vaccine to confirm the need for a reinforcing dose.

All travellers to enzootic areas should also be informed by their medical advisers of the practical steps to be taken if an animal bite is sustained.

Post exposure treatment

In the event of possible exposure, firstly, as soon as possible after the incident, the wound should be thoroughly cleansed by scrubbing with soap and water under a running tap for five minutes. Secondly, the name and address of the owner of the animal should be obtained and the animal observed for ten days to see if it behaves abnormally. If necessary, the assistance of local officials should be sought. Thirdly, advice should be taken from a local doctor. If the animal is wild or a stray and observation is impossible, the doctor will know if rabies occurs in the locality and if immunisation is advised.

For travellers returning to this country who report an exposure (break in skin or contamination of a mucosal surface) to an animal abroad, treatment, including cleaning the wound as above, should be started as soon as possible while enquiries are made about the prevalence of rabies in the country concerned and, where possible, the ownership and the condition of the biting animal. Information should be sought from the PHLS Virus Reference Division, London (0181 200 4400); in Scotland, the Scottish Centre for Infection and Environmental Health (0141 946 7120); in Northern Ireland, the Public Health Laboratory, Belfast City Hospital (01232 329241).

Subsequent treatment will depend on the risk of rabies in the country concerned and the immune status of the individual, and **each incident has to be judged on its merits. Points to consider include if the animal is indigenous (native) or not, its behaviour, the site and severity of the bite and whether the bite was provoked.**

Summary of post-exposure prophylaxis

Rabies risk in country of incident	Unimmunised/incompletely immunised individual*	Fully immunised individual
No Risk	None	None
Low Risk	5 doses HDCV	2 doses HDCV
High Risk	5 doses HDCV plus human rabies specific immunoglobulin	2 doses HDCV

*persons who have been immunised by the intradermal route, or who have received fewer than three doses of vaccine, or whose last dose of vaccine was given more than two years previously.

NO RISK: generally no rabies post-exposure prophylaxis needed, however, each incident needs to be judged separately.

The following countries are considered 'no risk':

Europe: Cyprus, Faroe Is, Finland, Gibraltar, Greece, Iceland, Ireland, Malta, Norway (mainland).
Mainland Spain exc N. African coast, Sweden, United Kingdom, Portugal, Italy (except the Northern and Eastern borders).

Americas: Bermuda, St. Pierre and Miquelon, Anguilla, Antigua and Barbuda, Bahamas, Barbados, Cayman Is., Dominica,

Guadaloupe, Jamaica, Martinique, Montserrat, Netherlands Antilles, St. Christopher and Nevis, St Lucia, St. Martins, St. Vincent and the Grenadines, Turks and Caicos Is, Virgin Is.

Asia   Japan, Singapore, Taiwan.

Oceania: American Samoa, Australia, Belau, Cook Is, Federated States of Micronesia, Fiji, French Polynesia, Guam, Kiribati, New Caledonia, New Zealand, Niue, Northern Mariana Is, Papua New Guinea, Samoa, Solomon Is, Tonga, Vanuatu, Western Samoa

LOW RISK: vaccine only required:

a. Previously unimmunised individuals should be given five doses of 1.0ml HDCV, one each on days 0, 3, 7, 14 and 30.

b. Previously immunised individuals should be given two doses of 1.0ml HDCV, one on day 0 and one between days 3 and 7.

Vaccine must be given by deep subcutaneous or intramuscular injection into the deltoid region (not gluteal) or, in a child, the antero-lateral aspect of the thigh.

The following countries are considered low risk:

France, Belgium, Germany, Luxembourg, Netherlands, Switzerland, Denmark, USA and Canada,
If the animal can be reliably observed and remains well for 10 days, immunisation may not be required

HIGH RISK

a. Previously un-immunised individuals should be given immunoglobulin as well as vaccine as follows:

    i.   Immunoglobulin: human rabies specific immunoglobulin 20 iu/kg body weight, up to half the dose infiltrated in and around the wound after cleansing and the rest given by intramuscular injection;

    ii   Vaccine: five doses of 1.0 ml HDCV by deep subcutaneous or intramuscular injection into the deltoid muscle (not the buttocks) or, in children, antero-lateral thigh, one each on days 0, 3, 7, 14. and 30.

b. Previously fully immunised individuals: two doses of 1. 0ml HDCV given as above, the first on day 0 and the second between days 3 and 7. Immunoglobulin treatment is not needed.

Countries considered at high risk are:

Parts of Mexico, El Salvador, Guatemala, Peru, Colombia, Ecuador, India, Nepal, Pakistan, Philippines, Sri Lanka, Thailand, Vietnam. Also most other countries in Asia, Africa and South America.

Up to date advice should be obtained from the Virus Reference Division, Central Public Health Laboratory, Colindale. London. (0181 200 4400), or in Scotland, from the Scottish Centre for Infection and Environmental Health (0141 946 7120) as the country -by-country risk groups may change.

Human rabies is a notifiable disease. In the event of a case of human rabies, the Consultant in Communicable Disease Control (in Scotland, the Chief Administrative Medical Officer) should be informed.

Adverse reactions

HDCV may cause local reactions such as redness, swelling or pain at the site of injection within 24-48 hours of administration. Systemic reactions such as fever, headache, muscle aches, vomiting and urticarial rashes have been reported. Anaphylactic shock has been reported from the USA and Guillain – Barré syndrome from Norway. Reactions may become more severe with repeated doses.

HRIG may cause local pain and low grade fever but no serious adverse reactions have been reported. Needless to state, suspected adverse reactions should be reported to the Committee on Safety of Medicines, using the Yellow Card system.

Contraindications

There are no absolute contraindications to HDCV, although if there is evidence of hypersensitivity subsequent doses should not be given except for post-exposure treatment. Pre-exposure vaccine should only be given to pregnant women if the risk of exposure to rabies is high.

For details of supplies of rabies vaccine. Consult the 'Green Book' Page 190.

Tick borne encephalitis

Vaccine

An unlicensed vaccine is available on a named patient basis. It is an inactivated whole cell virus vaccine containing a suspension of purified TBE virus grown in chick embryo cells and inactivated with formalin. It contains thiomersal as a preservative. The vaccine should be stored between 2-8 degrees C. Freezing or storage at a higher temperature must be avoided. An immunoglobulin preparation is also available for post-exposure prophylaxis

Recommendations

The vaccine is recommended for travellers who are to walk, camp or work in late spring and summer in warm heavily forested parts of Central and Eastern Europe and Scandinavia, especially if there is heavy undergrowth. Protection is also afforded by covering arms, legs and ankles and using insect repellents on socks and outer clothes. These measures are advised whether or not vaccine is given.

Route of administration and dosage

Two doses of 0.5ml (irrespective of age) given 4-12 weeks apart will give protection for a year. The injections must be given intramuscularly. A third dose 9-12 months after the second gives three years protection.

A further booster dose can be given up to six months later for longer protection. Booster doses are recommended at three yearly intervals for those at continued risk.

Adverse reactions

Reported reactions to tick-borne encephalitis vaccine are very rare. Local reactions at the immunisation site and some local lymphadenopathy may occur. Febrile reactions in children are described after the first dose.

General reactions such as fatigue, limb pain, fever, nausea and headache lasting up to 24 hours may occur occasionally and a transient pruritic rash may rarely occur.

Neurological symptoms have occurred on rare occasions following administration of the vaccine.

Contraindications

Allergy to the preservative thiomersal and to egg protein are contraindications.

For details of supplies of the vaccine see the 'Green Book' Page 216

Japanese Encephalitis
Vaccine

A formalin-inactivated whole cell vaccine derived from mouse brains is available in the UK but is unlicensed and must therefore be given on a named patient basis. The vial contains a single dose of vaccine which should be reconstituted with 1. 3 ml of sterile water for injection.

Recommendations

Immunisation is recommended for travellers to South East Asia and the Far East who will be staying for a month or longer in endemic areas, especially if travel will include rural areas. The risk to an individual traveller is difficult to assess, but areas where rice growing and pig farming coexist and journeys towards the end of the monsoon season (roughly June to September) are likely to increase the risk. Occasionally immunisation should be considered for shorter trips where there is a high risk of exposure, e. g. extensive outdoor activities in endemic areas. More detailed country by country information is contained in the UK Health Department's book, 'Health Information for Overseas Travel'.

Precautions against mosquito bites should be taken by all travellers to SE Asia.

Route of Administration and dosage

The recommended vaccine schedule is three doses of 1ml by deep subcutaneous injection on days 0, 7-14, and 28. Full immunity takes up to a month to develop. A two-dose schedule at 0 and 7-14 days is said to give short-term immunity in 80% of vaccinees.

One additional subcutaneous dose of 1 ml is recommended a month after the initial course for those over 60 years of age. For children under three years of age, the dose for each injection is 0.5ml by deep subcutaneous injection.

The duration of protection is not known. Neutralising antibody persists for at least two years after a 3-dose primary course. A booster may be given at this time.

Adverse reactions

Local reaction at the injection site may persist.

Allergic reactions, mainly urticaria, but also angioneurotic oedema and dyspnoea, occur occasionally within minutes or up to two weeks after receiving the vaccine. Caution is therefore required with the use of this vaccine; it is recommended that recipients are kept under observation at the immunisation centre for about 30 minutes after being given the vaccine and that the course is completed at least ten days prior to departure. Remember the yellow card notification to the CSM of any suspected adverse reaction. Also, inform the supplier. **For details of whom see** 'Green Book' Page 216.

Contraindications

Fever or acute infection.

History of anaphylactic hypersensitivity.

Immunisation is not advised in pregnancy or in those with cardiac, hepatic or renal disorders, leukaemia, lymphoma or other generalised malignancy because of the lack of data on its efficacy and adverse reactions in these conditions.

The vaccine should be stored below 10 degrees C prior to reconstitution and exposure to direct sunlight should be avoided. The reconstituted vaccine should be used immediately and not stored

Meningococcal vaccines

Meningococcal meningitis and septicaemia are systemic infections caused by the Gram negative diplococcus, *Neisseria meningitidis*. There are several distinct antigenic groups, the commonest of which in the UK are B, C, A, Y and W135. They are then further divided by type and sulphonamide sensitivity.

Group B strains account for approximately two thirds of all isolates submitted to the PHLS Meningococcal Reference Laboratory. Group C strains contribute about one third, but some years can be higher. Group A strains are rare in this country (less than 2%) but are the epidemic strains in other parts of the world.

Vaccine

Currently available meningococcal vaccine is a purified, heat stable lyophilised extract from the polysaccharide outer capsule of Neisseria meningitidis, effective against serogroup A and C organisms. Vaccine contains 50mcg each of the respective purified bacterial capsular polysaccharides. **There is no available vaccine against Group B organisms.**

A serological response is detected in more than 90% of recipients and occurs five to ten days after a single injection. The response is strictly Group specific and confers no protection against Group B organisms. Young infants respond less well than adults with little response to the Group C polysaccharide below 18 months and similar lack of response to group A polysaccharide below three months. Vaccine induced immunity lasts approximately three to five years;in younger children a more rapid decline in antibody has been noted. Conjugated vaccines on the same lines as Hib vaccines are presently being investigated for suitability for infant use to protect against Group C meningococcal infections.

Vaccine must be stored at 2-8 degrees C and the diluent must not be frozen. Vaccine should be reconstituted immediately before use with the diluent supplied by the manufacturer.

Route of administration and dosage

A single dose of 0.5ml is given by deep subcutaneous or intramuscular injection to adults and children from two months of age.

Recommendations

Routine immunisation with meningococcal vaccine is not recommended as the overall risk of meningococcal disease is very low. Group B organisms are the major cause of disease in the UK and a considerable number of cases of meningococcal disease from Group C organisms occur in children too young to be protected with presently available vaccines.

Asplenic children and adults, irrespective of age or the interval from splenectomy, should receive a single dose of meningococcal vaccine before travelling to areas where there is an increased risk of Group A infection. Otherwise the vaccine should be restricted to groups for whom it is otherwise specifically recommended.

Contacts of cases: Close contacts of meningococcal meningitis have a considerably increased risk of developing the disease in the subsequent months, despite appropriate chemoprophylaxis. The recommended schedule for prophylaxis is rifampicin 600mg every 12 hours for two days in adults, 10mg/kg dose for children over one year of age and 5mg/kg for children less than one year. (Remember the warnings with regard to contact lens wearers and those taking oral contraceptives). Ciprofloxacin as a single dose of 500mg is an alternative for adults but is not yet licensed in the UK for this purpose. Ceftriaxone 250mg intramuscularly can be given to pregnant contacts, but is not licensed in the UK for this purpose. Immediate family or close contacts of Group A or Group C meningitis should be given meningococcal vaccine in addition to chemoprophylaxis. The latter should be given first and the decision to offer vaccine should be made when the results of typing are available. Vaccine should not be given to contacts of Group B cases.

Local outbreaks: In addition to sporadic cases, outbreaks of meningococcal infections with Group C organisms tend to occur in closed or semi-closed communities such as schools and military establishments. Immunisation has been shown to be effective in controlling epidemics, reducing infection rates but not carriage rates.

Advice on the use of meningococcal vaccines is available from the PHLS Communicable Disease Surveillance Centre (0181 200 6868), the PHLS Meningococcal Reference Laboratory, 0161 445 2416, the Scottish centre for Infection and Environmental Health (0141 946 7120), and the Scottish Meningococcal and Pneumococcal Reference Laboratory (0141 201 3836).

Meningococcal vaccine has no part to play in the management of outbreaks of Group B meningococcal meningitis.

Travel: In some areas of the world, the risk of acquiring meningococcal infection is much higher than in this country particularly for those visitors who live or travel 'rough', such as backpackers, and those living or working with local people. Immunisation is recommended for longer visits (generally a month or more), especially if back-packing or living with local people, to:

(i) Sub-Saharan Africa:

Epidemics, mainly Group A infections, occur throughout tropical Africa particularly in the Savanna in the dry season which varies from country to country and can be unpredictable. More detailed country by country information is contained in the UK Health Department's book 'Health Information for Overseas Travel'.

(ii) the area around Delhi, and Nepal, Bhutan and Pakistan.

(iii) Since 1988, following an outbreak of Group A meningococcal meningitis in 1987, Saudi Arabia has required immunisation of people coming to the Haj annual pilgrimage.

Meningococcal vaccine may be given to HIV positive individuals in the absence of contraindications.

Adverse reactions

Generalised reactions are rare although pyrexia occurs more frequently in young children than in adults.

Injection site reactions occur in approximately 10% of recipients and last for approximately 24-48 hours.

Serious reactions should be reported on the yellow card to the CSM.

Contraindications

Immunisation should be postponed in individuals suffering from an acute febrile illness.

Although there is no information to suggest that meningococcal vaccine is unsafe during pregnancy, it should be given only when this is unavoidable, ie when there is a true risk of disease. During an epidemic of meningococcal meningitis in Brazil, no adverse events were reported in pregnant women receiving vaccine.

A severe reaction to a preceding dose of meningococcal vaccine is a contraindication to further doses.

For information about supplies of meningococcal Vaccine See the 'Green Book' page 153.

Pneumococcal disease

Invasive pneumococcal disease (pneumonia, bacteraemia, and meningitis) is a major cause of morbidity and mortality, especially among the very young, the elderly, those with an absent or non-functioning spleen and those with other causes of impaired immunity. The pneumococcus is the commonest cause of community acquired pneumonia. Pneumococcal pneumonia is estimated to affect 1/1000 adults each year and has a mortality of 10-20%. The pneumococcus is also one of the most frequently reported causes of bacteraemia and meningitis. During 1995, 3,897 laboratory isolates from blood or CSF were reported to the PHLS. Recurrent infections may occur associated with abnormalities such as fractures of the skull.

Streptococcus pneumoniae (the pneumococcus) is an encapsulated Gram positive coccus. 84 capsular types have been characterised, of which 8-10 cause two thirds of the serious infections in adults and about 85% of infections in children. Immunity to infection is complicated, but depends greatly on type specific anti-capsular antibodies. However, the level of antibody required for protection is not currently known.

Antimicrobial resistance among *S.pneumoniae* is increasing in the UK and world-wide and susceptibility to penicillin, cephalosporin and macrolide antimicrobials can no longer be assumed. In1994, 2.5% of bacteraemia and meningitis isolates reported to the PHLS in England and Wales showed full or intermediate resistance to penicillin and 11.2% were resistant to erythromycin.

Pneumococcal vaccine

Pneumococcal vaccine is a polyvalent vaccine containing 25 microgrammes of purified capsular polysaccharide from each of 23 capsular types of pneumococcus which together account for about 90% of the pneumococcal isolates causing serious infection in Britain. It is supplied in a single dose vial.

Most healthy adults develop a good antibody response to a single dose of the vaccine by the third week following immunisation. Antibody response is not so reliable in young children, those with immunological impairment (including an absent or dysfunctional spleen) and those being treated with immunosuppressive therapy. Antibody response in children under two years of age is likely to be poor.

Many studies in efficacy have found it difficult to reach firm conclusions, but overall efficiency in preventing pneumococcal pneumonia is probably 60-70%. The vaccine is less effective in children under two years of age and those with immunosuppression. It has been relatively ineffective in patients with multiple myeloma, Hodgkin's and non-Hodgkin's lymphoma, especially during treatment, and in chronic alcoholism. It does not prevent otitis media or exacerbations of chronic bronchitis, and since so much pneumococcal meningitis is in young children and those with skull defects, its scope for preventing this disease is limited.

Antibody levels usually begin to wane after about five years, but may decline more rapidly in asplenic patients and children with nephrotic syndrome.

The vaccine should be stored unopened at 2-8 degrees C and inspected before being given to check that it is clear, colourless and without suspended particles.

Recommendations

Pneumococcal vaccine is recommended for all those aged two years or older in whom pneumococcal infection is likely to be more common and/or dangerous, ie those with:

i   Asplenia or severe dysfunction of the spleen, including homozygous sickle cell disease and coeliac syndrome.

ii Chronic renal disease or nephrotic syndrome.

iii   Immunodeficiency or immunosuppression due to disease or treatment, including HIV infection at all stages.

iv   Chronic heart or lung disease

v   Chronic liver disease including cirrhosis.

vi   Diabetes mellitus.

Where possible, the vaccine should be given, together with advice about the increased risk of pneumococcal infection, four to six weeks (but at least two weeks) before splenectomy and before courses of chemotherapy. If this is not practicable, as in traumatic splenectomy, the vaccine should be given as soon as possible after recovery from the operation, and before discharge from hospital. If not given before chemotherapy and/or radiotherapy, immunisation should be delayed until at least six months after the completion of therapy.

Additional measures for asplenic and hyposplenic patients

Haemophilus influenzae b, influenza, and in some circumstances meningococcal vaccines are additionally recommended and antibiotic prophylaxis (usually phenoxymethyl penicillin) is advisable at least until the age of 16 years. New guidelines have recently been published and a patient card and information sheet are available from the Department of Health. (BMJ 1996 312 430-4)

It is recommended that medical practitioners actively identify and contact unimmunised asplenic patients to offer them advice and to immunise them and also, that they identify patients on their lists in the other groups for whom vaccine is recommended and wherever possible, take opportunities to immunise those who have not been previously immunised, e.g. at routine consultations or whilst immunising against influenza.

Pneumococcal vaccine may be given at the same time as influenza vaccine, at a different site, but note that whereas influenza vaccine must be given annually, for most patients pneumococcal vaccine is given once only and re-immunisation may cause adverse reactions.

Route of administration and dosage

A single dose of 0.5ml. is given subcutaneously or intramuscularly preferably into the deltoid muscle or lateral aspect of the mid-thigh. Intradermal injection may cause a severe local reaction. The vaccine must not be given intravenously. The vaccine is used as supplied: no dilution or reconstitution is necessary.

Re-immunisation

Re-immunisation is not normally advised except, after 5-10 years, in individuals in whom antibody levels are likely to have declined more rapidly such as those with no spleen, with splenic dysfunction or with nephrotic syndrome. A few centres are able to measure antibody levels in cases where there is doubt about the need for re-immunisation. This should first be discussed with a local haematologist.

Adverse reactions

Mild soreness and induration at the site of the injection and, less commonly, a low grade fever may occur.

Re-immunisation with the earlier 12 and 14 valent vaccines produced more severe reactions in some recipients, especially if less than three years had elapsed since the first injection. Reactions correlated with high levels of circulating antibodies. The same considerations are likely to apply to re-immunisation with the 23-valent vaccine.

Contraindications

Pneumococcal vaccine should not be given during an acute infection. The vaccine is not recommended in pregnancy or in women who are breast feeding.

Re-immunisation within three years of a previous dose of pneumococcal vaccine is contraindicated.

For details of supplies of this vaccine refer to the 'Green Book. ' Page171

References

(1)   Slater P. E., et al. (1995). Absence of an association between rubella vaccination and arthritis in under immune post partum women. *Vaccine*: 13 (16): 1529.

(2)   Chen, R. et al. (1991). Adverse events following measles-mumps-rubella and measles vaccinations in college students. *Vaccine*; 9: 297.

(3)   *Immunisation against Infectious Disease* (1996). Page 81. HMSO. London.

(4)   Beck S. A., Williams I. W., Shirrell M., Burks A. W. (1991) Egg hypersensitivity and measles /mumps/ rubella vaccine administration. *Paediatrics*: 88:5: 913.

(5)   James J. M, Burks A W, Robertson P K, Sampson H A. (1995) Safe Administration of the Measles Vaccine to Children Allergic to eggs. *N. Eng. J Med* 332: 19. 1226.

(6)   Jacobs R. L., Lowe R. S., Lahier B. Q. (1992) Adverse reactions to Tetanus Toxoid. *J. A. M. A*. 247: 40-4

Anaphylaxis

Fisher M. (1995) Treatment of acute anaphylaxis. *Brit. Med J*; 311 :731

Treatment of acute anaphylaxis (1995) *Brit Med J*. 311: 1434.

Fisher M. (1995) Treatment of acute anaphylaxis *Brit Med. J*. 312: 637.

Fisher M. (1992) Treating anaphylaxis with sympatheticomimetic drugs. *Brit. Med. J* 305;1107.

The use of adrenaline for anaphylactic shock (for ambulance paramedics) Resuscitation Council (UK) and the Joint Royal Colleges and Ambulance Liason Committee. March 1996.

NB See also the notes on 'Peanut Allergy' in Chapter 6.

Chapter 5

CHILDHOOD AND ADOLESCENCE

There are several excellent texts available detailing the changes which take place during growth from infancy to physical and sexual maturity, to which the reader is referred. (See after the references at the end of the chapter.) Since April 1990, general practitioners have been undertaking surveillance of children under five, experience of which has given many doctors a pleasurable means of acquiring a sound background of early child development and an appreciation of the many variations in the 'normal.' This has facilitated the early detection of abnormalities of growth and development thus allowing children to enter school with many of their problems at least partially assessed, if not fully evaluated. Also, perhaps any necessary treatment will have been commenced and be continuing.

The Physical Changes of Puberty

From the age of five years until the beginning of the adolescent growth spurt the growth rate of children is fairly constant. The adolescent growth spurt in the 'average' girl begins at about ten and a half years and reaches a maximum at about twelve years with the menarche occurring at about twelve and a half years: the whole process taking just about three years.

In the 'average' boy, puberty occurs eighteen months to two years later and lasts slightly longer. These figures conceal individual variations, so that any sizable group of twelve year old girls or fourteen year old boys will include a whole range of individuals from the prepubertal, to the virtually mature. As mental capacity develops parallel with physical size, the differences between the sexes and the individual variations have important applications for teachers as well as for games instructors.

Most measurements of the body increase at the same rate as body height, in both sexes, with some exceptions. The brain and the skull develop earlier than other parts of the body whilst, after puberty, lymphatic tissue diminishes in size. (See Figure 1, page 112). The eyeball keeps pace with brain development, but a small increase in the axial length of the eye, probably accounts for the observed fact that myopia so often develops at the time of puberty. Hence the need for regular vision testing. Facial measurements change rapidly in adolescence and so do facial expressions, especially in boys.

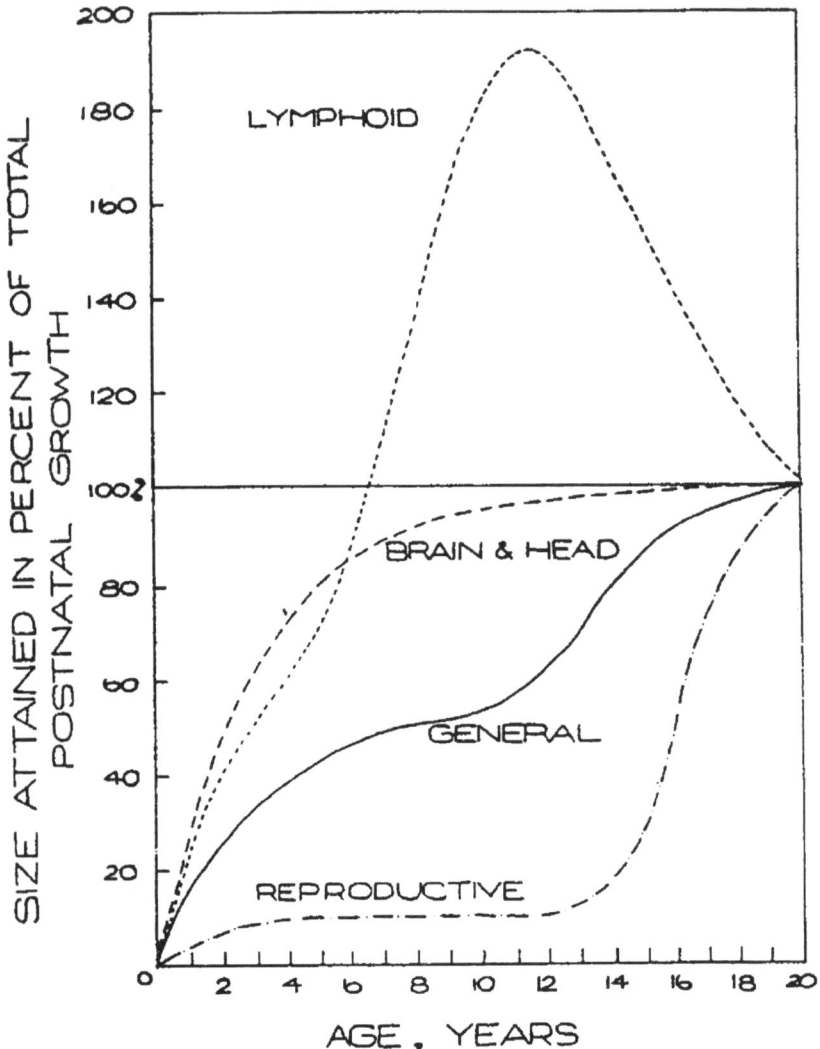

Figure1: Growth curves of different parts of the body – from 'The Measurement of Man' being Fig 73 from 'The Measurement of the Body in Childhood' by R. E Scammon, in J. A. Harris *et al.*, *The Measurement of Man* (University of Minnesota Press, 1930), p. 193.

The hands and feet are next after the skull to reach adult size, after which, leg length begins to increase rapidly, but most of the growth spurt in height is due to subsequent trunk growth. Girls have a particularly large growth in hip width whilst boys increase most in shoulder breadth. Muscle, including heart muscle grows rapidly in mass and strength, more so in boys than in girls, followed by a considerable increase in athletic ability.

The increased secretion of gonadotrophins from the pituitary leads in turn to the development of the sex organs in the following stages: (Sequences of events at adolescence for boys and girls, are illustrated, later, in Figures 2 and 3, page 115).

Stages of Genital Development

From 'Growth at Adolescence' (1962) by J. M. Tanner, and published by kind permission of Blackwell Science Ltd., Osney Mead, Oxford. OX2 OEL

Boys: Genital Development

Stage 1   Pre-adolescent. Testes, scrotum and penis are of about the same size and proportion as in early childhood.

Stage 2   Enlargement of the scrotum and testes. Skin of scrotum reddens and changes in texture. Little or no enlargement of penis at this stage.

Stage 3   Enlargement of penis, which occurs at first mainly in length. Further growth of testes and scrotum.

Stage 4   Increased size of penis with growth in breadth and development of glans. Testes and scrotum larger; scrotal skin darkened.

Stage 5   Genitalia adult in size and shape.

Girls: Breast development

Stage 1   Pre-adolescent. Elevation of papilla only.

Stage 2   Breast bud stage: elevation of breast and papilla as small mound. Enlargement of areola diameter.

Stage 3   Further enlargement and elevation of breast and areola, with no separation of their contours.

Stage 4   Projection of areola and papilla to form a secondary mound above the level of the breast.

Stage 5   Mature stage: projection of papilla only, due to recession of the areola to the general contour of the breast.

Both sexes: Pubic Hair

Stage 1   Pre-adolescent. The vellus over the pubes is not further developed than that over the abdominal wall, i. e. no pubic hair.

Stage 2   Sparse growth of long, slightly pigmented downy hair, straight or slightly curled, chiefly at the base of the penis or along the labia.

Stage 3   Considerably coarser, darker and more curled. The hair spreads sparsely over the junction of the pubes.

Stage 4   Hair now adult in type, but area covered is still considerably smaller than in the adult. No spread to the medial surface of the thighs.

Stage 5   Adult in quantity and type with distribution of the horizontal or classically 'feminine' pattern. Spread to medial surface of thighs but not up linea alba or elsewhere above the base of the inverse triangle. (Spread up linea alba occurs later and is rated Stage 6.)

Menstruation

It will be seen from Figure 3 that the menarche generally follows the onset of breast development by about two years. The enlightened attitude to menstruation which is now normal amongst girls and in schools was first widely documented over sixty years ago by Dr A. Sanderson Clow, medical officer to Cheltenham Ladies' College. This enlightened attitude is still undermined occasionally by mothers and even some boarding school house mothers, who cling to the old idea of 'unwellness' or 'poorly times' and the need to take extra care. School doctors can do much to encourage a more realistic approach to what is, after all, a natural function. If women are to take their full place in life, whether in work or sport, the variation of the menstrual cycle cannot be allowed to interfere with their lives. On the other hand, spasmodic dysmenorrhoea can be very disabling, and its management is discussed in Chapter 6.

Internal protection for the menstrual flow is now widely used and assists in the maintenance of normal activity. The use of tampons by school girls should no longer be discouraged and, indeed, most girls cope remarkably well. If, however, a girl in her late teens is worried or distressed by being unable to insert tampons, expert help should be sought. Vaginismus, or anatomical abnormality, e.g. a vaginal septum, may be the cause and can usually be corrected. It is worthy of mention here, that any woman who has failed to insert tampons should seek expert advice and the difficulty corrected promptly, otherwise non-consummation may wreck any relationship or marriage.

Forgotten tampons produce a very offensive vaginal discharge, but removal is all that is required.

Toxic Shock Syndrome

During the last decade, the toxic shock syndrome (TSS) has been recognised, initially in the USA, as a very serious and potentially fatal condition. There can be a variable onset of confusion, high fever, diarrhoea, vomiting and hypotension, producing shock and a generalised erythematous rash, which may be followed by peeling of the skin of the palms and soles several days later. Additionally, there may be muscle pains, sore throat, hallucinations, dry mouth, vaginal dryness in females and coma. The illness can occur in both sexes by a common bacteria, e.g. staphylococcus aureus, gaining entrance to the body via an open wound and producing a toxin which overwhelms the

Figure 2: Diagram of the sequence of events at adolescence – boys, showing the average and the range of ages at which each stage is reached. (from Tanner, J. M. (1962) 'Growth at adolescence' by kind permission of Blackwell Science Ltd., Osney Mead, Oxford. OX2 OEL.

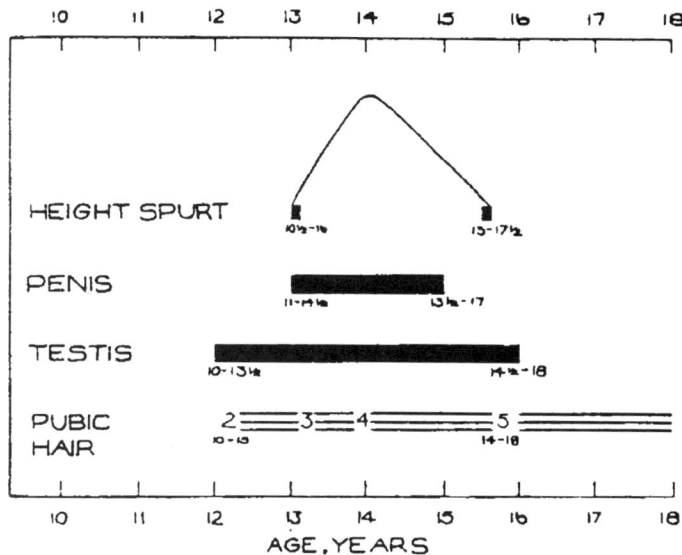

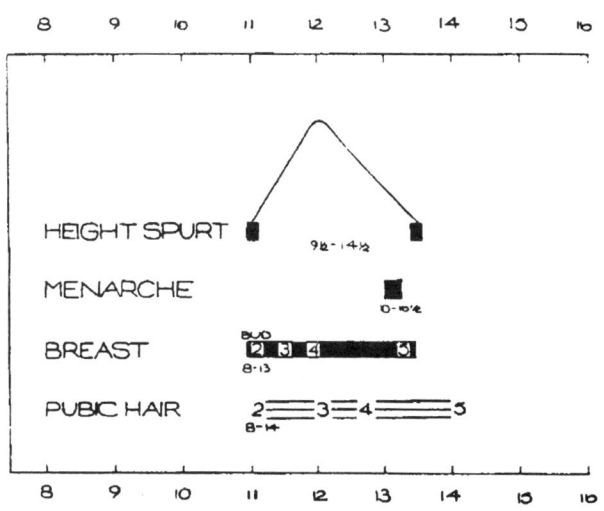

Figure 3. Diagram of the sequence of events at adolescence – girls, showing the average and the range of ages at which each stage is reached. (from Tanner, J. M. (1962) 'Growth at adolescence' by kind permission of Blackwell Science Ltd., Osney Mead, Oxford. OX2 OEL.

immune system, leading to the above signs and symptoms, and possible major organ failure or even death.

Initially, most of the known cases were found to occur amongst women, usually in the 15-25 year age group, who were menstruating and using tampons. Clearly, school medical officers require to be aware of this condition and if it is suspected, then because of the potentially rapid onset of hypotensive shock, hospital admission is mandatory.[1,2,3]

The charity, 'Tampon Alert', founded by Peter Kilvert, whose 15 year old daughter, Alice, died from the condition, has issued the following guidelines for continued tampon usage, in order to minimise the risk of TSS from this cause. Further information and leaflets are available from Mr. Kilvert at 16, Blinco Road, Urmston. Manchester. M41. 9NF. Tel: 0161 748 3123.

i   Use the lowest absorbency at each stage of the period. (Highly absorbent tampons dry-out and traumatise the vaginal walls, thus facilitating the entry of bacteria.)

ii   Alternate tampons with sanitary pads especially at night and at the end of a period.

iii Change tampons at least every four to six hours.

iv   Do not use tampons if you have had any unusual discharge.

v   Wash your hands before and after use and handle the tampon as little as possible.

vi   Alert your family and friends to the symptoms and emergency action required.

vii Read the TSS information on the packet and the enclosed leaflet.

Symptoms of TSS
Usually begin AFTER the start of a period.

Early symptoms may include headache, sore throat, aching muscles and high temperature. Vomiting, watery diarrhoea, rash, confusion and dizziness may follow. Only one or two symptoms may occur and they may not necessarily occur at once and may not continue.

What to do
Remove the tampon and seek **immediate** medical attention. Tell the doctor that you are menstruating and have been using tampons. Take a TSS leaflet with you.

For women who survive, there can be prolonged weakness and permanent disability of many kinds, depending on the tissue and organ damage sustained. These women are more likely to get TSS again, compared with women who have never suffered from it, so tampon use should be discontinued. It is thought inadvisable for women with staphylococcal infections to use tampons.

In the UK from 1990 to 1995 there have been 16 deaths due to tampon-related TSS. The Department of Health has reported 10 cases of tampon-related TSS per year, but these have been severe cases requiring hospitalisation. Undoubtedly, many other cases go unreported.[4] The highest risk is in the 15-25 year age group.

Emotional Changes in Adolescence

The progression from dependent childhood to that of a fully mature adult, capable of sustaining an independent existence is subjected to many influences, eg, cultural, socio-economic, genetic, etc.

These influences can react on the teenager in such a way as to produce uncertainty and anxiety in someone who, on account of the rapid physiological changes he is already undergoing, may make him feel even more insecure. His rapid growth phase will perhaps make him clumsy and uncontrolled and the accompanying hormonal changes initially may produce feelings of bewilderment. These changes may produce moodiness, disgruntled feelings and senses of low-worth and low self-esteem, especially if he has some minor 'imperfections'. A bit later on, of course, the burgeoning sexuality will produce further bodily and psychological changes, e.g. erections, nocturnal emissions, menstruation, which may engender further confusion and perhaps guilt, especially if there have been no preparatory explanations. As noted in Chapter 6, teenagers may become disproportionately concerned about their few spots of acne. Similarly, if they require to wear dental braces or spectacles. They cringe when unthinking persons call them names based on their perceived minor 'imperfections' and require sensitive handling by parents and teachers. In the absence of an explanation that what she is experiencing is part of normal development, a teenage girl with differential breast growth will be most upset, and understandably so.

Teenagers with feelings of low self-esteem and inferiority require to conform and to be accepted by their friends and peers. If a boy is endowed with athletic prowess, this is helpful, but if the reverse is the case then he may feel worse and even more unwanted. Similarly, with young girls who may find peer approval easier if they have athletic ability.

In their desire for acceptance and approval, they can be subjected to peer group pressure, which may incur disapproval from parents and teachers, especially if the peer group in turn, is yielding to the influence of the sometimes shameless exploitation of them by the media. Recent examples of this have been the production of attractively packaged drinks ostensibly for youngsters, but containing alcohol.

As they get older, their physical maturity outstrips their emotional maturity, but soon they begin to express their identity and often give parents and teachers the benefit of their views on society! Most youngsters have an innate sense of fairness and can fairly quickly detect and condemn hypocrisy, although they do tend to see things in 'black and white' and have difficulty in conceding reasonable points in an argument or even arriving at a compromise.

With the establishment of their identity, they feel the need to experiment and perhaps in so doing, challenge the authority of parents or teachers. The need to do this however, is different from the bravado which might induce an insecure youngster to do foolhardy things.

Either way, it is well known that teenagers take risks, usually with motor vehicles, alcohol, tobacco, drugs and sex. As far as sex is concerned, their emotional immaturity is thought to be responsible for their 'cognitive lapses.' Despite the fact that they have the physiological information and the contraceptives, they fail to use them.

Although the name adolescence frequently conjures up a popular view of unremitting turmoil and disruption, such is really not the case and this was borne out by a (by now) classical study in the Isle of Wight by Rutter, the conclusion of which was that 'Normal adolescence is not characterised by storm, stress and disturbance. Most young people go through their teenage years without any significant emotional or behavioural problems.'[5]

Some Problems of Adolescents at School
Anorexia nervosa and Bulimia nervosa
These are two related eating disorders, which present school doctors with problems.

Anorexia nervosa
This multifaceted disorder, with physical, emotional and behavioural characteristics, causes problems for the school doctor. The incidence is difficult to determine but it is thought to be of the order of one per 150 or 200, over 90% of whom are girls. Although cases as young as eight and as old as the early twenties, are known, it is commonest in the 15 to 17 year age group.

Reasons for the perceived increase in the incidence are probably social and peer group pressures, plus the difficulties of modern society and the media, where thinness is portrayed as being desirable. Part of the increase however, may be due to an increased awareness of the condition by parents, medical and nursing staff, teaching and house staff, resulting in more youngsters being brought forward or seeking help. The condition has been variously described as 'The Relentless Pursuit ofThinness'-(Bruch), 'Weight Phobia' – (Crisp) and 'A Morbid Fear of Becoming Fat' – (Russell). (6.7.8.)

The term anorexia is something of a misnomer, for initially the appetite exists and often the young people suffering from the condition may have been teased because of being plump or even overweight. Then they become pre-occupied with their weight and commence dieting, initially in an acceptable way, only to progress to unreasonable measures involving exclusively low calorie meals, missed meals and vigorous exercise.

The school doctor must be alert to a wide range of presenting symptoms and signs. Recognition in schools is often difficult as the girl (usually), and her family deny the existence of any problem. Early intervention by school medical officers, nursing and house staff, working well together, can often prevent the need for referral.

Precipitants include: vegetarianism, food-fads, including an avoidance of carbohydrate and fatty foods, chaotic eating patterns, obesity, (either in the child or the parents), overconforming, sexual naiveté or experience, puberty, obsessionality, family eating patterns and some hysterical features.

In school, awareness of these precipitants in girls who are losing weight is important, especially if associated with the following types of behaviour: – dieting, excessive exercising, vomiting, purging and diuretic misuse. When assessing these girls it is important to seek the following family features which are commonly associated with the development of anorexia:

Outside features emphasised, eg, high academic expectations – spoken or unspoken.

Difficulties with dependence and independence-enmeshment.

Poor generation of self-esteem.

Conflict avoidance.

Marital problems.

Alliance within the group.

Blurred generational boundaries.

'Protective' function of anorexia.

In the UK the most commonly used diagnostic criteria for anorexia nervosa in adolescents are those of the American Psychiatric Association's Diagnostic and Statistical Manual of Mental Disorders (DSM111R) and those of the International Classification of Diseases. (ICD9).

DSM 111R

Refusal to maintain body weight over minimal normal weight for age and height, (for example, weight loss leading to a body weight 15% below expected weight) or failure to make expected weight gain during the growth period leading to body weight 15% below expected weight.

Intense fear of gaining weight or becoming fat, even though underweight.

Disturbance in the experience of body weight, size or shape: (e.g. claiming to feel fat when emaciated, believing that one area of the body is too fat when actually underweight. i. e. distorted body image.

The absence of at least three consecutive menstrual cycles, when otherwise expected to occur.

(Primary or secondary amenorrhoea).

ICD 9

Persistently active refusal to eat and marked loss of weight.

Characteristic high level of activity and alertness in relation to emaciation.

Typical onset in teenage girls, sometimes before puberty. Rarely in males.

Amenorrhoea is usual.

Other possible physiological changes

- slow pulse and respiration with hypotension.

- low body temperature.

- dependent oedema.

- breast atrophy and sparse pubic hair.

- small stature due to premature fusion of epiphyses in patients suffering from early pubertal onset of anorexia.

Typical unusual eating habits and attitudes towards food. Sometimes starvation follows or alternates with periods of over eating .

Diverse accompanying psychiatric symptoms

These are not ideal when applied to prepubertal children, however the similarities between children with the condition and older patients are greater than the differences. Anorexia occurs in children of both sexes as young as eight years old. Differences which are specific to the younger patient include, a higher proportion of male patients, the absence of amenorrhoea as a readily available diagnostic criterion, a higher incidence of depression associated with the eating disorder, the dangerous tendency of children to refuse fluids as well as food and the severity of even modest weight loss.

As previously noted anorexia can occur as early as eight years but is commoner around 15-17 years: the diagnosis is made as previously described. Other symptoms and signs include preoccupation with body weight or energy intake, self-induced vomiting, excessive exercising and laxative abuse. Other emotional pointers include irritability, the tendency to be easily upset or frustrated, inability to tolerate unplanned events (especially those involving food), withdrawal, moodiness, temper outbursts, loss of enjoyment and tearfulness. It is important to be alert and remember that presentation may be with secondary effects such as constipation or complications of poor circulation. Often, especially at very low weights, there is body wide distribution of the very fine downy hair (lanugo) often seen in small pre-term babies.

The main role of the general practitioner or the school doctor is to make a prompt diagnosis and a swift start to management as this may prevent the eating disorder from becoming well established and more resistant to treatment. In making the diagnosis however, especially in severe or resistant cases, it is wise to consider other possible medical conditions such as thyrotoxicosis, insulin dependent diabetes mellitus, severe infections including tuberculosis, alone or in association with HIV infection, and mal – absorption syndromes.

Having made a diagnosis of anorexia nervosa, treatment involves regaining and stabilising weight at an agreed safe level, which allows restarting menstruation and gradual exercise if it has been excessive and stopping diuretics and purgatives.

It is important for a rapport to be gained with the boy or girl and for family and other issues to be looked at in psychotherapy (individual group or family therapy) as well as an emphasis on normal eating behaviour and improving physical health. For moderately severe cases, a target weight, based on a mean matched population weight should be set and must not be negotiable. Lacy recommends a usual school diet supplemented by two rounds of cheese sandwiches daily as a good source of extra calories.[9]

The general UK view is that drug therapy is unhelpful.

This work may be with the medical officer, a counsellor, a psychologist or a psychiatrist, depending on the stage the anorexia has reached. Very severe and resistant cases, may have to be excluded from school and admitted to hospital, voluntarily if possible, but very occasionally by compulsory detention under section 3 of the Mental Health Acts, for severe cases of this condition do carry a significant mortality, due to inanition or suicide.

Many of the precipitating factors can be spread within the school environment eg, chaotic eating, food fads, laxative abuse and vomiting. This must be recognised and opportunities found to educate pupils and staff, also giving support and individual counselling where appropriate. The general levels of stress and pressure in the whole school may need to be addressed.

Most schools will have, or have had, one or more cases and it is important to recognise and treat these early, for as noted earlier, anorexia can be a life threatening condition and it is also important to recognise the distress that even early or mild anorexics can cause to their fellow pupils, who also will need support.

Bulimia nervosa

This is another eating disorder, first described in 1979 and which may occur singly or in combination with anorexia nervosa. Again, there is a marked female preponderance, usually affecting the late teens or early twenties. Sufferers from bulimia have a 'morbid fear of becoming fat' and have distorted body images. At the same time, they have irresistible urges to indulge in secret binges after which they feel guilty and ashamed. To avoid putting on weight, they then induce vomiting by a variety of methods ranging from exercise, putting their fingers down their throats, abuse of diuretics and finally purgatives.[10]

Compared with anorexia, bulimia is more difficult to diagnose because usually, there is no weight loss. Physical signs can be swelling of the parotid glands and erosion of enamel from the teeth. The presence on the dorsal aspects of the hands and fingers of callouses and lacerations, is highly suggestive of the condition.[11,12,13] Sometimes girls themselves or their friends will volunteer information on what is happening. Treatment is difficult and it is better if cases are picked up early. Psychotherapy and counsell ing may help.

The approximate incidence is 3% of women between the ages of 16 and 40. However, no social class predominates. It is very rare in males. Treatment with drugs is disappointing. Psychotherapy and counselling offer the best hope. Menstrual disorders are common in bulimia and recent work has indicated a possible relationship between bulimia nervosa and polycystic ovaries[14]). Perhaps the school doctor could look for evidence of bulimia whilst investigating menstrual difficulties in older girls.

Obesity

There is a need to monitor obesity in schools, especially where there are girls. It is estimated that 5% to 10 % of young children are overweight, and about 15% of teenagers, compared with 30% of the adult population.[15] General education on sensible eating and nutrition may be helpful, perhaps allied to advice on a sensible diet from the dental health point of view. However, care is required so as not to trigger off any potential cases of anorexia.

Adolescent adjustment and serious mental illness

There is no serious psychiatric disorder which is unique to adolescence, and adolescents are unlikely to have any real mental problems. The distinction would have to be made of course, between age appropriate behaviour and psychopathology. However, adolescents are likely to suffer from mental anguish simlilar to adults at times of anxiety, like, for example, A level and scholarship examinations. Post traumatic stress disorder and eating disorders occur in this age group and can be helped by early recognition. Depression accounts for 25% of adolescent psychiatric cases, with a female to male ratio of four to one. Also, depression acounts for 25% of adolescent suicides (second most common cause of death). Look for changes in behaviour and mental state, frequent evasiveness, persisting abnormality and physical disease.

Chronic Depression in Adolescence
(Differentiate from 'depressed mood' and 'permanent depression')
Major clinical depression
Watch for a pervasive low mood ('emptiness and absence of feelings'), declining academic work, poor sleep – usually early morning awakening, but feeling better as the day progresses, feelings of guilt, feelings of helplessness regarding the future, loss of weight and appetite for food, self neglect, suicidal ideation, self-inflicted wounds and a family history of affective disorder. Major depression in an adolescent may represent the first episode of severe depression or of schizophrenia. However, usually, modern psychotropic drugs can restore normality.

Mild depression ('Dysthymia')
The risk factors for this are bereavement – especially with the death of a parent before the child is 12, relationship difficulties (parental divorce), academic failure and poor self esteem.

The classical features include restlessness and boredom, fatigue, bodily preoccupation and physical symptoms, which can include uncharacteristic behaviour, e.g. drug taking, promiscuity and risk taking behaviour. It is important to note that drug misuse is not always due to peer pressure. Drugs are often misused by adolescents with low self esteem.

NB Beware of schools with a punitive expulsion policy for drug misuse. If a pupil is being considered for expulsion following illegal drug taking, make sure that there is no evidence of an underlying depressive illness (or even anxiety). If such a pupil is expelled, then make sure that there is continuity of care in case of an underlying psychiatric disorder.

Suicide
This is the second most common cause of death in the 15-24 year age group. Also, suicide is increasing in young males in the 14-24 year age group. In the decade 1980-1990, male suicides were up by 78%, (thought not to have been related to unemployment), whilst female suicides in the same age range were down by 50%. 90% of successful suicides were found to have had mental health problems. Also, there has been an increase in affective disorders in adolescence, but whether this is a true increase or due to improved methods of diagnosis is not quite clear. Despite a high rate of potentially affective disorders and despite communication of intent, there is only a minority of necessary help at the time of death. ('No one hears!')

Risk factors for suicidal adolescents
Antisocial behaviour, verbal expression of suicidality (may raise a flag), previous attempts at suicide, mood disorder, (studies of suicides have shown 50%-60% have had clinical mood disorder), alcohol and drug misuse and male sex. Girls are more likely to indulge in 'self harm' (parasuicide).

Parasuicide

This is deliberate self harm: victims act impulsively. The rate is increasing in girls and static in boys. 50% use paracetamol. 9% repeat the exercise within a year and 3% have a psychiatric disorder. Thus there could be tragedy if a girl is expelled for attempting suicide and there has been no passing on of information to her new doctor and /or school.

Prevention of suicides

This is related to the detection of mental disorders. Do not assume that depressive moods are not serious and do not be afraid to enquire about suicide. ('Have you thought of this before?"Have you attempted this before?', or 'Do you know anyone who has killed themselves?'or even'How would you do it now?') A family history of suicide is a potent predictor and there requires to be a clinical assessment of the patient's memory. Then there should be an exploration of the patient's problems, a mood assessment and a psychiatric referral.

Mania

This is rarely seen in adolescents. The prevalence rate being 0.6%.

Clinical Features

Elevation of mood, infectious optimism, irritability, rough and outrageous activity, uncharacteristic promiscuity, self-important ideas, possible development of psychosis with hallucinations and delusions. There may be a switch from mania to depression within hours. There may be a family history of manic depression. This is a highly familial condition, especially in creative and successful writers and composers: the other side of the coin to creativity.

Schizophrenia in adolescents

As stated earlier, there is no psychosis unique to adolescence. However, schizophrenia occurs typically in young adults, but *may* occur from the age of 12. The younger the onset, the more severe the illness is likely to be. The condition afflicts all races and all social classes of adolescents from the brightest to the dullest. ('Everyone Everywhere')

Schizophrenia is predominantly a brain disorder and is not *caused* by family or social problems. It is a neurodevelopmental·organic illness, demonstrated after puberty and is thought to have some relationship to myelination. Modern drugs, e.g. Clozapine, have given new hope to patients with refractory schizophrenia, especially with the symptoms of school refusal, being watched and hearing voices. Early diagnosis is very helpful, and reluctance to consider a diagnosis of schizophrenia to thus 'label' a patient, might be the means of adding years of suffering. Psychiatric referal is therefore mandatory if suspected.

Clinical problems in schizophrenia in early adolescence

These are depression, poor concentration, failing, a socially dead past, incoherence and bizarre action ('can't think straight'), preoccupation with morbid thoughts, neglect of appearance and (may be fleeting) hallucinations or delusions.

What to do

Devise a simple interviewing scheme.

1. General psychiatric adjustment: – iritability, poor concentration, etc.

2. Anxiety and worries: physical worries, tension, phobias, etc.

3. Symptoms of depression; depressed mood, low self esteem, early morning wakening, suicidal thoughts.

4. Details of parents, home life, etc.

Serious adolescent psychiatric disorders or psychotic states are largely undetected. These disorders have a very poor public perception.

School Refusal

School refusal is a form of separation anxiety in which a child refuses, or is very reluctant, to go to school. Sexes and social classes are equally affected, and the child has an accompanying plethora of psychosomatic symptoms, such as abdominal pain, headaches, nausea and diarrhoea, usually, but not always, at school times. Less definite, unexplained symptoms occur, with no obvious association with school, raising the possibilty of early organic disease and this is sometimes referred to as the 'masquerade syndrome'.[16] Berg has suggested that the condition may be thought to be ME.[17]

The psychopathology usually lies in the mother-child relationship, and the longer the absence from school is allowed to continue, the more difficult the problem becomes to resolve. The child needs to be returned to school, firmly, by the parents, with the active, sympathetic assistance of the school staff, social worker or psychotherapist. Family psychotherapy is required to explore the underlying reasons for the child's anxiety. In boarding schools, separation of this kind can result in pathological homesickness and running away. The family requires professional help. A contract of week-ends at home at increasing intervals is often successful, but in a few resistant cases there is no alternative to the child's withdrawal from boarding school. Preferably such a move could be followed by continuing family psychotherapeutic support.

There is a legal obligation for children to attend school which can be enforced via the magistrates' courts.[18] Drug therapy has no value in this condition.

Truancy

Whilst 'school refusers' make no attempt to conceal their problem from parents, the reverse is the case with truanting children, who elect to stay off school illegally, often to further their antisocial behaviour, eg. stealing, vandalism, and usually without the knowledge of their parents or guardians. However, in some cases, parental collusion is suspected. This is a burgeoning social problem which requires the combined approach of the home and many agencies (social services, education welfare services, etc.)since truancy is a predictor of adult antisocial tendencies.[19]

Bullying and Mobbing

A comprehensive definition of bullying appears in a questionnaire based on the work of the Norwegian, Dan Olweus, an international expert, who has studied bullying for many years and is quoted thus:'We say a child is being bullied or picked on, when another child, or group of children say nasty or unpleasant things to him or her. It is also bullying when a child is hit, kicked, threatened, locked inside a room, sent nasty notes, when no one ever talks to them and things like that. These things can happen frequently and it is difficult for the child being bullied to defend himself or herself. It is also bullying when a child is teased repeatedly in a nasty way, but it is not bullying when two children of about the same strength have the odd fight or quarrel'.[20]

In one of his studies of bullying in schools, Olweus found that about 5% of a boys' school population could be classed as bullies and 5% as whipping boys. The two groups were quite distinct: neither were below average in academic achievement. The whipping boys tended to be weaker in physical strength and often they had over-protective parents, but did not differ from a control group in other respects. Bullies were characterised by a strong need to dominate and often had weak relationships with their parents. Although the personality types were determined before school age, Olweus concluded that there was no place for a tacitly permissive attitude and teachers were advised to be authoritative but firm.[21]

In 1991, mobbing was defined by Heinemann as 'a form of aggression exercised by groups against smaller groups or individuals. This requires no great intellectual or emotional involvement and the actors involved often have only a hazy awareness that their actions are experienced as devastating attacks by the victim, who can be psychologically and even physically devastated by this apparently organised collective rejection.'[22] Heineman states that individual conflicts or the aggression of one individual (a bully) should not be confused with the group dynamics of mobbing. He states that bullies comonly exploit and direct their peers' predisposition to mobbing. A bully and followers must always be treated differently: the bully by a child psychiatrist. The victim must be protected immediately: often too with treatment by a child psychiatrist. The followers need the educational treatment and training as suggested by Pikas.[23]

The Norwegian work quoted above is part of the work funded by the Norwegian government almost twenty years ago. This contrasts markedly with the situation in the UK, where, had it not been for the sustained efforts of some voluntary organisations over the last few years, it is doubtful whether even the present degree of progress would have been made in the recognition of the extent of bullying, let alone attempting to control it.

It is very sobering to learn that in the UK in the1990s, some youngsters have met their death because of bullying. In 1991, a teenage girl committed suicide beause of prolonged bullying and a few years later a two year old boy was bullied and killed. (Later, two ten year old boys were convicted of his murder). These two tragedies received national media coverage, but other deaths due to bullying occur. One of the charitiable organisations campaigning for the recognition and abolition of bullying has estimated that there are about

10 suicides a year due to bullying, in addition to many more children who are severely traumatised by verbal and physical abuse at school.[24]

Now, increasing numbers of local authorities and schools are establishing anti-bullying policies, so a very welcome start has been made to try and control this source of danger, misery and unhappiness to so many children.

ALCOHOL, TOBACCO AND ILLEGAL SUBSTANCES

The widespread use of both legal and illegal drugs is now established as part of youth culture throughout the United Kingdom, in all social classes and racial groups, by both sexes and in all schools, state and independent. Drug misusers are a heterogeneous group of people ranging from children and adolescents experimenting with drugs to illicit drug users whose lives are dominated by their habit and who are likely to be drug dependent.[25]

Alcohol

Ethyl alcohol, a central nervous depressant, produces the well known effects of disinhibition and impaired skills and judgment. It is an offence under the Licensing Act 1964 to sell intoxicating liquor without a licence. This prevents the sale of alcohol at school events unless an occasional licence has been obtained under the Licensing (Occasional Permissions) Act 1983. It is also an offence to sell alcohol to any person under the age of 18 and, under Section 6 of the Children and Young Persons Act 1933, to give any child under the age of 5 intoxicating liquor. Despite this, all types of alcoholic drinks are available from a variety of commercial outlets at various times of day.

Most youngsters have their first taste of alcohol around the age of ten and are introduced to it by their parents, usually to celebrate a special occasion. By 16 years of age, about 90% have tried alcohol. Alcohol is thought to be important in adolescent development and socialisation as it helps young people to integrate with their peers and to negotiate their passage into the adult world. Although most young people drink moderately and sensibly, many, however, have experience of intoxication and a considerable minority drink heavily. Anecdotal evidence suggests that with hundreds of primary school children consuming alcohol, a significant number of 11 year olds are arriving at school with hangovers.

Although not causally linked, adolescent intoxication is associated with accidents, certain crimes and risky behaviour, including unsafe sexual encounters. The quantity of alcohol being consumed by teenagers during a typical drinking occasion is increasing, leading to an increase in the occurrence of intoxication. The amount of alcohol consumed and the frequency of drinking increases with age, as does the tendency for drinking to move from the parental home and into more public places where it is often done in the company of friends. Heavy drinking, while not a predictor of alcohol problems later in life, is associated with the use of illegal substances and poor performance at school.

In 1992, 12% of 11-15 year olds were regular drinkers and in an average week 4% of under 16 year olds consumed alcohol in excess of the levels considered sensible for adults – formerly not more than 21 units a week for men and 14 units a week for women, but increased, rather controversially, in late 1995, to 28 units and 21 units respectively.

Dr John Balding of the Schools Health Education Unit at Exeter University in a yearly survey of 11-18 year olds' attitudes to health related issues reported in 1995 that more than half of 15 and 16 year old boys had drunk an average of four pints of beer or lager in the week preceding the survey. Girls also drank more than the recommended alcohol limit for adults in a week and 10% of boys and 8% of girls drank more than the equivalent of 10 pints of beer for males and seven pints for females.

Hughes *et al* studied 824 12-17 year olds in Scotland and drew attention to the so called 'designer drinks', a new range of fortified fruit wines and strong white ciders. Their study found that 2% of 12 year olds drank once a week and 4% had taken more than 15 units in their last session. 19% of the 12 year olds who said they had been drinking in the previous six months claimed to have been 'really drunk'. Contrary to the claims by the manufacturers that such drinks are aimed at young adults over the age of 18, the brand imagery of designer drinks matched the perceptions and the expectations of drinking of many 14 and 15 year olds; by the age of 17 the young drinkers wished to appear grown up by choosing conventional beers and spirits instead.[26]

Tobacco

Despite the incontrovertible evidence of the health hazards of tobacco smoking, this activity in young people, like drinking, continues to increase. In 1993, a total of 10% of 11-15 year olds were regular smokers and this figure rose to 12% in 1994. Balding found that by 16 years of age, one in three girls and one in four boys were already smoking 40 cigarettes a day. World-wide, there are growing indications that even in countries with the most aggressive tobacco control policies, teenage smoking has stopped declining. While et al surveyed 1,450 children aged 11 and 12 years and found a relationship between awareness of the most advertised cigarette brands and the heightened risk of taking up smoking, especially by girls.[27] It is widely accepted that cigarette advertising plays a part in childrens' decisions to smoke and While's data contradicts tobacco industry claims that its advertising is intended to encourage brand switching in adults who are already smokers. Correlations between higher experimentation with tobacco by teenagers and sports sponsorship by tobacco companies have been found and, outwith any educative progress made by school doctors, nurses and teachers, an immediate ban on tobacco advertising would be an extremely helpful step in reversing the trend.[28,29]

There is evidence that the children of smokers are more likely to take up the habit themselves and one of the main contributions that parents and teachers, not to mention doctors and nurses, can make is not to smoke themselves. The establishment in some schools of smoking rooms is to be deplored as this merely condones the habit. It is vital that children are educated about the harmful effects of tobacco and this should be covered in schools in appropriate science or PSHE lessons. Young people are unlikely to be persuaded to give up smoking by the health risks, and education should emphasise the cost and unattractiveness of smoking. Mentioning to young men the risks of impotence from the circulatory effects of nicotine can be quite effective!

Illegal substances

The use of illegal substances, as opposed to alcohol and tobacco, by young people is increasing and Balding's 1995 survey revealed that 33% of 15-16 year old boys and 27% of girls had smoked cannabis, and 13% and 11% respectively had taken hallucinogenic drugs such as LSD.

Miller and Plant in a study in 1995 of 7,722 pupils aged 15 and 16 years in 10 independent and 59 state schools found even greater evidence of cannabis use with 38% of girls and 43.6% of boys using the drug. Their survey also revealed that higher levels of drug use were associated with poorer school performance and that levels of illegal substance use tended to be higher in Scotland than in England, Wales or Northern Ireland.[30]

Comparing Miller and Plant's figures with data from a Health Authority study in 1989 reveals the dramatic increase in drug experimentation in this age group.

15 and 16 year olds who have used illegal drugs:

	Boys		Girls	
	1989	1995	1989	1995
	%	%	%	%
Cannabis	22.0	43.6	15.0	38.0
Glues and solvents	4.0	19.7	2.0	21.0
Amphetamines	4.0	14.5	1.0	12.3
Ecstasy	3.0	9.2	2.0	7.3
Tranquillisers	1.0	6.9	1.0	9.5
Cocaine	1.0	2.8	1.0	2.4
Heroin	0.5	1.7	0.5	1.5

'Drug Misuse' is defined as the non-medical use of drugs that are only intended for use in medical treatment, and the use of drugs that have no accepted medical purpose. Such drugs are controlled by the Misuse of Drugs Act 1971 and it is an offence under this Act

- to supply or to offer to supply a controlled drug to another.

- to be in possession of, or to possess with intent to supply to another.

- for the occupier or someone concerned with the management of any premises knowingly to permit or suffer on those premises the smoking of cannabis or the production, attempted production, supply or attempted supply or offering to supply, of any controlled drug.

Solvent misuse is not covered by the Act and possession of volatile substances is not illegal. However, it is an offence in English Law to supply or attempt to supply a substance to a person under 18 knowing, or having reasonable cause to believe, that the substance or its fumes are likely to be used by that person for the purpose of causing intoxication.

Cannabis (marijuana, dope, grass, hash, pot, high)

Cannabis is a Class B drug under the Misuse of Drugs Act and the most widely used illegal substance in the United kingdom. It is derived from various parts of the cannabis plant and is usually smoked, often with tobacco, or taken by mouth. It has depressant and hallucinogenic effects and its use results in euphoria, excessive relaxation, lack of co-ordination and inappropriate giggling. Users may have blood-shot eyes, dilated pupils and increased heart rates. Because of the effects on co-ordination and reaction times, road accidents and accidents in the work place are more likely and chronic users may develop paranoia and psychological disturbances not unlike schizophrenia. Smoking cannabis with or without tobacco, may result in respiratory illnesses and permanent lung damage.

Following recent reports that the drug may be of therapeutic benefit in a few instances, e.g. relieving the painful muscular spasms of multiple sclerosis, there is now quite a vocal lobby for the decriminalisation of cannabis.

Solvents and Glues

Solvent misuse has become increasingly common over the last 25 years and many commonly available domestic substances are inhaled. Aerosols, lighter fuels, typewriter correction fluids, glues, paint strippers, nail polish remover and petrol are some of the fluids which are misused with, usually, the substance being poured on to a rag, or into a bag, and inhaled. The effects depend on the substance used and the duration of exposure, and range from euphoria and intoxication, not unlike the effects of alcohol, to hallucinations, drowsiness and unconsciousness. The user may have a rash around the mouth and nose and an obvious chemical smell about his person and /or clothing, may be detected. He may complain of stomach cramps and display unco-ordinated movements and slurred speech. Dangers may arise from asphyxia, due to the inhalation of vomit or from the plastic bag adhering to the face, (especially if the user is inhaling alone). Long-term damage to the heart, lungs, liver, kidneys and nervous system may take place. The death rate from solvent misuse, which rose steeply from 1984 to 1990, fell again in 1994 when there were 57 deaths. In the mid 1980s, the UK government introduced the Intoxicating Substances Supply Act, which made it an offence for the shopkeeper to supply to any person under the age of 18, any substance which he believed might be used in this way. It was a start, but there have been few prosecutions.

Amphetamines (speed, whiz, billy, uppers, sulph, bennies, black bombers, meths, crystal, dixies)

These Class B drugs come in powder or tablet form and can be taken by mouth, dissolved in water and injected, or sniffed up the nose – 'snorting'. Their effects are euphoria without the aggression, restless and hyperactive behaviour with increased energy, loss of appetite and insomnia. These effects can last for four to six hours and are often followed by a 'come down' with, often, profound depression. Regular use will interrupt sleep patterns and eating habits, and can lead to extreme paranoid delusions and other psychotic behaviour. Most 'street' 'speed' contains amphetamine sulphate and is 'cut' or adulterated with other substances, such as brick dust, dried milk powder, chalk etc, so that the purity can be as low as 5%.

Ecstasy (E, XTC, white dove, playboy, dollars, bulldogs, strawberries, hug drug, dennis the menace, rhapsody, disco biscuits)

Ecstasy is a Class A drug containing an amphetamine analogue, MDMA, and it has both stimulant and hallucinogenic effects. Despite recent well-publicised deaths from ecstasy use, it is increasingly popular among young people. It is estimated that there are more than one million users a week and it is readily available at parties, night clubs and raves. Taken orally it causes increased energy, thirst, sleeplessness, depression and paranoia, but occasionally, it is accompanied by a feeling of 'togetherness' (the 'hug drug'). It interferes with the body's temperature regulating mechanisms, (causing the need to 'chill out') and the need to drink excessive fluids, especially water and soft drinks. As a consequence, water intoxication can occur with cerebral oedema, collapse, coma and death.

Recent research has shown that long-term users may be prone to panic attacks, depression and psychotic illness and that the drug may cause direct damage to the heart and liver. Poisons experts are still unable to explain why many people use the drug and receive no more than a hang-over, yet other people receive (often fatal) liver and kidney disease and vascular disturbances. People suffering from diabetes mellitus, epilepsy, liver disease, glaucoma hypertension, hyperthyroidism, or any mental or heart disorder are advised not to take ecstasy since it has been observed that they would be particularly at risk of complications.

Benzodiazepines (bennies)

Benzodiazepines have anxiolytic, sedative and anticonvulsant properties. Usually, they are available in tablet form but occasionally, they are injected, particularly temazepam. (jellies, norries, green eggs.) They cause sedation, inco-ordinated movements and sleepiness: these effects being enhanced by alcohol, a common form of misuse. Long term use affects memory and cognitive function.

Cocaine (coke, flake, charlie, ice, snow)

A powerful, short acting stimulant, cocaine has many similar effects to amphetamines causing heightened alertness, excitation and euphoria. These last for about 30 minutes and are followed by a compulsion to take more to avoid 'coming down'. In the form of a white crystalline powder, cocaine may be smoked, injected or snorted from a piece of glass or mirror using a straw or rolled up paper. Prolonged and repeated sniffing can damage the nasal mucosa or even perforate the nasal septum. 'Street' cocaine is usually adulterated or 'cut' as occurs with amphetamines. (See above).

Regular cocaine use produces distorted sleep patterns, anxiety and paranoia although there is no physical dependence. High doses may produce convulsions or even psychotic states.

A smokable cocaine derivative, made by heating cocaine with baking powder, known as 'Crack' (so called because of the cracking sound produced on burning), is extremely short acting and produces even more intense effects than cocaine. It is smoked using a pipe and causes agitation, aggressive behaviour and toxic psychosis. It has a high addiction potential and can sometimes have a direct toxic effect on the myocardium which may be fatal. With a rock of smokable cocaine costing £15 – £20, it is possible to use several hundred pounds worth of the drug in a few hours. Other names for crack, are 'rocks', 'wash', 'stones'.

Heroin (H, horse, smack, skag, junk)
The most abused narcotic in the UK, heroin, is an opiate derived from the poppy. It is a brown or white powder which can be injected, smoked or sniffed and which causes drowsiness, feelings of warmth and relaxation and a sense of well-being. Regular use rapidly produces tolerance and dependence whilst someone withdrawing from the habit is likely to experience several unpleasant symptoms including sweating, anxiety, muscle cramps, nausea, diarrhoea and fever as well as an intense craving for the drug.

It is smoked by placing the powder on tin foil and then heating it with a match or a candle. The fumes are then inhaled or sniffed through a tube – 'chasing the dragon'. Some users progress to injecting the drug, thereby running the risk of overdosage, septicaemia and exposure to HIV and hepatitis B and C infections. Like cocaine and the amphetamine drugs, heroin can be 'cut' i. e. adulterated with inert substances, and, since it is not very soluble in water, the addition of lemon juice assists the solubility for intravenous injection. The mixing of heroin in the same syringe with cocaine produces a dangerous, but superior state of euphoria, known as 'speedball'.

Other Opiates
Morphine, codeine, dihydrocodeine, Diconal and buprenorphine are other opiates which may be misused.

LSD (acid, trips, blotters, microdot, white lightning)
Another Class A drug, the hallucinogen LSD is taken as a powder or tablets, or impregnated on a square of blotting paper about a quarter the size of a postage stamp. Its effects begin about one hour after ingestion and may last for up to 48 hours. Initially, the user will feel disorientated following which he will become giggly, confused or anxious. Feelings are enhanced and perceptual distortions, especially of sight or sound, or hallucinations occur. Someone using LSD may be come less aware of risks from the environment and accidents are common. 'Bad trips', rather like a nightmare, can be experienced and 'flashbacks' may occur in the form of previously experienced hallucinations many months after the last dose was taken.

Naturally occurring hallucinogens are found all over the world. Many types of mushrooms, grow wild in the UK:perhaps the best known one being the Liberty Cap mushroom, (Psilocybine semilanceata).

The active principles, psilocybe and psilocybin, are heat stable, thus permitting the mushrooms to be eaten raw, dried, or brewed into drinks or stews. Bad 'trips' can occur. Another indigenous UK plant, called 'morning glory', contains alkaloids, which produce effects similar to those produced by LSD, after oral ingestion.

Ketamine (Special K, bump, cat Valium, LA coke)
There is now much anecdotal evidence that more and more young people are abusing the anaesthetic, Ketamine – 'K-holing'. Ketamine was first manufactured as an analgesic and anaesthetic and has dramatic hallucinogenic effects. It comes in a liquid form but is boiled and baked into crystals which are then ground into a powder and snorted.

It is now becoming popular at raves and parties and its effects have been likened to taking amphetamine, an opiate and a hallucinogen at the same time. It can become as addictive as crack and some addicts display the features of catatonic schizophrenia.

Anabolic Steroids

Although there is no reliable estimate of the extent of anabolic steroid misuse in the United Kingdom, these substances are widely available to young people. They are said to bring about an increase in strength, speed, aggression and competitiveness and, by reducing recovery time, to enable more intensive training of longer duration to take place. Preparations misused commonly include stanozolol, nandrolone, testosterone and clembuterol.

Misusers include not only those who wish to succeed in competitive sport but also those whose motivation is cosmetic, to improve their body image and muscle contours. There is a wish to emulate role models and be attractive and well-liked.

However, prolonged use has a range of adverse effects for young people including hypertension, diabetes, restricted growth, menstrual irregularities, deepening of the voice and hirsutes and a degree of psychological dependence. Profound depression may follow withdrawal of anabolic steroids. The young sportsperson runs the risk of this habit being detected by anti-doping measures which are now increasingly employed at representative sporting events.

Drugs Misuse and Schools

Given the widespread and increasing use of drugs among young people there is a clear need for schools to provide appropriate education, to share the mutual concerns of parents and to exercise proper care and control when pupils are under the jurisdiction of the school. It is therefore necessary for every school to have a drugs policy or charter which states in an unequivocal fashion how that school will deal with drugs education and the problems of drug misuse, and how it will seek to deter its pupils from using drugs. It is suggested that the policy is drawn up by the headteacher, appropriate members of the governing body and academic staff and even one or two senior pupils. Consideration should be given to parental involvement in the process and the final policy should reflect the ethos of the school and the wishes and beliefs of governors, staff, parents and pupils.

A drugs policy should include the following elements:

- the school's stance in relation to the use of tobacco, alcohol and illegal substances.

- the stated aims of discussing and sharing the problem with parents, and inviting their support.

- an outline of the school's PSHE (personal, social and health education) programme, with special reference to education about drugs.

- a clear statement about drugs and the law, including police actions.

- a clear statement of the school's rules about drugs and the procedures for dealing with drugs-related incidents in the school.

- consideration of using drugs testing as part of the educative process and, if testing is deemed appropriate, the exact methods to be employed.

- who is to be tested, when, and the methods of dealing with positive and negative results.

- a range of appropriate punishments for those testing positive and the need to establish a 'contract' for them to remain in the school.

These elements encompass the school's commitment to the health and safety of its members and the fact that it neither condones the misuse of drugs by its pupils nor the illegal supply of such substances. The importance of the school's pastoral role in the welfare of its pupils is acknowledged, as well as its duty to inform and educate its young people about the consequences of drugs use and mis-use. Also, it is suggested that, eventually, the main objectives of the policy should appear in the school prospectus so that the School's position with regard to drugs is absolutely clear and available to all.

Drugs Testing
Over the past three or four years a number of schools, predominantly in the independent sector, has instituted drugs testing and in 1995 MOSA produced guidelines for this.

MOSA Guidelines for testing for substance misuse in schools
1. The use of illegal substances by young people is increasing.

2. All schools, both day and boarding, independent and state, must appreciate that they will have a number of illegal drug users amongst their pupils. No school is immune.

3. Every school should have a drugs policy or charter which states in an unequivocal fashion the way in which that school will deal with the problem of drugs misuse.

4. Such a policy must include statements about drugs education, detection of illegal drug use, drugs testing and the handling of positive and negative results.

5. Drugs education should be part of a comprehensive PSHE programme. The school doctor should have an input into this.

6. Drugs testing should be viewed as a useful tool in this drugs education programme. It should also be regarded as part of the educative process and not something carried out for purely punitive reasons.

7. Awareness of drugs misuse – change in demeanour, change in personal appearance, declining academic performance, reports from others – peers, parents, staff. Consideration should be given to raising staff awareness but beware of the normal adolescent personality.

8. 'For cause' testing rather than 'random' testing i. e. testing is carried out where there is cause to suspect the misuse of drugs. Random testing is considered unethical, cost ineffective and likely to offend the innocent.

9. Testing is performed on urine samples collected using recognised procedures – the 'chain of custody'. There must be absolute certainty that the sample is from the person it is claimed to be from and that it is not interfered with in any way between the donor and the testing laboratory. Chain of custody allows a second aliquot to be available for testing by the donor if required. A good rapport should be established with the laboratory so that help is readily available in interpreting questionable results. Testing is also possible using hair or blood samples although both these methods have disadvantages.

10. Written informed consent is required before a sample is collected but the pupil does not have to be 16 years of age or over to give valid consent. 'Competency' i. e. the ability to understand the nature of the test and the consequences of refusing to provide a sample, is the yardstick. It is not necessary to have parental consent but it is very desirable that parents are informed at some stage that testing is taking place. Sample collection must not be delayed by the school trying to contact a parent. e. g. one abroad.

11. The results of tests should be considered to be confidential information with their ownership resting with the school authority requiring the test. The school medical officer should only be involved in 'interpretation', should this become necessary.

12. The school drugs policy will have decided how positive and negative results are to be handled and consideration will have to be given to a scale of punishments including expulsion or internal rustication. As part of the 'contract' for the pupil to remain at the school there may be a requirement for repeat testing in the future at intervals determined by the school – and this might involve 'random' testing i. e. random in time rather than in person.

13. There is no statutory requirement to inform the police of a positive result and using illegal substances is not an offence in itself. The actual offence is possession and in the case of a school – 'allowing' its premises to be used for drugs misuse. Discussions should take place with the local police as to whether or not they would expect to be informed of every positive result but it is worth taking the line that the school will inform the police every time.

14. Wherever possible the school medical officer and the school nurses should be outside the testing process. It is important that their caring, supportive role should be respected and not compromised by being involved with the testing. Ideally, the collecting officer should be an outsider who is paid a retainer by the school and is called in when sampling is required.

15. Who pays for the test – school or parent? It is suggested that the school pays for the first test and the parent for any future tests, required in accordance with the 'contract' whereby the pupil remains at the school.

It is emphasised that testing should be used as part of the educative process, and not for purely punitive reasons. Although any school must reserve the right to expel any pupil who has been found misusing drugs, it is hoped that expulsion will be the exception rather than the rule. Many schools agree with the view that it is neither morally nor educationally acceptable to 'write off' a young person for experimenting with drugs and on that basis, testing may be employed with the aim of detecting, and the subsequently helping, those pupils who are misusing drugs.

Who To Test?

Both the Medical Officers of Schools Association and the Head Masters Conference are in favour of 'for cause', rather than 'random' testing. The latter is considered to be unethical, cost ineffective and liable to offend the innocent. 'For cause' testing implies that an individual is asked to provide a sample of urine when there is good reason to suspect that he has been misusing drugs. Staff, parents and pupils should be aware of the warning signs that might suggest drug misuse:

- decline in school performance.
- unwillingness to take part in activities previously enjoyed.
- unusual outbreaks of temper, marked mood swings, restlessness and irritability.
- staying out more, perhaps with a new group of friends.
- excessive spending or borrowing of money.
- reduced interest in personal appearance.
- excessive tiredness without obvious causes.
- lack of appetite.
- heavy use of scent, aftershave etc., to hide drug odours.
- wearing sunglasses to conceal dilated or constricted pupils.

It must be emphasised however, that many of these features might reflect normal teenage behaviour or demeanour.

How To Test?

Testing may be carried out on samples of :

- urine
- hair
- blood

Of these, urine testing is the most practical as blood sampling is too invasive and requires the skills of trained personnel. Drug detection in hair (DDH) is a useful alternative but does have some disadvantages. It is more expensive, currently does not detect cannabis and does not conform to the 'chain of custody' (vide infra). However, samples can be collected easily and hair analysis can give retrospective information about an individual's use of drugs over a period of several months.

Urine testing detects the metabolites of the drugs and it is possible to test for the following substances:

- alcohol.
- amphetamines.
- benzodiazepines.
- barbiturates.
- cannabis.
- cocaine.
- methadone.
- methaqualone.
- opiates.
- phencyclidine.
- propoxyphene.
- (LSD)

Various laboratories in the UK offer a testing as well as an advisory service. Obviously, there are differences between individual laboratories but in general, a screening test for amphetamines, benzodiazepines, cannabis, cocaine and opiates, using radioimmuno-assay techniques, is employed first, Any positive results are confirmed by gas chromatography and mass spectrometry (GC/MS). Each laboratory will have its own quoted cut-off levels for both the screening and GC/MS confirmation tests although some-times more sensitive tests may be carried out on request. Detection of LSD by urinalysis, although possible, requires more complex technology than that used for other drugs.

The clearance times from the urine of the various metabolites differs but as a rule of thumb, are between 24 and 72 hours for the most commonly abused drugs.

The following are the clearance or drug detection times for one-off doses but the greater the abuse, the longer the clearance takes

Drug	Clearance Time
Amphetamines	24 – 48 hours
Ecstasy group	24 – 48 hours
Opiates	48 hours
Cocaine	2 – 4 days
Barbiturates – long acting	2 – 3 weeks
Barbiturates – short acting	24 hours
Benzodiazepines	3 days
– chronic use for more than 1 year	4 – 6 weeks
Cannabis – 1 joint	48 – 72 hours
– oral ingestion	1 – 5 days
– 4 joints a week	5+ days
– heavy smoker	10+ days
– more than 5 joints a day	14 – 18 days
Phencyclidine	14 days
– chronic user	30 days
Methaqualone	14 days
Methadone	3 days
Propoxyphene	6 – 48 hours

Clearly, knowledge of the clearance time will determine the chances of detecting that particular drug and it might be less productive to test at the end of the school week, during which time the pupil may not have had the chance to misuse any drug, than on the day after a long week-end at home when drugs might have been ingested and it could be anticipated that a positive result will be obtained.

The urine sample must be collected under a system known as 'chain of custody', by a so called collection officer. 'Chain of custody' ensures that the sample is collected from the correct donor and is not tampered with between the donor and the laboratory. There are several ways in which the donor can attempt to adulterate the urine sample or influence the result and to overcome this the sample must be collected in a dedicated lavatory, in two tamper-proof containers which are sealed immediately after collection of the urine, with the seals being signed by both the collection officer and the donor. The second sample is available for the use of the donor personally, should he or she wish to arrange an independent, private analysis.

Prior to the collecting of the sample, the collection officer will record the personal details of the donor and take a drug history which gives the donor the opportunity to declare the recent use of any drugs, either prescribed or non-prescribed, which might influence the final result. Written, signed, informed consent is required before the sample is collected and it is important to emphasise that a pupil does not have to be 16 years of age or over in order to give valid consent. The yardstick is so called 'competency' which, in this context, is the ability to understand the nature of the test and the consequences of refusing to provide a sample. Although it is not necessary to have parental consent it is important that the parents are informed as soon as possible, both of the test and of the result.

The urine samples are sent to the testing laboratory and the analyses are carried out. Both dilution and adulteration checks are made and the results are returned to the school within a few days.

Ideally the collection officer is someone who is independent and outside the school but in practice many schools require that the sampling is carried out by a school nurse or, less commonly, a member of the academic staff. In this situation there is concern that the nurse's or teacher's relationship with the pupil could be compromised and MOSA recommends strongly that wherever possible, both the school doctor and the school nurses should not be involved in the testing process.

The Management of Drugs-related incidents

It is vital that all young people are helped to understand the dangers of drug misuse and dependence but however effective any school's health education programme may be, there will be some pupils who will choose to experiment with illegal substances, sometimes on school premises.

Although the possession and use of illegal drugs will be regarded as serious disciplinary matters, the majority of schools will wish to give continuing support to all at risk, including pupils guilty of misconduct. Further education programmes, effective pastoral care and counselling will be important parts of

this support and it may be necessary to consider liaison with outside professionals such as community psychiatric nurses, social workers or specialist
counsellors from local drug action teams. The school medical officer, with
particular knowledge of available local services, is in an ideal position to
advise the head teacher and other staff.

Contraception

One of the five key areas in the 'Health of the Nation 1992, 'in relation to the
health of adolescents was concerned with teenage pregnancy and a target was
set for the year 2000, of reducing by at least 50%, to no more than 4.8 pregnancies per 1,000, the rate of conceptions amongst the under 16s. Regrettably,
there has been only a slight improvement overall and from a figure of 9.5 pregnancies per 1,000 in 1989, peaking at 10.1 per 1,000 a year later, the conception rate fell to 8.1 per 1,000 in 1993. In 1994 there was a slight increase to 8.3
per 1,000 with a total of 7,754 pregnancies, of which 53% ended in abortion.

Using figures from the Office of Population Censuses and Surveys (OPCS)
for conception rates in women aged 15 to19 years in England and Wales and
for the number of teenage mothers in the same age group, a similarly worrying
picture emerges. In 1983 the conception rate per 1,000 women in this age group
was 56, rising to 61.7 in 1992 and dropping back to 59.6 a year later – with a
total number of pregnancies in 1993 of approximately 86,700. There were 37.4
teenage mothers per 1,000 women aged 15 to19 years in 1983, a figure which
rose to 40.4 in 1992 and fell slightly to 38. 6 in 1993. In general the pregnancy
rate fell in the 1970s, only to rise through the 1980s and early 1990s.

In the mid 1960s 4% of young women had experienced sexual intercourse
by 16 years of age. Ten years later this figure had risen to 9% while, currently,
19% of girls report having had intercourse before their 16th birthday. For
young men and women the average age of their first sexual experience, but not
necessarily intercourse, is 13 years and 14 years respectively while more than
50% of 16-19 year olds have had intercourse. Over the past four decades, the
median age of first intercourse has fallen by four years for women and three
years for men.

The reasons cited by youngsters for having intercourse for the first time
include curiosity, being in love, peer pressure and a natural follow-on to less
intimate sexual contact. Furthermore, in adolescence, sex is part of a wider
spectrum of risk taking behaviour in which substance abuse, smoking, alcohol
consumption and underage sex are more likely to occur in combination.
Cognitive immaturity is thought to explain the well-documented tendency of
this age group to avoid preventive action, in spite of being aware of the risks
involved. There is considerably increased physical and psychiatric morbidity
with early teenage sexual activity including pregnancy, cervical dysplasia,
sexually transmitted diseases and an increased risk of depression and suicide.
A survey of 16-24 year olds showed that 15% of men and 36% of women felt
that they had had sexual intercourse too soon.

In the developed world the lowest teenage pregnancy rates are to be found
in Holland while world-wide the highest rates are to be found in the USA
where nearly 1 million American teenagers become pregnant annually. It is

salutary that the age of consent in Holland is only 12 years and undoubtedly, a more open attitude to sexual matters and an assurance of confidentiality in all contraceptive services in that country are key factors in reducing the teenage pregnancy rate to one seventh of that in England and Wales.

Therefore, there is justifiable concern about teenage sexual behaviour and a clear need exists for the provision of contraceptive advice which is effective, confidential and non-judgmental. The school doctor and nurse have a vital role in promoting the sexual health of young people, in reducing teenage pregnancies, in minimising the risks of sexually transmitted diseases and in providing contraception, including emergency contraception, when appropriate. The aim should be to enable young people to remain sexually healthy and to retain the ability to have children when and if they wish. Of an estimated 52,000 sexually active 15 year old young women in England in 1991, only a third visited family planning clinics. Some of the remainder sought advice from their general practitioner while many remained apprehensive about talking to any doctor for fear that confidentiality would not be respected.

In 1994 MOSA, produced the following guidelines for school doctors on contraception:

1. Every school doctor should be prepared to offer contraceptive advice and, if appropriate, provide contraception subsequently including emergency contraception, for any boy or girl of any age.

2. Contraception should only be provided after full and adequate counselling and discussion, with the pupil realising fully, the implications of his/her actions.

3. Pupils should be encouraged to discuss contraceptive matters with their parents or those acting in *loco parentis*.

4. The school doctor owes a duty of confidentiality to the boy or girl and must not break that confidentiality except in the most extreme circumstances.

5. If the school doctor finds it necessary to breach professional confidence, he must first discuss this with the boy or girl and then be fully prepared to justify his actions.

6. It is the duty of the school doctor to inform the school of his policy with regard to the provision of contraception.

7. The school doctor must be aware of the potential for conflict between his position and that of the school authorities and parents.

In fact these guidelines offer a framework for every school doctor and nurse to provide not only contraceptive advice, but also a sexual health service, within the school setting. It is so necessary nowadays for this service to be available that if any doctor has moral or religious objections, particularly with regard to contraception, then the question arises as to his or her suitability to fulfil the role of a school doctor. So that pupils are not thereby disadvantaged by the doctor with these objections, then at least, arrangements for this part of his work should be delegated to a partner or other medical colleague.

Teenagers have serious concerns, perhaps inappropriate, but nevertheless real, about confidentiality in sexual matters. Also, they have perceived views of the doctor who, in the general practice setting, is perhaps a family friend or who in schools may be regarded as part of the establishment, and of the practice or health centre receptionist who is often the youngster's first contact with the medical services. In providing sexual health advice the doctor must assure pupils, regardless of their age, of confidentiality. To that end, consideration should be given to displaying a poster about this in the waiting area of the medical centre or the sanatorium, or inserting a paragraph in the school's medical policy or in other written information which is provided for parents of new pupils. In the boarding situation particularly, pupils must be allowed to attend the school doctor's or nurses's outpatient sessions without having to explain their reasons for attendance to teachers or house staff. A friendly environment must be created and suitable leaflets and display posters made available. Helpful leaflets are available from the Brook Advisory Centres, the Health Education Authority or local health promotion units. School medical centre staff must be friendly and receptive as well as comfortable themselves discussing sex and sexuality.

Practical considerations

When discussing a pupil's request for contraception, the doctor will wish to cover a number of points such as their age, whether she is currently in a sexual relationship, or planning one, and whether or not any contraception is being used. The doctor will wish to make an assessment of the pupil's maturity, particularly if she is a girl under the age of 16 years. (See below). There should be a full and frank discussion about the pupil's intentions and wishes and it should be determined if she has discussed the matter with parents or, in the case of a boarding school, teachers, i. e. house parents, who are acting in *loco parentis*. The pupil should be encouraged to involve her parents, but the pupil's refusal to do so should not prevent the doctor from offering contraceptive advice or contraception and must never be the grounds for telling the parents or the school that contraception has been sought. The only possible exception to this, which could justify such a breach, is if the doctor considers the pupil is a victim of sexual abuse and decides that disclosure is for the pupil's own protection. The doctor should satisfy himself that the pupil has a full understanding of the implications of her actions and then, if appropriate, guide the pupil on the best method of contraception to be used.

It is quite likely that considerable time will be required for the discussion and the doctor might consider bringing the pupil back to another outpatient session or setting aside another time outside of normal consulting hours. The process is one that cannot be rushed and this is particularly important when discussing the use of the actual chosen contraceptive method.

Hormonal contraception

If it is decided that the pupil requires contraception, it is likely that a hormonal method, and particularly, a combined oral contraceptive, will be prescribed.

Combined oral contraceptives

Considering efficiency, convenience and safety, the combined oral contraceptive (COC) provides the most reliable method for a young woman. Such pills contain oestrogen – ethinyloestradiol (EO) – and a progestogen, e. g, levonorgestrol, norethisterone, norgestimate, desogestrol or gestodene. Used correctly the COC has a failure rate of only approximately 0.2% but as this is very much user-dependent; the quality of instruction and the use of appropriate leaflets can have a significant impact on efficiency.

During the assessment, a medical history must be taken which will include determining if there are any absolute contraindications to the use of a COC. A past personal history of thrombosis, liver disease, cancer of the breast or endometrium, focal migraine, porphyria or otosclerosis precludes a COC although many of these conditions will be very rare in the age group under consideration.

Diabetes mellitus and migraine are relative contraindications and should be noted; and details of the family history, particularly of venous thromboemolism (VTE) in close relatives, must be obtained. A menstrual history should be taken including period and cycle lengths and the presence of any irregular bleeding. It is important to enquire about smoking habits and perhaps take the opportunity for some health education.

Conventional advice is that a breast and pelvic examination should be carried out before provision of the pill and, of course, pregnancy must be excluded. However, in practice, a young woman's fear of such intimate examinations may prevent her seeking contraceptive help and it is reasonable to delay such checks until the second or the third follow-up visits. However, the blood pressure, height and weight must be recorded and from the last two observations, the body mass index (BMI) calculated.

As well as advice about smoking, it may be helpful for the doctor or nurse to discuss 'breast awareness', sexually transmitted diseases, the concept of 'safe sex' and the need for regular cervical smears, although some authorities are now suggesting that screening for cervical cancer in the under 20s is cost ineffective and likely to generate excessive anxiety.

The risks of taking the pill must be explained but also, it is helpful to mention its benefits. Pelvic inflammatory disease, benign breast disease, ectopic pregnancy, functional ovarian cysts, ovarian and endometrial cancer and endometriosis are all less common in pill – takers. The adverse effects of the COC are mainly cardiovascular ones although it should be acknowledged that, especially among young, healthy pill-users, the absolute risks are very small. Haemorrhagic and thrombotic strokes and myocardial infarctions are commoner in pill-users and in October 1995, the UK Committee on Safety of Medicines reported epidemiological studies showing a differential in the risk of VTE between pills containing the newer third generation progestogens – desogestrel and gestodene – and those with the older, second generation progestogens such as levonorgestrel. A doubling of the risk of VTE was found in users of pills containing the newer progestogens although this must be balanced against the risk of VTE in pregnancy which is doubled again and the risk inherent in normal, day to day activities such as driving a car or crossing the road.

The doctor must determine any risk factors for venous or arterial disease in the medical history and use this information when deciding which preparation to prescribe. The lowest acceptable dose of oestrogen should be used combined with one of the second generation progestogens for any young woman with or without any single risk factor for arterial or venous disease. Ovranette and microgynon 30 are examples of two commonly prescribed levonorgestrel-containing pills.

Young women with oestrogen-dominant symptoms such as nausea, pre-menstrual syndrome or breast tenderness might benefit from a more progestogenic pill such as Loestrin 30 while those with progestogen-dominant side effects such as acne, seborrhoea, hirsutism or mastalgia might find a pill with more oestrogen preferable such as Norimin or Brevinor. Dianette which contains 35 mcg of EO and the anti-androgen, cyproterone acetate, is particularly effective in those with acne.

Education about the use of the pill should include a detailed description of pill-taking, including a day 1 or a day 5 start, the '7 day rule', missed pills and emergency contraception. The effects of taking other medication, particularly antibiotics, and of diarrhoea and vomiting, must also be discussed. For a young woman starting her first packet of pills on day 1 of her period, there is no need for additional contraceptive precautions although she should be warned to expect some breakthrough bleeding in the first one or two cycles. A day 5 start may result in less breakthrough bleeding but there is the need for additional contraception for 7 days. If pill-taking is delayed by more than 12 hours, it should be considered that contraceptive cover has been lost and the '7 day rule' must be invoked. In such situations, the young woman and her partner must use extra contraception for the following 7 days and, if those 7 days extend beyond the end of a pack, the next pack of pills must be taken immediately without the usual 7 day break.

Progestogen only pill

The progestogen only pill (POP) containing norethisterone or levonorgestrol is an effective alternative to the combined pill, particularly when oestrogen is contraindicated. However, it has a failure rate of 0.3-4% and as it is more effective in older women, it is not as useful in the younger pill taker. Obsessive regularity in pill-taking is necessary as there is a loss of contraceptive effect if the POP is taken more than three hours late. In theory, additional contraception is only required for 48 hours but in practice, in order to avoid confusion with the COC, the '7 day rule' is recommended. Emergency contraception (See below) is recommended if unprotected intercourse takes place any time from missing a pill to 48 hours after restarting it.

The main side effect is irregular bleeding but other progestogenic side effects, such as acne and seborrhoea, are less common. It should be noted that the risk of an ectopic pregnancy is greater with a POP.

Barrier methods

In general the barrier methods, diaphragms and caps, and male and female condoms, are simpler but less effective. In the context of contraception for young people, their use should be encouraged as a way of reducing sexually transmitted diseases – the concept of 'safe sex' – including HIV and wart virus infections, in addition to the use of a more effective contraceptive method. Quoted failure rates in the world literature for barrier methods range from 2-15% and some authorities believe that with careful use the condom can be more effective than the diaphragm. Condoms are readily available while the cap or the diaphragm needs to be fitted by a family planning trained doctor or nurse. Although without side effects, many couples find the use of barrier methods unacceptable although the protection they offer against infection cannot be over emphasised. For both boys and girls of an appropriate age, sex education talks in schools should include explicit instruction about the correct application of condoms.

Intrauterine contraceptive devices

IUCDs have become more effective and compared with hormonal contraception there are no cancer or cardiovascular risks. However, for young people their use is extremely limited because of first: the technical difficulty of fitting such a device through a nulliparous cervix and second: the risk of pelvic infection subsequently leading to impaired or even permanent infertility. Failure rates for copper bearing devices range from 0.3-2% while the levonorgestrel-releasing IUCD, Mirena IUS, is over 99.5% effective. IUCDs have a place in emergency contraception. (See below.)

Depot contraceptives

Depot contraceptives provide a means of achieving a high level of contraceptive efficiency independent of the problems associated with patient compliance. They are designed to release a progestogen, levonorgestrel, medroxyprogesterone or norethisterone, over a prolonged period ranging from eight weeks to five years, depending on the device and the formulation. Depot-Provera with 150 mg of medroxyprogesterone, is given by deep intramuscular injection during the first five days of the menstrual cycle, being repeated at 12 week intervals as required. Full counselling is necessary with regard to its long term action and potential side effects, and users should be warned that it is not possible immediately to reverse the injection's side effects. Irregular bleeding can be a problem initially, although most women develop amenorrhoea. This preparation can be quite useful for the young user but only if she is made aware of the side effects beforehand.

The subdermal implant, Norplant, is another effective progestogen-only method and consists of six flexible rods, which release levonorgestrel, implanted by means of a trocar. Insertion and removal can sometimes be difficult and this method is possibly too invasive for the younger user.

Other methods

Other contraceptive methods including the use of a spermicide alone, coitus interruptus or withdrawal, contraceptive sponges, C-film and 'fertility awareness' are all much less effective than other established methods and their use alone should not be encouraged.

Emergency contraception

It is important that both young men and young women should be aware that emergency contraception is available, where there has been contraceptive failure e. g. split condom or missed pills, or where no contraception at all has been used. The school doctor should make himself familiar with the methods available and be prepared to offer advice and treatment in the emergency situation.

Emergency contraception may be achieved by hormonal methods or the insertion of a IUCD. The use of the phrase 'morning after pill', although firmly established in lay language, should be discouraged as it creates the impression that it is for use 'after the night before' and is only applicable a short time after intercourse.

The Yuzpe regime, named after a Canadian gynaecologist, is the best known method and will be suitable for most young people. It can be given within 72 hours of intercourse and involves the administration of two pills each containing 50mcg of ethinyloestradiol and 250mcg of levonorgestrel at once and repeated 12 hours later. Four tablets of Ovran may be given or the Schering proprietary preparation 'PC4', which contains a useful instruction leaflet. For any couple having unprotected intercourse midcycle, there is a 10-30% risk of pregnancy; with the Yuzpe regime this risk is reduced to approximately 5% and to 1-2% if used at other times in the menstrual cycle. These failure rates are significant and it should be realised that repeated use of emergency contraception is less effective than the consistent use of other methods.

The young woman must be counselled fully and important clinical details such as the date of her last menstrual period, cycle length and day in the cycle when the unprotected intercourse occurred need to be ascertained. The risk of venous thromboembolism needs to be established and the use of any medication recorded. The risks and side effects of the method including the extremely unlikely teratogenic effects of the hormones must be discussed and the patient's attitude to failure and the subsequent, possible need for a termination of pregnancy needs to be explored.

The necessity for abstinence for the rest of the cycle, or at least the careful use of a barrier method of contraception if intercourse is contemplated, must be emphasised and the young woman should be advised to return after her next period to confirm that treatment has been successful and to arrange further contraception.

The only absolute contraindications to the use of this method are existing pregnancy and an attack of focal migraine. The young woman's weight and blood pressure should be recorded but as with the provision of COCs and POPs (as above) it may be considered inappropriate to insist on a breast and pelvic examination. It is useful for the doctor or nurse to oversee the administration of the first two tablets and the young woman should be told that if vomiting occurs within three hours of either of the two doses, she should return to receive a further dose together with, perhaps, an antiemetic.

In the Hoffman regime, a POP may be used with 20 of 30mcg of levonorgestrel, for example, Micro-val, being taken as a single dose within 12 hours of unprotected intercourse. In the Ho regime, 25 tablets containing 30 mcg of levonorgestrel are taken as a single dose and repeated 12 hours later, within 48 hours of unprotected intercourse. Because of the large numbers of tablets involved, these two methods are not practicable but might be necessary if the use of oestrogen is contraindicated.

If more than 72 hours has lapsed a copper bearing IUCD may be inserted within 5 days of unprotected intercourse or up to day 19 of a regular 28 day cycle. However, as already stated, this method may not be applicable for the young nulliparous patient in whom insertion of an IUCD may be painful and difficult.

Prescribing for young people under 16 years

One of the most difficult areas in providing contraceptive advice for young people concerns those under the age of 16 years and this is particularly pertinent in the school setting. The current legal position in England and Wales was established after the 1985 House of Lords ruling in the famous 'Gillick case'. Mrs Victoria Gillick, a mother of ten, sought to bring an injunction against the West Norfolk and Wisbech Health Authority preventing any employees of the Authority from prescribing the contraceptive pill to her daughters, then under the age of 16. Citing the Family Law Reform Act of 1969, which states that a child aged 16 or over is competent to consent to medical treatment with or without the knowledge or consent of either parent, Mrs Gillick argued that under 16s were unable to give valid consent. The case eventually reached the House of Lords where the Law Lords stated that the paramount concern was the health of the young girl and that young people under 16 who are able fully to understand what is proposed and its implications are competent to consent to medical treatment regardless of age. The House of Lords' judgment stated that it is not unlawful to treat a child who is under 16 without parental consent, and in the situation where contraception is requested by a girl under 16 who refuses to inform her parents or allow them to be informed, the doctor would be justified in providing advice and treatment if he was satisfied that:

- a young person could understand his advice and had sufficient maturity to understand what was involved in terms of the moral, social and emotional implications.

- he could neither persuade the young person to inform her parents or guardians, nor allow him to inform them, that contraceptive advice was being sought.

- the young person would be very likely to begin, or to continue having, sexual intercourse with or without contraception.

- without contraceptive treatment or advice, the young person's physical or mental health, or both, would be likely to suffer.

- the young person's best interests required him to give contraceptive advice, treatment or both without parental consent.

Competency to seek medical advice independently and give valid consent to medical treatment is understood in terms of the young person's ability to understand the choices and their consequences, including the nature, purpose and possible risk of any treatment or non-treatment. There is no specific lower age limit for the prescription of contraception or any other treatment, and the doctor must exercise his own clinical judgment in each individual case based on the child's competence to give consent and his or her physical and emotional maturity. It must also be emphasised that the child consenting to treatment is entitled to the same degree of confidentiality which the doctor is obligated to provide for any of his patients regardless of age.

Despite the school doctor's overriding duty to his patient he does have an obligation, by virtue of his appointment, to the school that employs him and to the parents. This potential conflict of interests may result in the doctor having to make some difficult judgments but it is important that the school is made aware of the doctor's policy with regard to the provision of contraception. The Children Act 1989 states that children are entitled to see a doctor of the same gender and the school doctor should be aware of the need to make the services of a female practitioner available for the female pupils. Patients also have the right of opting to register with another general practitioner for the provision of contraceptive services only, although in the boarding situation where it is recommended that all boarding pupils register with the school doctor, logistical difficulties could arise if a pupil has to be taken to another surgery or health centre. However, such problems should not detract from the young person's right to seek contraceptive advice from whomsoever they wish.

References

1. Eykyn, S. J. (1982) Toxic shock syndrome:some answers but questions remain. *Br. Med. J.* 284. 1585.

2. Williams, G. R. (1990) The Toxic shock syndrome. *Br. Med. J.* 300. 960.

3. Burke, A. (1996) Toxic shock syndrome. *Practice Nursing.* Vol. 7. No. 1.

4. *Tampon Alert* (1996). Womens' Environmental Network, Aberdeen Studies, 22, Highbury Grove, London N5 2EA. (Tel: 0171 354 8823.)

5. Rutter, M (1979) *Changing youth in a changing society.* (London: The Nuffield Provincial Hospital Trust.)

6. Bruch, H. (1973) *Eating disorders: obesity, anorexia nervosa and the person within.* New York. Basic Books.

7. Crisp, A. H., Callender, J. Halek, C. Hsu, L. K. G. Long term mortality in anorexia nervosa. A 20-year follow up of the St George's and Aberdeen cohorts. *Br. J. Psychiatry*, 16 104.

8. Russell, G. F. M., Szmukler, G., Dare, C., Eisler, N. An evaluation of family therapy in anorexia nervosa and bulimia nervosa. *Arch. Gen Psychiat.* 44. 1047.

9. Lacey, J. H. (1976) Anorexia Nervosa. *Nursing Times*, 71. 407.

10. Russell, G. F. M. (1979) Bulimia nervosa: an ominous variant of anorexia nervosa. *Psychol. Med.* 9. 429.

11. Levin, P. A., Falko, J., Dixon, K., Gallup, E. M., Saunders, W. (1980) Benign parotid enlargement in Bulimia. *Ann. Intern. Med.* 93. 827.

12. Burke, R. C. (1986) Bulimia and parotid enlargement – case report and treatment. *J. Otolaryngol*, 15: 49.

13. Simmons, M. S., Grayden, S. K., Mitchell, J. E. (1986) The need for psychiatric-dental liason in the treatment of bulimia. *Am. J. Psychiat.*

14. McClusky, S., Evans, C., Lacey, J. H., Pearce, J. M., Jacobs, H. (1991)Polycystic ovary syndrome and bulimia. *Fertility and Sterility*, 55. 287.

15. Buckler, J. M. H. (1987) *The Adolescent Years. The ups and downs of growing up.* Page 110. Castlemead Publications. Ware.

16. Waller, D., Eisenberg, l. (1980) School refusal in childhood – a psychiatric – paediatric perspective. In: Hersov, L., Berg, I. eds. *Out of School: modern perspectives in truancy and school refusal.* Chichester: John Wiley, Page 209.

17. Berg, I. (1997). Annotation. *Arch. Dis. Child.* Vol 6. No 2: 90.

18. Berg, I. (1996) Unauthorised absence from school. In: Berg. I., Nursten, J. eds. *Unwillingy to school.* 4th Ed. London. Gaskell. Page14.

19. Farringdon, D. (1995). The development of offending and anti-social behaviour from childhood. *J. Child Psychol. Psychiat.* 36: 929.

20. Lawson, S. (1995) *Helping Children Cope with Bullying.* Sheldon Press. SPCK. London. NW1 4DU. Page 10.

21. Olweus, D. (1978). *Aggression: Schools – Bullies and Whipping boys.* (New York: Hemisphere Publishing Corporation.)

22. Heinemann, P. (1991) Mobbing. Presented at the Congress of the European Union for School and University Health and Medicine. June 10-13, 1991. Turku. Finland. Abstracts, p. 9-11.

23. Pikas, A. (1989) A pure concept of mobbing gives the best results for treatment. *School. Psychol. International.* 10: 95.

24. Gerard, L. (1997) Bullied. In *The Independent* Magazine. Saturday 2 August 1997. Page 11 Newspaper Publishing plc. 1 Canada Square, Canary Wharf. London E 14 5DL.

25. Reid D. (1996) Leading Article. Juvenile Smoking – 'on the increase and clear links with advertising and sports sponsorship'. *Br. Med. J.* 313:375

26. Hughes, K, Mackintosh, A. M., Hastings, G., Wheeler, C., Watson, J. and Inglis, J. (1997) Young people, alcohol and designer drinks: quantitative and qualitative study. *Br. Med. J.* 314: 414.

27. While, D., Kelly, S., Wenyong, H., Charlton, A. (1996) Cigarette advertising and onset of smoking in children: questionnaire survey. *Br. Med. J.* 313: 398.

28. Vaidya, S., Naik, U. D. and Vaidya, J. S. (1996) Effects of sports sponsorship by tobacco companies on childrens' experimentation with tobacco. *Br. Med. J.* 313: 400.

29. Reid *et al.* (1995) Reducing the prevalence of smoking in youth in Western countries; an international review. *Tobacco Control.* 4: 266.

30. Miller, P. McC., Plant, M. (1996) Drinking, smoking and illicit drug use among 15-16 year olds in the United Kingdom. *Br. Med. J.* 313: 394.

Further Reading

Joint Working Group Royal College of Physicians and British Paediatric Association. (Now The Royal College of Paediatrics and Child Health) – *Alcohol and the Young.* London. (1995) The Royal College of Physicians.

Report of Drugs Guidelines Working Group. Headmasters' Conference. 1995

Drug Prevention and Schools. DFE (now DFEE) Circular. 4/95.

Tackling drugs together: a strategy for England 1995-1998. HMSO. London 1995.

Drug misuse and dependence. Guidelines on clinical management. HMSO. London 1991.

Health Education Authority. *A parent's guide to drugs and solvents*. London. 1995.

See Below – for details of The Health Education Authority

DoH. *The Task Force to Review Services for Drug Misusers*. Report of an Independent Review of Drug Treatment Services in England. 1996.

Forbidden Drugs. (Understanding drugs and why people take them) by Philip Robson Oxford Medical Publications. Oxford University Press

Risk Takers – Alcohol, Drugs, Sex, Youth by Martin Plant and Moira Plant. Routledge. London and New York.

Anorexia nervosa and the wish to change Crisp, Joughlin, Halek and Bowyer. Department of mental Health Sciences. St. George's Hospital Medical School. London. 1989.

Living with Anorexia and bulimia. J Moorey, Manchester University Press. Manchester. 1991.

Getting better bit(e) by bit(e). U Schmidt, J Treasure. Lawrence Erlbaum, Hove. 1993.

Growth Disorders in Children by J M H Buckler (1994) BMA Publishing Group, London, WC1H 9JR.

Adolescence – The survival Guide for Parents and Teenagers by Elizabeth Fenwick and Dr Tony Smith (1995). Dorling Kindersley, Henrietta street, London WC2E 8 PS.

ADHD *How to deal with VERY DIFFICULT CHILDREN* by Alan Train (1996) ISBN 0-285-63311-2 Souvenir Press (Educational and Academic) Ltd., 43, Great Russell street, London WC1B 3PA.

The Health Education Authority is a special health authority within the NHS to advise Government on health education issues. A 50 page catalogue of publications on Health Topics, Resures for Specific Groups, Community Health and Periodicals is available from: The Health Education Authority, Hamilton House, Mabledon Place, London, WC1H 9TX. Tel: 0171 383 3833 Fax: 0171 413 0339.

CHAPTER 6

SOME MEDICAL PROBLEMS OF CHILDHOOD AND ADOLESCENCE

Acne Vulgaris

This is the commonest skin disorder of adolescence for both sexes: the face, forehead, back and chest, being the usual sites. It's exact cause is still unknown: most cases are amenable to treatment. There is an androgenically induced excessive secretion of sebum, combined with keratin obstruction of the pilo-sebaceous glands. Thickening of the lining of the sebaceous ducts occurs, with the production of whiteheads and blackheads. Bacterial colonisation then occurs, leading to varying degrees of inflammation and occasionally, cyst formation with scarring. There may be a familial tendency to acne.

Exacerbating factors

Certain oral contraceptives, especially the high dose oestrogen and the combined oestrogen/progesterone varieties, fluid retention, as in the premenstrual phase, prolonged contact with certain oils – both mineral and vegetable, and certain drugs, eg, phenytoin, are considered to be exacerbating factors. The earlier belief that acne was made worse by the consumption of chocolate and other cocoa products is not now considered valid. Fresh air and sunshine are usually beneficial, but can be exacerbating factors in a few unfortunate children.

Treatment

Some adolescents seem disproportionately upset by the presence of a few mild lesions of acne: hence the need for sensitive understanding and sympathetic handling. They can be reassured that acne is not infectious, that it is usually self-limiting (normally without any sequelae) and that they, themselves, can do much to help in managing the condition. In discussing time-scales it is as well to be realistic, for often several months elapse, before any convincing improvement is noted. Whether local or systemic treatment is appropriate, careful, daily, local toilet of the acne area is most helpful. The use of a face flannel wrung out in hot soapy water and applied to the lesions, by means of a circular movement, for a few minutes each day, before the area is cleaned with plain water and patted dry with a smooth towel, will suffice.[1]

Local treatment

Local applications of benzyl peroxide, twice daily, combined with the local measures above will often be sufficient. A useful adjunct to benzyl peroxide is retinoic acid which acts by loosening the follicular plugs of keratin. Pustules respond to topical antibiotics and those preparations containing tetracycline, erythromycin or clindamycin may be helpful, although there is a risk of producing drug resistant organisms. Ultra violet light therapy, occasionally, is a useful adjunct to local measures.

Systemic antibiotic treatment

Sufferers from rather more severe or persistent acne will require oral antibiotic therapy, which may be combined with topical therapy as noted above. Oxytetracycline or erythromycin are usually used, initially each in the dosage of 500mg twice daily for a week, then 250mg twice daily, before food. Several month's oral therapy is often required before there is any really obvious improvement and youngsters must be encouraged to persevere with treatment. Care must be taken to avoid taking these drugs with milk, since the calcium in it will combine with the antibiotic, thus reducing its absorption. Also, it is very important to warn girls of the reduced efficiency of the contraceptive pill when taken with oral antibiotic therapy and to be prepared to arrange alternative or additional methods of contraception.

Hormone treatment

Severe acne in girls will occasionally respond well to hormone treatment, as in combination therapy of an oestrogen, ethinyl oestradiol, and an anti-androgen agent, e.g. cyproterone acetate. A suitable preparation should contain 2mg of cyproterone acetate and 0.035 mg of ethinyl oestradiol. This preparation, which of course is contraindicated in pregnancy, will also provide contraception and the usual procedures associated with the prescription of oral contraceptives should be observed. (See Chapter 5.)

Retinoid therapy

This form of therapy is reserved for very carefully selected cases of severe acne which have proved resistant to other forms of therapy. It is expensive, potentially dangerous and requires to be undertaken in hospital under strict dermatological supervision.

Allergic conditions

The allergies which most commonly cause problems amongst school children are hay fever and allergic rhinitis and it is unfortunate that the pollen season often coincides with school examinations when children require to be maximally alert. This should be considered before embarking on any therapy.

Allergen avoidance must be practised by keeping bedroom windows closed and wearing sunglasses out of doors during the hay fever season. The latest antihistamine preparations such as cetirizine and astemizole are usually free from unwanted daytime sedation, but it would be as well to ascertain the optimal antihistamine treatment regime for each child well in advance of the examinations, usually in the hay fever season of the preceding year. Consult up-to-date information from the manufacturers regarding the choice of modern oral antihistamine preparations, having regard to special precautions and contraindications, including concurrent medication with other drugs.

Troublesome eye irritation may be alleviated by the use of eyedrops containing antihistamines or preparations derived from cromoglycate, but these are contraindicated in wearers of contact lenses. Steroid containing eyedrops should be reserved for cases which do not respond to simpler preparations and of course, they are absolutely contraindicated in the presence of herpes simplex lesions because of the risk of dendritic ulcers.

Depot injections of steroids are now thought to carry some risk of adrenal suppression. However, if severe hay fever symptoms occur within the school examination period, despite appropriate local treatment, then high doses of oral prednisolone should be prescribed for the duration of the examination period and tailed off gradually as soon as is practicable on conclusion of the examinations.

Rhinitis is usually controlled by local sprays of antihistamines, cromoglycate or corticosteroids, an alternative being surgery, e. g. cautery to the turbinates. Skin testing may reveal a reaction to the house dust mite, in which case, plastic mattress covers, foam pillows instead of conventional ones and duvets for blankets, restriction of the use of, or frequent vacuum cleaning of, curtains and other soft furnishings, are measures which will usually bring about considerable improvement.

Hyposensitising injections are now completely contraindicated in schools, owing to the risk of potentially fatal allergic reactions.

Anaphylaxis

Anaphylaxis, or anaphylactic shock, is a severe, potentially fatal allergic reaction. It is rare but is very unpredictable and can follow the administration, either by injection, or, more commonly, by ingestion, of any food, (including peanuts), drug or vaccine, to which the patient (either knowingly or not) may be allergic.

Very occasionally anaphylactic shock can follow bee or wasp stings.

Identifying individuals at risk

The medical histories of all new pupils should be carefully searched to identify possible cases of allergy sufferers and any medical questionnaires not returned at the commencement of the school year should be vigorously pursued. Thus children with allergies and other significant medical conditions are examined very early after their admission to school. (See Chapters 2 and 11.)

A widespread urticarial rash, swelling of the inside of the mouth, tongue or throat, and wheezing after eating the allergen suggest a potentially serious sensitivity. The following factors have been associated with a lethal outcome: (i) allergy since early infancy. (ii) co-existing asthma. (iii) young age.

The observed strength of the reaction is the most reliable guide to the seriousness of the condition. Blood tests for IgE antibody can identify other potential allergens (see below) *but are not a reliable guide to the degree of risk.* As with all laboratory test results, they must be interpreted in the light of the clinical picture. If there is a clear history of anaphylaxis, even a weak IgE reaction is significant.

Advice to sufferers

Avoiding the allergen is the mainstay of prevention. At risk individuals must be aware that peanuts, for example, may be found 'hidden' in a variety of unlikely foods. These include cooking oils, sweets, puddings, gravies, ice-cream, confectionery, pie cases and crusts and sauces. In very sensitive individuals, the reaction is so strong, that merely licking the food or touching it to the lips produces a noticeable reaction – and this can be a useful screening test for suspect foods.

What other foods might cause concern?

Although peanuts are actually peas (légumes) and not nuts, serious allergy to true nuts, like walnuts, almonds, brazil nuts, etc., also occurs, sometimes in association with peanut allergy. Fish and shellfish can also cause anaphylaxis. There is sometimes cross-sensitivity between peanuts and soya, but in such cases soya products do not carry the risk of serious anaphylaxis.

Egg sensitivity occurs in younger children but this is not a problem with teenagers. Many other foods, including strawberries and some mushrooms, can cause unpleasant urticarial reactions but fatal anaphylaxis is not seen.

Advice to the school

1   *The presence in the school of a susceptible pupil must be made aware to all those who need to know*, including, especially, the catering staff.

2   *Consideration might be given to asking caterers not to use the known allergen.* This is certainly feasible in the case of, for example, peanuts, if there is a pupil at high risk and it is known to be the only allergen. In the case of fish however, a total ban seems impractical.

3. *Label foods in which the presence of the responsible ingredient is not obvious* – this would include dips, casseroles, soups, stews, meat dishes, puddings, etc. It is not necessary if the presence of the food is obvious, e.g. fried fish, whole peanuts in biscuits, etc. Labelling as a routine would also cover the school against the risk of a visiting sufferer dining as a guest.

4. *Consider keeping adrenaline at strategic locations* eg. dining hall, sports pavilion, boarding house.

5   Sanatorium staff must be fully up to date with resuscitation procedures and the treatment of anaphylaxis. There should be a written protocol for anaphylaxis treatment, readily to hand; few of us have had recent first – hand experience and it is easy to get rusty. Drugs should be regularly checked and changed before they go out of date. Oxygen and other resuscitation equipment should be regularly checked, serviced and replenished. Training in basic cardiopulmonary resuscitation should be offered to other school staff.

NB See references at the end of this chapter.

Treatment of an attack

This is a summary. For fuller details see in Chapter 4 on Immunisation.

Give adrenaline. 0.5ml-1.0ml of 1:1,000, s.c., repeated after 5-10 mins according to response.

If collapsed, lie flat, elevate legs and give intravenous fluids to restore B.P.

Treat bronchospasm with nebulised salbutamol (or other beta-agonist), intravenous aminophylline, and oxygen.

Cardiopulmonary resuscitation and emergency tracheotomy maybe needed. Laryngospasm may be intense and, hence intubation difficult.

To prevent relapse after successful treatment, give intravenous or oral steroid and antihistamine.

Prednisolone 20-30mg and chlopheniramine 8mg by mouth **OR** hydrocortisone 200mg intravenously and chlorpheniramine 10mg intravenously diluted in the syringe with blood and given slowly over one minute.

Self administration of adrenaline

It is recommended that susceptible individuals should carry adrenaline in a disposable syringe. Min-I-Ject is available as either 0.5mg or 1. 0mg of 1:1000 adrenaline. EpiPen is an auto-inject syringe and has the advantage of being very easy to use. EpiPen contains 0.3mg 1:1000 adrenaline so that at least two are needed for initial treatment. Also, the shelf life of two years is longer than standard adrenaline. At present it is made only in the USA but can be obtained in the UK on a doctor's prescription for an individually named patient. An alternative to an injection is an adrenaline inhaler, Medihaler – Epi. The dose is 20 puffs but, obviously, it is less effective than the injection.

Useful addresses and contacts

The father of one of the teenage girls who died has started a self-help and pressure group for anaphylactic sufferers and their families. This is: Anaphylaxis Campaign, David Reading, 8, Wey Close, Ash, Aldershot, Hampshire.

Professor Jonathan Brostoff, Centre for Allergy Research, Department of Clinical Immunology, The Middlesex Hospital, London W1N 8AA. (Tel: 0171 380 9351/9359 Fax: 0171 380 9357) would be happy to offer advice as would Dr. Philip Bosworth, MO to Bryanston School, Dorset. (Tel: 01258 452411 (school), 01258 452501 (surgery) or 01258 454605 (home)

Asthma

This is a very common condition affecting all ages, but, as yet, the cause is incompletely understood. In the light of current research, it is a state of chronic inflammation of the intrapulmonary airways, rendering them hyper-irritable, so that they react to a wide variety of common stimuli by constricting rapidly. This then causes cough, dyspnoea and a tight feeling in the chest. This constriction of the airways is usually reversible, giving variable degrees of airways obstruction and there is an associated intraluminal exudation of inflammatory cells and mucus. In time, the smooth muscle of the walls of the airways may undergo hypertrophy.

There is no accepted universal definition of asthma, neither is there any specific diagnostic test for the condition, although respiratory function tests are very useful in augmenting the clinical diagnosis and also in monitoring treatment. Asthma tends to be under diagnosed and still carries unacceptably high mortality and morbidity rates. The diagnosis must be a clinical one, having due regard to the family history.

While most sufferers have a wheeze at some time, the absence of wheeze does not preclude a diagnosis of asthma and the child with a chronic cough, especially at night, for which no other cause can be found may well have asthma. Children who are more than ordinarily short of breath during or after P. E. and games, or who are habitually late returning from a cross country run, may well have exercise induced asthma. An important view of asthma, after a consensus statement, is that it is a condition of 'episodic wheeze and/or cough in a clinical setting where asthma is likely and other rarer conditions have been excluded.' However, asthma is a common condition and there is no reason why it should not co-exist with relatively less common conditions such as cystic fibrosis. Respiratory function tests would be required to confirm the diagnosis.[2]

Childrens' asthma may be precipitated by exercise, the inhalation of cold air or seasonal pollens, active or passive cigarette smoking, and respiratory infections, either viral or bacterial. There may well be a constitutional factor in the production of asthma, which may be aggravated by emotional factors. Thus, an emotional upset or crisis may precipitate an asthmatic attack. However, emotion does not cause asthma and, contrary to earlier views, sedatives and tranquillisers have no part to play here especially as these drugs may depress the sensitivity of the respiratory centre. Antibiotics have a very limited role in the treatment of asthma and should be considered only after treatment for the airways obstruction has been commenced.

For optimum management, co-operation is required from patients, parents and house parents. Care must be taken to see that children with asthma do not acquire an attitude of mind where, tacitly, they settle for less than their true potential, especially with regard to physical activity. By thoughtful, expectant and pro-active management it is possible for the majority of children with asthma to lead normal lives. School doctors, however, must be aware of the problem of nocturnal cough and/or wheeze and the damage that this can do to the child's school progress. Chronically disturbed nights lead to broken sleep and tiredness the following day, producing inattention in lessons. Other children sleeping in the same school dormitory as a child with asthma may have their sleep disturbed as well. Similarly, asthmatic children at home and their parents and siblings, can suffer from the consequences of broken sleep due to nocturnal cough and wheeze. If information about nocturnal cough and wheeze is not volunteered, then it should be enquired about specifically, since it is such an important feature of asthma.

A very small proportion of children have severe, chronic asthma, associated with chest deformity, growth retardation and constant wheezing. Such children are resistant to most forms of therapy and they should be managed with the aid of a hospital or a community paediatrician.

Peak flow meters have revolutionised the management of asthma and after their technique in using them has been checked and approved, children should be encouraged to record their peak flow readings frequently and over different parts of 24 hour periods in order to establish their individual reference values and to bring the charts to consultations with the doctor.

Parents, house parents and, as they acquire more maturity, children (including sufferers, siblings and class-mates) can now join with the school doctor in providing 'shared care'. They may supervise lifestyle and environment, (particularly with regard to cigarette smoking and punctuality in taking medication), vary the asthma medication within agreed limits and, most importantly, they should know when to call for assistance and to know how to do so when necessary.

Treatment of chronic asthma for schoolchildren over 5 years of age and adults

The British Thoracic Society has issued the following guidelines on asthma management, (1997), which are reproduced here, with grateful acknowledgement. A stepwise approach is suggested, starting treatment at the step indicated by the initial severity of the asthma, by selecting the most appropriate inhaler and where possible, eliminating any trigger factors.[3]

Step 1

For occasional relief of bronchospasm, use inhaled short acting beta agonists, e. g. salbutamol, as required, but if, after checking inhalation technique, therapy is required more frequently than once daily, move up to step 2

Step 2

In addition to the inhaled beta agonists taken as required, regular inhaled anti-inflammatory agents are introduced. These are beclomethasone dipropionate, or budesonide 100-400mcg twice daily or, fluticasone propionate 50 – 200mcg twice daily. ALTERNATIVELY sodium cromoglycate or nedocromil sodium, can be used in preference to the steroids, but if control is not achieved start inhaled steroids.

Step 3

In addition to the inhaled beta agonists taken as required, high-dose inhaled steroids OR low-dose inhaled steroids plus long-acting inhaled beta agonist bronchodilator are prescribed.

Either: beclomethasone dipropionate or budesonide increased to 800-2,000mcg daily or fluticasone propionate 400-1,000mcg daily via a large volume spacer.

Or: beclomethasone dipropionate or budesonide 100-400mcg twice daily or fluticasone propionate 50-200 mcg twice daily PLUS salmeterol 50mcg twice daily.

NB In a very small number of patients who experience side effects with high dose inhaled steroids, either the long-acting inhaled beta agonist option is used or a sustained release theophylline may be added to Step 2 medication. Cromoglycate or nedocromil sodium may also be tried.

Step 4

In addition to inhaled short-acting beta agonists, as required, high-dose inhaled steroids and regular bronchodilators are prescribed. These are inhaled beclomethasone dipropionate or budesonide 800-2,000 daily, or fluticasone propionate 400-1,000mcg daily via a large volume spacer. **PLUS** Sequential therapeutic trial of one or more of the following:

> inhaled long-acting beta agonists
> sustained release theophylline.
> inhaled ipratropium or oxitropium
> long-acting beta agonist tablets
> high-dose inhaled bronchodilators
> sodium cromoglycate or nedocromil sodium.

Step 5

In addition to inhaled short-acting beta agonists as required, the following are suggested. Beclomethasone dipropionate or budesonide 800-2, 000 mcg daily or fluticasone propionate 400-1,000 mcg daily via a large volume spacer. PLUS One or more long-acting bronchodilators. PLUS Regular prednisolone tablets in a single daily dose of 0.6mg/kg. The latter can be reduced gradually, according to progress, and hopefully tailed off after a few days. The prophylaxis must then be reviewed and the appropriate 'step' determined.

In the light of progress, patients can step down as well as up and they should ordinarily be reviewed at monthly intervals and if stable, the dose of inhaled steroid can be reduced by 25-50% every month. The doctor should familiarise himself with the prescribing details of these drugs and have a knowledge of their side effects and interactions with other drugs.

Occasional asthma

The child with the occasional asthmatic attack should respond to occasional inhalations of beta agonists, e. g salbutamol or terbutaline via a pressurised aerosol up to once daily up to thrice weekly, according to need. Most children can be relied upon to carry their inhalers on their person, but with very young children, ideally, the teacher should keep the inhalers and ensure their constant availability. Exertional asthma can be anticipated and usually prevented by one or two inhalations of the inhaler just before games or P. E.

In asthma which remains difficult to control, sustained-release xanthine preparations may be added to beta agonists and inhaled steroids. (See steps 2-4 above). Not all children are able to take xanthines because of the narrow margin between the optimal therapeutic effects and unwelcome side effects, such as nausea, irritability and occasionally, cardiac arrhythmias. Care must be taken to maintain serum levels of xanthines between 10 and 20 µg/ml. Also, xanthines react adversely with viral infections and certain antibiotics, e.g erythromycin and ciprofloxacin, which should be avoided.

Also as noted in Step 4, inhaled ipratropium or oxitropium bromide are suggested. These are anticholinergic drugs, which act by blocking the vagally mediated parasympathetic bronchoconstriction. Their action is slow, but safe and lasting.

Finally, if indicated and at any of the above, 'stages' oral prednisolone may be given in addition to inhaled therapy, as a 'rescue' procedure. In children over five years of age, the dose is in the range of 20-40mg per day, for up to five days, according to response and to be progressively reduced thereafter, again, according to response. After the 'rescue' the existing regime must be reviewed and, modified if necessary.

When control is achieved treatment must be reviewed regularly, preferably every three months and therapy gradually 'stepped down' in the light of clinical progress.

Management of acute severe asthma in those aged 5-15 years

Most of the 2,000 people who die from asthma each year are adolescents and young adults. All patients, parents and carers must be able to recognise the signs of incipient severe deterioration and call for help. Written instructions, reinforced verbally at frequent intervals, should be available.

In a severe asthmatic attack, the child may be too breathless to talk or feed and pulse and respiratory rates will be 120 and 40 per minute or more, respectively. The PEF will be equal to or less than 50% of the predicted or best. The immediate treatment is as follows:

1. High flow oxygen via a face mask.

2. Salbutamol 5mg or terbutaline10mg via an oxygen driven nebuliser (half doses in very young children)

3. Prednisolone 1-2 mg/kg body weight orally (maximum 40 mg).

In a life threatening attack there may be cyanosis, no wheeze, poor respiratory effort, grossly reduced PEF (Less than 33% of predicted or best) and agitation and reduced consciousness.

If these features are present, give, or do the following:

1. Give intravenous aminophylline 5mg/kg over 20 minutes followed by maintenance infusion, 1mg/kg: omit the loading dose if the child is already receiving oral theophyllines.

2. Give intravenous hydrocortisone 100mg 6 hourly.

3. Add ipratropium 0.25 mg to nebulised beta agonist (0.125mg in very young children)

4. Pulse oximetry is helpful in assessing response to treatment. An oxygen saturation equal or less than 92% may indicate the need for chest radiography. (Oximetry and X rays unlikely to be available in schools.)

In the school situation, it is hoped that a child with severe asthma, as described above, already would have been transferred to hospital, urgently by ambulance, before further deterioration. But, recognising that occasionally long distances may be involved, the above recommendations for life-threatening attacks have been given, so that the patient is correctly managed pending the arrival of the ambulance and on the journey. The accompanying doctor should be prepared to intubate if there is:

1.   Deteriorating PEF, worsening or persisting hypoxia or hypercapnia

2.   Exhaustion, feeble respirations, confusion and drowsiness

3.   Coma or respiratory arrest.

NB It is suggested that all school doctors should be familiar with The British Guidelines on Asthma Management, as detailed in Thorax, February 1997. Volume 52 Supplement 1, the assistance from which is gratefully acknowledged here.[3]

Address: National Asthma Campaign, 300, Upper street, London N1 3XX. Tel: 0171-226 2260.

Attention-Deficit-Hyperactivity Disorder (ADHD)

This condition now seems to be receiving media attention and school doctors appear to be seeing more children with the condition, although it has been known, under a variety of different names, over the last century. Down the years it has been variously ascribed to lead poisoning, defective parenting and minimal brain disorder, to mention a few. The term 'hyperkinetic syndrome' was introduced in the latter 1950s and occasionally is still diagnosed, although now this would equate to ADHD with excessive hyperactivity. The condition is said to affect between 3% and 5% of children and boys outnumber girls by 3:1. The main symptoms are inattention, and impulsivity, with or without hyperactivity.

Easy distractibility, poor, unsustained concentration on the task in hand, apparent inattention and reluctance to complete tasks constitute the inattention. The impulsivity is easily recognised. The child acts before thinking; 'he shoots from the hip!' In butterfly like manner, he shifts from task to task, rarely completing any of them and is disinclined to queue or to take turns. The hyperactivity, if present, just cannot be ignored or fail to be recognised. The child is always 'on the move', 'he'can't sit still'. He fidgets excessively so that he is reluctant to keep in his place in class, which of course is very disruptive.

There are varying degrees of the condition and the diagnosis is made after considering all the facets of the child's behaviour over several months. It can vary from being just containable in a classroom to being extremely disruptive, to such a degree as to make it impossible for the rest of the class to work. At home, it may be worse, with the familiarity of the situation causing the child to abuse, verbally or physically, the siblings and parents, thereby creating much family disharmony and anxiety.

Clinical examination, with investigations, should be done to exclude treatable organic conditions like juvenile thyrotoxicosis, inborn metabolic errors like phenylketonuria, or toxic states from drug misuse, say barbiturates. If the hyperactivity is absent and the child's inattention is marked, it might just be worthwhile having an EEG done, to exclude subclinical seizure discharge. (See under 'Epilepsy' in this Chapter)

Management

Help is needed not only for the child, but for the teachers and the parents, with whom counsellors and selected, trained social workers should liaise, in order to work out plans of management. Several sessions will be required.

Drug therapy has a limited place in the management of this condition, but methylphenidate, 'Ritalin' has acquired a reputation of being very helpful and several authorities testify to this now being the drug of choice.[4] It is contra-indicated in epilepsy and where there is a family history of Tourette's syndrome.

The commencing dose is 5mg in the morning, increasing by weekly incre-ments of 5mg alternately at midday and early mornings until the child is tak-ing 10mg at midday and early morning. The duration of treatment may need to be several months or even years, yet 'drug holidays' can be organised dur-ing school holidays to suspend treatment to assess progress and see if therapy requires to be continued. Parents can be reassured that the drug is not addictive but on long term therapy, annual blood and platelet counts need to be done.

On long term therapy the appetite tends to be suppressed, so in addition to the blood tests, children require to be weighed from time to time to check that weight gain is satisfactory. Sometimes, it may be worth-while giving the drug at the conclusion of the meal. There is occasional nausea and abdominal pain. Consult the manufacturer's literature for further information regarding side effects.

Alternative drugs are dexamphetamine 5-40 mg daily in divided doses and possibly, low doses of haloperidol, 0.025-0.05 mg/kg daily in divided doses, but beware of Parkinsonian side effects.

The prognosis should be guarded, for the symptoms may continue well into adult life.

Diabetes Mellitus

Most children with diabetes mellitus cope with school life very well. The school doctor must advise the various departments in school about the special needs of the diabetic child, particularly with regard to the recognition and immediate management of hypoglycaemia. Preferably, the child should have been allowed to have had a few 'hypo' attacks whilst under supervision in hospital, so that he is able to recognise their onset and take some carbohydrate, which he would have with him, always. Staff and senior pupils should know the location of the emergency supplies of glucose, (dextrosol tablets), jam or honey, (for rubbing on to the gums if the patient is unable to swallow), and the pre-packed injection kits of 1mg of glucagon, (or 0.5mg if the child is under the age of six.)

Members of staff could be instructed in how to recognise hypoglycaemia and the indications for immediate treatment, which may involve giving dextrosol tablets, rubbing jam or honey on to the gums, or actually administer-ing the intramuscular injection of 1mg of glucagon into the thigh or upper outer arm.

Games and P. E. masters should discreetly ensure that children with diabetes should have some extra food before undertaking any vigorous exer-cise, especially swimming. Also, schools should be appraised of the inadvisa-bility of these children taking part in sponsored fasts (in aid of various charities) and that the successful management of the child's condition may require the consumption of snacks at times when eating is normally forbidden.

The school catering department should be advised that diabetic children require their carbohydrate in high fibre foods and not the usual sweets and puddings. Diabetic sweets and fruit drinks should be taken instead of the usual tuck shop fare. Liaise with the tuck shop manager!

If the child is able to inject his own insulin, using the newer pen systems of delivery, then life will be easier. Injection techniques and the care and safe disposal of syringes and needles can be checked from time to time by the school doctor or the nursing staff.

Monitoring of urine and blood glucose is now much easier using the modern reagent impregnated sticks and automated devices. A periodical, say termly, estimation by the doctor of the child's glycosylated haemoglobin will provide valuable information of the diabetic control over the preceding three months. A glycosylated haemoglobin value of 10 to 12 is acceptable for a growing child or adolescent. Depending on age and maturity, the child should be encouraged, under medical and/or nursing supervision to carry out urine and blood testing, to record the results and bring the chart to consultations with the doctor.

The child should know when to seek medical advice, particularly if feeling unwell, and certainly if there is any vomiting or if the blood sugar readings should be abnormally high. In these circumstances, the urine must be tested for ketones. Menstruating girls or even pre-pubertal girls with diabetes, may have cyclical episodes of loss of diabetic control. A full clinical examination should be carried out without delay and the possibility of infection, especially of the urinary tract, must always be considered. In any case, an annual test for albuminuria and urinary infection should be undertaken.

When children with diabetes go on holiday, it is essential that they take ample supplies of insulin, spare disposable syringes and needles, and all their other diabetic equipment, including dextrosol tablets and even glucagon, with them in their hand luggage, which should be accessible at all times. Incidentally, insulin should never be packed in luggage to be transported in the hold of the aircraft, since it may then freeze and become useless. A companion who knows about them, can carry the spares. If the child is travelling alone, especially on a long journey, it is essential that the airline should have his or her medical details. At all such times, it is advisable that the child wears an identity bracelet detailing the diagnosis, insulin dosage and any concurrent drug therapy. If indicated, any travel sickness tablets should be taken before the commencement of the journey and insulin dosages shall have to be adjusted on long flights where several time zones are crossed.

If several time zones are to be crossed, the doctor might find it helpful to consult the literature in order correctly to advise the child regarding adjustments to amounts of insulin and times of injection . The British Diabetic Association receives regular requests for advice with this problem. Gill and Redmond have done a survey of current advice from British Diabetic Clinics and report their findings with some helpful references.[5]

It is stressed that the insulin should continue to be taken during other illnesses, e. g diarrhoea, and that the necessary carbohydrate should be taken in an easily assimilable form, initially, by fluids. If the diarrhoea does not settle, or particularly, if there is significant vomiting, then the insulin and the fluids must be continued and hospital admission urgently sought.

Membership of the British Diabetic Association is strongly recommended, as well as the Juvenile Diabetic Foundation. Both organisations provide useful information and the former organisation produces a booklet on travel and arranges holiday camps for children, with expert residential diabetic care.

Children and (especially) adolescents with diabetes often, understandably, rebel against the restrictions in their lives and a sympathetic school doctor is usually able to help by being available for the discussion of their problems. These youngsters also require careers advice, since people with diabetes are not permitted to do certain jobs, e. g. LGV and PCV driving.

As stated earlier, it is advisable for identity bracelets to be worn, giving details if insulin and any other drug therapy.

Addresses: The British Diabetic Association, 10, Queen Street, London W1M OBD. (Tel: 0171 323 1531)

The Juvenile Diabetic Foundation, 12, Great Portland Street, London W1N 5PF. (Tel: 0171 436 3112).

Medicalert, 1 Bridge Wharfe, 156 Caledonian Road, London N1 9UU. (Tel: 0171 833 3034).

Eczema

There is usually no difficulty in diagnosing or treating eczema. Dry eczema and ichthyotic skin respond to ointments whilst creams are better for flexural and exudative eczema. Use topical steroid preparations with care, and use low potency preparations on the face. Do not use fluorinated steroids on the face. The associated pruritus can be troublesome and oral promethazine or trimeprazine are helpful, especially at night when their sedative action is useful.

If the eczema is infected, then mupirocin 2% is useful and if a systemic antibiotic is indicated, then erythromycin is the one of choice, but should not be used with terfenadine. In any case, terfenadine is not now advised, due to potential cardio-vascular effects.

For extensive eczema or ichthyosis, then the use of bath oils can be soothing and simple emollient ointments can be used as soap substitutes. The old fashioned coal tar preparations may be used instead of steroids and they have antipruritic properties. Nowadays, a severe exacerbation of eczema, even if not obviously infected, is assumed to be so and antibiotics are prescribed orally.

Enuresis and Soiling (Encopresis)

90% of children are dry by the time they are five and 95% by the time they are eight. A small proportion continue to have nocturnal enuresis into their adult life and the condition can occur in families suggesting that primary enuresis is due to late maturation of bladder control. Emotional factors may make matters worse. Common organic causes, such as diabetes mellitus and urinary tract infection, should be excluded and in resistant cases, other causes should be considered, including diabetes insipidus, congenital abnormality of the urinary tract and even undiagnosed epilepsy, since some forms of epilepsy, e. g. occasional cases of temporal lobe epilepsy may start with exclusively nocturnal attacks. If any of these diagnoses are feasible, then appropriate investigations should, of course, be undertaken. Needless to state, the urine should be examined initially and during the management of the condition.

Exclusively daytime and certainly, diurnal enuresis merit prompt consultant referral, but nocturnal enuresis continues to be regarded as a functional disorder and since children vary a great deal in the time they take before achieving night time dryness, active management is not usually started until the age of eight years. A calendar with stars and a system of rewards may sometimes be effective, especially if the calendar is commenced after at least a few scattered dry nights, so that the child does not become dispirited at having to render another 'nil return.' Dry nights should be praised and wet ones ignored. If, after several months, this fails, then an enuresis alarm bell or buzzer provides the best hope of success.[6,7] This is despite the cynical views that for the alarm to work the child must already be wet, that it is preferable to change the bed after a night's sleep and that often, such is the depth of the enuretic child's sleep, that he or she, (usually he) sleeps on whilst everyone else in the house or dormitory is roused by the alarm.

In fact, the child need only pass a few drops of urine before the circuit is completed and the alarm is activated. This wakes most children, who switch off the alarm, visit the toilet to void urine, change the top sheet and their pyjamas and then go back to sleep. This 'conditioning', whereby the act of micturition is inhibited by the sound of the alarm is quite effective, especially in an intelligent and well-motivated child. Of course, the children who do respond to this method will vary greatly in the times in which they achieve complete dryness. Raising the foot of the bed may assist in some cases.

Drug therapy, of which there have been many examples in the past, is usually unhelpful, apart from the tricyclic antidepressants, imipramine and amitryptiline, or, very occasionally, intranasal vasopressin, derived from the antidiuretic hormone. The usual nocturnal doses of imipramine and amitryptiline are 25mg and 10 mg respectively, which may be doubled after two or three weeks if there is a disappointing response. These drugs are usually well tolerated by children and there seems little risk at the above dosages, of their masking depressive symptoms, as has been suggested in the past. However, the dose could be reduced in the event of daytime sleepiness. Imipramine and amitryptiline should not be given to children with epilepsy, since the tricyclic drugs can precipitate fits. The dose of vasopressin is 20 micrograms intranasally, at night, for up to three months after which, the efficacy should be assessed by cessation of therapy for a week.

The tricyclic drugs are effective for the duration of the therapy, but there is a marked tendency to relapse when they are withdrawn. One way of tackling this, is to give the drugs in liquid form and over a period of several weeks, progressively reduce the dose, whilst keeping the volume of fluid constant.[8]

In dealing with these children parents and house parents need optimistic encouragement, for the condition is almost always self limiting and most children are dry at night by the time they reach puberty. Most enuretic children want to be dry and a punitive approach to the management of enuresis is not only unkind, but is counterproductive.

ERIC stands for the Enuresis Resource and Information Centre, which is a registered charity providing advice and information for children, parents and medical and nursing staff on enuresis. The address is: 65, St. Michaels Hill, Bristol. BS2 8DZ. Tel: 0117 926 4920.

Encopresis

As in the case of enuresis, most children who soil wish to be clean. Often, the condition is spurious diarrhoea, caused by overflow incontinence which, in turn, is caused by liquefaction of faeces in chronic constipation. Perhaps initially, a hard stool causes an anal fissure and painful defaecation. The child then ignores the call to stool and a large faecal mass accumulates in the rectum, causing loss of tone and the above sequence of events. Treatment consists in emptying the rectum by a series of enemata, giving adequate fluids and, concurrently, a faecal softener, such as lactulose, and a drug to stimulate peristalsis, such as a senna product. The doses of these preparations have to be worked out for each child by trial and error and not discontinued prematurely.

Rarely, the constipation is caused by Hirschsprung's disease, due to an aganglionic segment of gut near the rectosigmoid junction and this condition should be suspected if there is a long history of constipation, perhaps even since birth. This is usually not accompanied by peri-anal faecal staining, which is almost always noted in cases of simple overflow incontinence. If this rare condition is suspected, then referral to a paediatric surgeon is indicated, as it may well be possible for the aganglionic segment of gut to be resected, with beneficial results.

Soiling, may of course occur as part of an emotional disorder, in which case psychiatric advice may be sought.

Epilepsy

The incidences of epilepsy and diabetes mellitus are roughly equal (about 1 in 200) and in children and adolescents suffering from these conditions, sympathetic understanding and readily available support are required, to a greater extent perhaps, than with other long-term disorders. Apart from and in addition to their occasionally rebellious attitudes towards the restrictions placed on them by their respective medical conditions, e. g. diet, injections, restrictions on activity, the need for constant therapy, career limitations, etc., sufferers from both these conditions are subject to episodes of irritability, over which they have no volitional control. Patients with diabetes are prone to varying degrees of hypoglycaemia which can cause irritability and confusion and children and adolescents with epilepsy may have similar episodes caused by their cerebral dysrhythmias and even, occasionally, by unwanted effects of their anticonvulsant drugs.

Epilepsy is a clinical diagnosis which should be made with great care and circumspection, lest a child should acquire an erroneous diagnosis of the condition, with all that that implies. It should be differentiated from conditions such as simple vaso-vagal faints (in which tonic/clonic movements and cyanosis may be noted), night terrors, masturbation, benign paroxysmal vertigo, reflex anoxic seizures, cardiac arrhythmias, migraine and even some cases of child abuse, as in the Munchausen syndrome by proxy.[9,10] Many children referred to hospital with an diagnosis of 'known' or 'established' epilepsy do not have the condition.[11] Betts has described 'pseudoseizures': seizures that are not epilepsy.[12]

Although an epileptic attack (fit, seizure or convulsion) may occur in anyone at any age or time, it is only after a tendency to recurrent attacks has been established that epilepsy can justifiably be said to exist. In making the diagnosis, eye-witness accounts are invaluable and these may be sought not only from parents, but from teachers, youth leaders, scout masters or even intelligent class-mates. If a child has his first fit in school, then it should be investigated in hospital, and, unless the first attack is an episode of status epilepticus (see later), then drug treatment should not be commenced until at least after the second attack has occurred.

The generalised tonic/clonic seizure is perhaps the commonest manifestation, with a cry and loss of consciousness, followed by convulsions, cyanosis, frothing at the mouth, bitten tongue and loss of bladder and/or bowel control. (The 'grand mal' attack) Care in these attacks is limited to placing the patient on his left side, clearing his mouth (of food or dental appliances), and shielding him from traffic, water or other hazards. Do not place anything in his mouth, other than an airway, do not cover with blankets, or attempt to restrain the convulsing limbs. These attacks usually last up to two or three minutes, after which care is still required, because of drowsiness, confusion and disorientation. There may be a residual temporary hemiparesis (Todd's palsy), lasting up to 36 hours and sleep for an hour or so, usually follows the fit.

If the generalised tonic/clonic attack does not stop after ten minutes, or there are several similar shorter attacks with intervening deep unconsciousness as distinct from several similar attacks with return to consciousness between them (i. e. serial epileptic fits), then the potentially fatal condition of status epilepticus exists. Diazepam is the drug of choice for this condition, given either intravenously (0.25 to 0.5 mg/kg) slowly over 3 to 4 minutes or rectally: this, by means of disposable plastic enema packs, 5mg up to 4 years of age and 10 mg for older children.

There is a slight risk of respiratory depression, requiring assisted respiration with the intravenous preparation, especially if the child is receiving barbiturate or related drugs prophylactically. Intravenous diazepam should not be used if the child has diabetes mellitus or any other form of disordered carbohydrate metabolism.[13] If the status persists, the child must be admitted urgently to hospital, the IV or rectal diazepam can be repeated 20 minutes after the initial dose and oxygen and oral suction should be continued during the ambulance journey.

Before considering any drug therapy régime for epilepsy it is important to realise that good seizure control depends on a settled life style with the avoidance of hunger, thirst, sleep deprivation, constipation, boredom and alcoholic excess. Children who are known to have photosensitive epilepsy should take care at discos, should not go too close to the screen of a working TV set and should wear polaroid spectacles on visits to the seaside on a sunny day. The last named precaution is suggested in order to avoid flicker induced convulsions due to reflections of bright sunlight on an agitated sea. If the child has to be exposed to a source of flickering light, the covering of one eye by the palm of one hand will minimise the risk of a convulsion. Also, it is preferable that photosensitive children should do their televiewing from the opposite end of the room to the TV set and certainly should not sit or lie directly in front of it.

Drugs for generalised tonic/clonic (i. e. 'grand mal') seizures and partial, e. g. focal seizures – seizures, which are either simple, if there is no associated impairment of consciousness, or complex if there is such associated impairment, (N.B. psychomotor absence seizures are in the latter category), are carbamazepine, sodium valproate and lamotrigine: the last named, for children over 12 years of age.

The drug of choice for generalised absence seizures (i.e. 'petit mal epilepsy)' with a pathognomonic 3 per second spike and wave discharge on the EEG, is ethosuximide. If this is ineffective, or, as can rarely happen, it precipitates the appearance of latent tonic/clonic seizures, then sodium valproate is indicated. 'Petit mal' epilepsy is almost exclusively confined to the school child and, if undiagnosed, or inadequately treated can lead to under achieving, apparent disobedience or even behaviour problems. Just occasionally, it can exist in a sub-clinical form, i. e. the child having episodic impaired attention due to the cerebral dysrhythmia yet showing no outward sign of the seizure, and this diagnosis is worth considering if a previously able child should start to underachieve. The EEG would be the means of making the diagnosis of 'sub-clinical petit mal seizure disorder' and this is perhaps an exception to the definition that the diagnosis of epilepsy should be made on purely clinical grounds. Other drugs, such as clonazepam and clobazam are useful for the less common myoclonic epilepsy.

Great efforts should be made to secure early seizure control with minimal or no side effects from drugs, thus making it less likely that the child will develop chronic epilepsy.

Serum levels of anticonvulsant drugs are occasionally useful in monitoring therapy, especially with carbamazepine and phenytoin, but other than in suspected toxic levels, or checking compliance with therapy, they tend to be overused. If a child with an accurate diagnosis of epilepsy is happy, seizure free, performing optimally in school and without any obvious untoward side effects, then serum levels are not required and do not require routine 'checking'.

Children on long-term carbamazepine therapy should have their folate levels checked from time to time and all school doctors should be aware of the slight risk of thrombocytopenia with sodium valproate. All rashes and abnormal bleeding should receive prompt attention.

Monotherapy is the aim of the drug treatment of epilepsy, largely to avoid drug interactions due to polypharmacy, but this is not always possible. However, the newer anticonvulsants lamotrigine, gabapentin and vigabatrin, are licensed for monotherapy and 'add-on' therapy, according to seizure types. Doctors are advised to consult manufacturers' literature for further information.

Small changes in the bioavailabilty of anticonvulsants have resulted in loss of seizure control when some patients have had their therapy switched from generic to proprietary brands or vice versa, or between different manufacturers' brands of the same preparation. It is now advised that anticonvulsants are prescribed by brand name and not altered unless there is a good reason and then only after a proper evaluation.

Liver enzyme induction takes place when drugs like oral contraceptives, antifungal preparations, some antibiotics, e.g. rifampicin, and the anticonvulsants, carbamazepine, phenytoin and the barbiturate group of drugs are given concurrently. The result is increased drug metabolism and reduction in serum concentrations of the drugs. Hence contraceptive failures may occur with low dosage oestrogen oral contraceptive pills. Vigabatrin does not induce liver enzyme activity so that reactions with other drugs are unlikely. Recent reports however have described visual field restriction in some patients taking vigabatrin. No causal relationship has yet been established and it has been pointed out that disturbances of retinal function have been noted in patients with epilepsy receiving other anticonvulsant drugs. Harding has confirmed the findings of visual field restriction, advanced four possible explanations and advised that further studies will be required.[15]

Lamotrigine has its metabolism enhanced by phenytoin, carbamazepine, phenobarbitone and primidone (a manipulated barbiturate), but there is no effect on the clearance of oral contraceptives. Lamotrigine metabolism is inhibited by sodium valproate, so a reduction in the lamotrigine dose by half is recommended when these two drugs are used together. Just recently, it has been reported that with lamotrigine therapy, the incidence in children of side-effects in the form of a skin rash is higher than was previously thought. New data suggests that between 1 in 100 and 1 in 300 children could be affected. Treatment must not be stopped without medical advice. Report any adverse reaction to the CSM.

Activity

Careful assessment of risks must be carried out and they should be reviewed in the light of clinical progress, remembering that even if a child does have an aura, which he may be able to describe in great detail retrospectively, fear at the time it is experienced may prevent his 'taking cover.' Lone fishing or swimming should be discouraged. Swimming in a group should be encouraged, but with dedicated supervision, initially on a one to one basis, which may be relaxed as seizure control improves. Other pursuits, except boxing and mountain climbing may be encouraged. There should be no unaccompanied cycling, especially on busy roads. A personal identity bracelet or medallion should be worn at all times, giving details of the diagnosis, any allergies and current drug therapy. Discreet observation is also required in laboratories and craft rooms.

Careers Advice

This should be discussed with the child, parents and teachers. Epilepsy precludes entry into HM Forces. Any convulsions occurring after the age of five mean that Passenger Carrying Vehicle and Large Goods Vehicle licences cannot be granted. When a patient of driving age reaches a period of freedom from daytime fits for two years, (whether taking medication or not) it will entitle him to apply for a licence to drive a private car for his own use. That is, he will not be able to earn his living as a driver, (Taxi, private hire car, delivery van etc.)Encouragement should be given for the child to become a member of the British Epilepsy Association, who will provide information on drugs, legislation and advice about employment and insurance.

Address: The British Epilepsy Association, Anstey House, 40, Hanover Square. Leeds LS3 1BE. Tel: 0113 2439393.

Epilepsy Freephone Helpline 0800 309030. Also Medicalert (see page 161).

Headaches and Migraine

Spontaneous headaches in otherwise healthy children tend to be unusual, although headaches are commonly a feature of other conditions, especially many of the common infections of childhood, particularly if there is fever or dehydration. Even in epidemics of upper respiratory tract infections and influenza when headaches are very common, it is as well constantly to bear in mind the possibility of meningitis and to take special notice of any associated features like vomiting or rashes, remembering that in meningococccal infections a non-specific erythematous rash may precede the petechial one.

Of the non-febrile causes of headaches, perhaps so called 'tension' headaches are the commonest, with migraine coming second. Cerebral tumours are rare, but this diagnosis must be considered if the child persistently complains of waking from sleep with a headache and also, if the headache is made worse by coughing or sneezing. Such symptoms warrant a detailed neurological examination and urgent referral . If the headache gets worse as the day wears on, then one should think of tension headache, or perhaps, sinusitis. Tension headaches are often associated with an anxiety state and the pain results from contraction of the muscles round the head and neck. Sometimes, the patient describes a feeling of a 'tight band' round the head. Studious youngsters working for their examinations occasionally have this type of headache.

Migraine is the other common condition, which is defined as a headache coming on at intervals, lasting for periods of variable length, and then remitting completely until the next attack. The basic pathology is thought to be constriction, followed by dilatation of the cerebral blood vessels, although the underlying mechanism producing these changes, is not yet known. Most migraine sufferers have 'common' migraine, consisting of a headache, usually over one cerebral hemisphere ('hemi-crania') nausea and sometimes vomiting. 'Classical' migraine affects fewer people, in whom the headache, nausea and vomiting are often accompanied by visual symptoms like partial loss of vision, everything seeming smaller, flashing lights and some zig-zag shapes, known as fortification figures, and other forms of visual distortion. Associated abdominal symptoms, including anorexia, diarrhoea and vomiting can occur and last for quite long periods of time, even to the extent of producing dehydration.

Some migraine sufferers may have their attacks triggered off by various factors, including food, chocolate, cheese, coffee, citrus fruits and alcohol.

Occasionally, girls will describe premenstrual exacerbations of their attacks, perhaps due to cerebral fluid retention.

Often there is a family history of migraine and occasionally a history of travel sickness, or a history of cyclical vomiting in early childhood (the periodic syndrome). Abdominal migraine, in the form of episodic abdominal pain, with or without vomiting, has been described, and this pain tends to be centred around the umbilicus. Possible trigger factors must be discussed with youngsters, because they may not appreciate their existence, or their role in the causation of attacks of migraine. During a migraine attack, which may actually be heralded by the visual disturbance or irritability, (often misconstrued as bad behaviour or disobedience in children) the sufferers are further disturbed by bright lights and loud noises and appreciate a quiet and darkened room.

If trigger factors have been eliminated and if pain relief is required the best remedy for children is soluble paracetamol given as early as possible in the attack, preferably in a syrup in case there is a hypoglycaemic factor in the production of the attack. The addition of metoclopramide to control any associated vomiting, is contraindicated in children because of the rather disturbing dystonic reactions which may be produced.

Provided the diagnosis of migraine is accurate however, teenagers may find some benefit from metoclopramide if they are vomiting. If the attacks occur so frequently that some form of prophylaxis is indicated, then pizotifen (depending on age and weight) up to 1.5 mg daily in divided doses or as a single dose of 1.0mg at night can be given. This drug may be associated with weight gain and drowsiness in some patients however. Other drugs which may be tried are the non-steroidal group of drugs, such as diclofenac, or small doses of tricyclic antidepressants such as amitriptyline or the beta blocker, propranolol.

There is a long standing medicinal herb remedy for migraine prophylaxis, called feverfew. It is claimed to be safe and non-addictive and in 1988, a randomised double-blind placebo-controlled trial of feverfew was carried out in Nottingham.[15]

If, however, further pain relief is required, or the attacks of migraine are too frequent or the associated symptoms are of a disturbing nature, then referral for a paediatric or neurological opinion is suggested.

Address: The British Migraine Association, 178a, High Road, Byfleet, West Byfleet, Surrey, Tel;01932 352 468. The Association has some very helpful and relevant literature available on request. (SAE and donation preferred.)

Haemoglobinopathies

Worldwide the haemoglobinopathies thalassaemia and sickle cell disease are the most common autosomal genetic disorders affecting human populations. The WHO estimates over 250 million people carry a haemoglobinopathy gene and at least 250-300,000 affected homozygotes are born annually. Sickle cell disorders are most common in the African and Caribbean populations in the UK where in some inner city areas their birth prevalence reaches 1 in 300 (cf 1 in 2000 for cystic fibrosis). The alpha and beta thalassaemias are more widely distributed and affect children from ethnic minorities which originate from the Mediterranean, Middle East, Africa, Indian sub-continent and Far East. Because of their special and life-long medical needs, all children with sickle cell disease and thalassaemia should be registered with a clinic under the direction of a paediatrician and/or haematologist with expertise in this field. In areas of low prevalence this may be facilitated by sharing care between local and specialist centres. As with other chronic illnesses, cumulative loss of schooling may impact upon educational and social attainment. In some cases this is coupled with difficulties of culture and language to which the school doctor must be sensitive.

Over the past two decades there has been a dramatic improvement in the outlook for children with thalassaemia and sickle cell disease. Reassurance may need to be given to families whose preconceptions are shaped by experience outside the UK where the childhood mortality of haemoglobin – opathies remains high. Bone marrow transplantation now offers an excellent chance of cure to children with thalassaemia who have a suitable donor and is an emerging option for selected patients with sickle cell disease.

Thalassaemia major.

In its most severe form, homozygous beta thalassaemia results in the development of profound anaemia after birth due to an inability to produce adult haemoglobin. (haemoglobin A; $\alpha2$ $\beta2$). This is aggravated by surplus alpha globin chains which precipitate the red cell precursors and cause ineffective erythropoesis. With optimal medical management most children with beta thalassaemia major attain normal growth and development. Treatment involves regular blood transfusion every three or four weeks to prevent the haemoglobin level falling below 10.0 g/dl. This ensures normal growth and prevents abnormalities of the facial bones and dentition and hypersplenism due to expansion of erythropoesis in the marrow and spleen. With appropriate transfusion, physical activity need not be restricted unless there are specific contraindications such as cardiac disease. Blood is fully matched to prevent red cell alloimmunisation and leucodepleted to minimise the risk of non-haemolytic transfusion reactions and cytomegalovirus transmission. It is recommended that all newly diagnosed cases of thalassaemia and others who are non-immune receive hepatitis A and B vaccination. Children with thalassaemia major, particularly those transfused prior to the introduction of donor screening for hepatitis C virus in 1991, should be tested for antibodies to HCV. If sero-positive further investigation is indicated to exclude chronic hepatitis which develops in up to 60% of cases and may benefit from treatment with alpha interferon. Although the risk of transmission of human immunodeficiency virus (HIV) by transfusion has been reduced in the UK to less than 1/100,000 units, children transfused outside the UK in countries without effective donor screening programmes are at greater risk. In such cases HIV counselling and screening are indicated (See Chapter 11).

An inevitable consequence of long-term transfusion is iron overload (siderosis) which if untreated leads to endocrine, cardiac and liver failure. This is avoided by regular administration of the iron chelating drug Desferrioxamine (Desferal). This is usually given subcutaneously over eight to ten hours via a portable syringe pump five nights a week. Most children with thalassaemia in the UK will have begun Desferal therapy well before school age, generally within one year of starting transfusion. Oral vitamin C is given to promote urinary iron excretion. Children and their families often find Desferal therapy burdensome. Painful lumps may develop at the site of injection, usually the anterior abdominal wall, and sleep may be disrupted. More serious side effects of which the school doctor should be aware are ocular and ototoxicity. Ophthalmic and audiological assessment should be performed annually. If recognised early, hearing loss usually recovers on withdrawal of Desferal. Another important complication related to iron chelation therapy is Yersinia infection. This species of bacteria requires iron for growth and children with thalassaemia on Desferal are particularly susceptible. The diagnosis should be suspected in any child receiving iron chelation who develops abdominal pain, diarrhoea or vomiting and fever. Appropriate antibiotic therapy must be initiated without delay.

Sickle cell disorders

Sickle cell disease embraces a group of disorders whose clinical effects may be attributed to the production of a structurally abnormal type of haemoglobin. The most common form of sickle cell anaemia (HbSS) is caused by homozygous inheritance of sickle haemoglobin. Interaction with beta thalassaemia or other structural haemoglobin variants for example haemoglobin C, which is common in some West African populations, results in the sickling disorders HbSbeta thalassaemia and HbSC disease which often display milder effects than HbSS. On deoyxgenation, sickle haemoglobin depolymerises forming crystals which lead eventually to irreversible distortion and rigidity of red cells. These sickled cells which lack normal rheological properties become entrapped in the microvascular circulation leading to vaso-occlusion with tissue and organ damage. The clinical consequences are protean and vary in severity considerably amongst affected children. They include painful 'crises' due to infarction of the bone marrow, hyposplenism, stroke, avascular necrosis, lung disease, leg ulcers and renal failure.

The introduction of newborn screening with from early life, prophylaxis against pneumococcal sepsis in the form of twice daily penicillin and immunisation with poylvalent pneumococcal vaccine has resulted in a decline in mortality of children with sickle cell disease in the developed world. Compliance with prophylaxis with respect to which the school doctor should be vigilant, is vital. Acute complications of sickle cell disease are unpredictable and may be life threatening. A list of medical emergencies is included in Table 1. Cold, dehydration and exhaustion may trigger sickling and signal the need to avoid strenuous outdoor games in cold or wet weather. Swimming should only be permitted if the pool and changing room are adequately heated. Occasionally 'crises' develop despite these precautions in which case swimming should be discouraged. Because of impaired renal tubular function, children with sickle cell disease are prone to dehydration and must maintain a higher fluid intake than normal. It is important that teachers are aware of this

Table 1 Some medical emergencies in sickle cell disease

Symptoms	Possible Diagnosis
Respiratory distress	Acute chest syndrome
Chest/girdle pain	Pneumonia
Fever (greater than 38 degrees C and unwell)	Overwhelming pneumococcal sepsis
Focal weakness	Cerebral infarction
Headache	Intracranial haemorhage
Photophobia	Meningitis
Abdominal pain + /distension	Acute splenic or hepatic sequestration
	Mesenteric crisis
	Acute cholecystitis
	Salmonella infection (risk of subsequent osteomyelitis warrants treatment of primary infection).
	Yersinia enterocolitis (if on Desferal)
Pallor	Severe anaemia due to parvovirus
Lassitude	induced aplastic crisis or sequestration
Dyspnoea	(see above).
Priapism	

and the likely need for the child to visit the toilet more frequently. Although sickle cell disease is associated with anaemia, due to chronic haemolysis (the Hb in sickle cell anaemia is typically between 6.0 and 8.0g/dl), compensatory changes in red cell metabolism improve oxygen delivery and in most cases effort tolerance is not severely restricted. Affected children can participate in most sports except where there is a risk of hypoxia. e.g. scuba diving, and high altitude mountaineering. Mild to moderate jaundice due to shortened red cell survival is frequently seen in children with sickle cell disease, particularly during a painful 'crisis' or an intercurrent infection. Fluctuation in the degree of the icterus is common but sudden worsening may signal hepatic sequestration, cholecystitis, transfusion associated hepatitis or acute haemolysis. The latter in some cases may be due to glucose-6-phosphate dehydrogenase deficiency.

Of special importance to the school doctor are those manifestations of sickle cell disease which cause neurological or cognitive impairment and may determine special needs provision. These range from stroke which occurs in 5% of children with sickle cell disease, usually between the ages of five to ten years, to more subtle neuropsychological defects. Though scholastic attainment may be normal, recent research suggests some affected children have small IQ deficits. The basis for this is likely to be multi-factorial. On average children with sickle cell disease miss 2% of schooling due to pain. Children with significant learning difficulties or psychological problems should be referred for detailed assessment including neuro-imaging to exclude cerebral vasculopathy. If present, transfusion therapy may be considered to arrest further ischaemic cerebral damage. Sickle cell disease may result in growth delay, the deficit in weight typically exceeding that in height and delayed puberty. This may lower self-esteem and impact upon a child's psychological and social adjustment. Painful priapism is a particular problem in adolescent males though it can occur before puberty and if prolonged for more than a few hours, may lead to permanent impotence.

In addition to prophylactic penicillin, some children with sickle cell disease receive oral folic acid supplements to meet the requirements of increased bone marrow erythropoesis. Its value in the developed world where dietary intake of further folic acid is plentiful is controversial. For the inital management of pain crises, oral paracetamol or ibuprofen alone or in combination are suitable. If effective analgesia is not achieved quickly advice must be sought. Sickle cell patients travelling to parts of the world where malaria is endemic are at particular risk of severe malarial infection due to hyposplenism and vigorous anti-malarial prophylaxis is essential. Specific advice on travel precautions for people with sickle cell disorders may be obtained from the Sickle Cell Society, 54, Station Road, London NW 10 4UA. Tel: 0181 961 7795/4006.

Kawasaki Disease

This is a rare disease, primarily affecting infants and young children up to the age of about five years, although cases can occur in older children and present to the school doctor. Early diagnosis really is vitally important and recently, doctors have been criticised because they did not know about the disease. It is thought to be an inflammatory condition, but so far, no infecting organism has been identified and it is diagnosed if any five out of six of the following criteria are present: (1) high temperature present for five days or more and un-responsive to antibiotics, (2) red eyes, (3) mouth changes, including cracked, red lips, and a 'strawberry tongue', (4) a generalised erythematous rash, (5) cervical lymphadenopathy – often unilateral, (6) swelling and redness of the hands and feet with – often – extensive peeling of the skin.

There are other non-specific signs and symptoms, e.g. irritability, mood changes, diarrhoea and vomiting, but the most frequent (and serious) com-plication is the production of aneurysms of the coronary arteries, which may rupture and it is thought that early diagnosis and treatment (with aspirin and immuno-globulins) may prevent these. Urgent early referral to hospital, even on suspicion, is indicated.

The National Co-ordinator is Sue Davidson who operates the National Telephone Help-Line on (01203) 612178.

Orthopaedic Problems

There are three areas in which significant non-traumatic orthopaedic problems are likely to occur: the back, the hip and the knee.

Scoliosis

Apart from rare causes due to underlying lung disease or congenital vertebral abnormality, adolescent scoliosis is of the idiopathic variety, 80-90% occurr-ing in girls. There is painless lateral deviation of the spinal column at any age which progresses quickly during a growth spurt. The 'forward bending' test has already been described (Chapter 2). This should reveal the presence of a scoliosis if the scapulae are viewed first along the line of the spine and then at right angles to it. In severe cases, bunching of the ribs may be present on the side of the concavity of the spinal column. This condition requires prompt orthopaedic referral, for there is a risk of permanent deformity and a brace or an operation may be required. Further help may be obtained from The Scoliosis Association (UK), formerly the Scoliosis Self Help Group, 380 – 384, Harrow Road, London W9 2HU. Tel 0171 289 5652.

Osteochondritis

Osteochondritis or avascular necrosis occurs in several well known sites in the growing child. In the spine, it can occur in one or more vertebral bodies, which are not necessarily adjacent. This leads to backache and limited forward flexion. (The child is unable to touch his toes with knees straight). The avoidance of vigorous spinal flexion and extension exercises and the substitution of a firm mattress for a soft one, will provide comfort until spontaneous resolution takes place.

Hip

There are several disorders of the hip which can affect the growing child and all of them require prompt diagnosis. Congenital dislocation of the hip is usually diagnosed at, or soon after birth but in some cases the diagnosis is delayed. (16). Very young infants can get a serious septic arthritis of the hip, which is associated with marked systemic signs, requiring prompt referral. In the older toddler, or young school child, avascular necrosis of the femoral head can produce Perthe's disease, which, if not diagnosed early, can lead to destructive changes in the femoral head predisposing arthritic changes later in life. A limp may be the first sign. Less commonly, avascular necrosis of the navicular bone produces pain in the foot and a limp. Special insoles will help here. Older children and some young adolescents get a painful hip, known, for want of a better term, as the irritable hip. There is pain on hip movement, but minimal systemic signs and normal ESR values. The condition usually settles quickly, with simple analgesics and has no sequelae. A slipped upper femoral epiphysis should always be considered. (See below).

NB. See Table 6 in Chapter 9 on 'Sports Injuries' for a differential diagnosis of 'The Irritable Hip'.

Knee

School doctors are reminded that in dealing with all cases of pain in the hip or the knee in an older child or adolescent, they should have a high index of suspicion of a slipped upper femoral epiphysis A lateral X-ray of hip is advisable and urgent orthopaedic referral is mandatory, if suspected.

Anterior knee pain due to other causes is a fairly common condition of youngsters, especially girls. Causes may be due to pathology within the knee joint or to extra-articular causes. Osgood-Schlatter's disease is a painful swelling of the tibial tubercle occurring in adolescents of both sexes and is a combination of avascular necrosis of the tibial tubercle and a traction epiphysitis. It is a self limiting condition and resolution can be helped by the avoidance of kneeling and of exercises involving knee flexion. Occasional simple analgesia may be required. Subject to the above, no restriction in activity is usually necessary.

Menstrual difficulties
Dysmenorrhoea

Mild – sympathy and understanding.

Primary (spasmodic) – usually pain is caused by prostaglandin release: rarely due to uterine abnormality. Examination is usually not useful. The need for this can be assessed at history taking.

Treatment: reassurance and simple analgesia, or non steroidal anti inflammatory drugs, e.g. mefenamic acid (Ponstan). Then review after three or four cycles. If there is no improvement then consider low dose oral contraceptive pill or referral for gynaecological opinion. If the girl is sexually active, smear status should be checked and advice on safe sex should be given. Pelvic inflammatory disease should be considered. Low dose oral contraceptive pills may be used electively for examinations, interviews, field trips, etc.

Secondary dysmenorrhoea may occasionally be present in the older girl.

Mittelschmertz. The onset is usually sudden with pain in either iliac fossa, or the rectum, seldom lasting more than a day and possibly accompanied by a slight degree of vaginal bleeding, mid cycle. Explanation is important. Simple analgesia is occasionally necessary.

Menorrhagia – may occur just after the menarche. There may be heavy bleeding associated with clots. The early cycles are usually anovulatory. Non-hormonal therapies, e.g. mefenamic acid, naproxen or ibuprofen or anti-fibrinolytic drugs, e.g. cyklocapron (tranexamic acid) or dicynene (ethamsylate) are useful, together with reassurance. Treatment with these drugs can be confined to menstruation. If the cycles are ovulatory, then norethisterone can be used.

Very occasionally, really serious bleeding can occur, perhaps requiring blood transfusion. An urgent gynaecological opinion should be sought.

Irregularity. Irregular periods are common and part of growing up. No treatment is necessary.

Amenorrhoea. The age range of the menarche is from 10 to 16 and should be investigated if delayed beyond the normal range or when the girl displays concern. If the other signs of puberty are well in evidence, then always keep in mind the rare condition of haematocolpos, due to an imperforate hymen. This condition requires prompt surgical intervention in order to avoid psychological upset and damage to the fallopian tubes.

Secondary amenorrhoea should be investigated, always remembering the possibility of pregnancy, and more than one pregnancy test and pelvic examination may be required to exclude it. Other underlying causes which should be borne in mind are anorexia nervosa, thyroid dysfunction, tuberculosis, and diabetes mellitus. Girls who are vigorous athletes may have secondary amenorrhoea and possibly develop osteoporotic fractures round their femoral heads if the exercise is particularly strenuous.

Premenstrual tension tends to affect older girls, due to the retention of fluid in the premenstrual week. Oil of evening primrose might be tried first.

Myalgic Encephalomyelitis. 'M. E. Syndrome' or 'Chronic Fatigue Syndrome'

Most doctors are aware that it is usual to have varying periods of debility in the convalescent stages of many illnesses, especially those of viral origin. Glandular fever, adult chicken pox and infective hepatitis A, are examples of this.

The 'ME' syndrome, or as it now tends to be known, the 'Chronic Fatigue Syndrome', has come into the news in the last decade or so, although it has been around for a very long time beforehand, with a variety of names. This condition is characterised by persistent fatigue, lasting several months, usually following a viral upper respiratory infection or an intestinal viral infection (Coxsackie, Epstein-Barr or cytomegalovirus) and accompanied by extreme muscle weakness and tenderness. There are several associated symptoms and Cleare and Wessley have described a recent consensus criteria for other features of the condition, as follows: fatigue must be severe enough to cause a 50% loss of physical and social function for a minimum of 6 months; and four of the following symptoms must also be present: sleep disturbance (usually hypersomnia), impaired concentration, muscle pain, multijoint pains, headaches, post-exertional exacerbation of fatigue, sore throat and tender lymph nodes.[17]

'ME' or 'CFS' is now thought to be a condition of 'multifactorial aetiology' and a viral illness figures high on the list of causes or precipitating factors. Perhaps this view is conditioned by the fact that the Royal Free Hospital outbreak in 1955, was thought to have followed a viral (perhaps Coxsackie) infection. The other possible causes of the condition are psychological causes, stress, certain personality traits and cerebral biochemical abnormalities.

There is no specific laboratory test, so the diagnosis of CFS is made on clinical grounds. However, it must be remembered that the symptoms of CFS can be the early ones of serious disease, so that all individuals presenting thus, especially the articulate ones with a self-diagnosis, require a detailed history and a full clinical examination, with some base-line investigations. These are not to 'confirm' the presence of CFS, but to attempt to exclude serious disease. All persons deserve a FBC and ESR, urea and electrolytes, thyroid function tests, blood sugar and urinalysis, initially.

Programmes of continuous and graded realistic exercise and cognitive behavioural therapy, as opposed to rest, seem to be favoured at present, for adults. (June 1997, Ed)[18] Marcovitch claims that experience suggests that a similar result would be likely with children. Also, he has suggested that a good way of managing children with the condition is to have case discussions at school, with parents present, which can do a great deal to ensure that all parties work together, even if, as he says, 'they have differing perceptions of the underlying problem'.[19]

Patients and their parents require full explanations of the illness and a sympathetic consideration of their worries, which may include accusations of malingering. It is also helpful if the patient can keep a diary of symptoms and their changes, so that these can be discussed in the meeting with parents and teachers, thereby affording the patient more support.

Although there may be occasional anecdotal evidence to the contrary, drug therapy is not thought to be helpful.

A joint report of a working group of the Royal Colleges of Physicians, Psychiatrists and General Practitioners suggested that research should be directed to the management of the condition in children.[20] Further information can be obtained from the Director, The ME Association, PO Box No 8, Stanford-le-Hope, Essex. SS17 8EX. Also, a 14 page summary of the Report from the National Task Force on CFS, PVFS and ME, is available from Westcare, 155, Whiteladies Road, Clifton, Bristol BS8 2RF. Tel: 0117 923 9341, Fax 0117 923 9347. The full report, 137 pages, is available from the same address.

Psoriasis

Psoriasis is a common scaling condition of the skin. Different types run a chronic course of remissions and exacerbations. There is a constitutional factor and a peak incidence at puberty. Children can also develop guttate psoriasis following streptococcal sore throats.

Those who suffer from psoriasis often endure their symptoms for a long time before seeking advice. When they do so, it is because they are exasperated by the itching, embarrassed at showering or changing for games in front of their peers or perhaps they are upset about their perceived distortion of their body image. Lesions can occur on any part of the body but are frequently on the elbows and knees. Always remember to examine the nails for pitting and separation of the nail plate from the underlying nail bed, (oncholysis). Part of the reluctance of children to seek advice may be because of reports about the unaesthetic acceptability of some of the earlier topical skin preparations used for the condition.

The various local preparations of dithranol, in the form of dithrocream are helpful now, especially if treatment commences with the lower strengths, which can then be increased in the light of clinical progress. Initially, the dithrocream is applied direct to the plaque lesions and left in place for an hour before being washed off. As treatment progresses, the milder forms may be left on overnight.

An alternative is calcipotriol, or 'Dovonex' in cream or ointment form, which does not produce burning of the skin or staining of the clothes. No more than 100g should be used in a week and it should not be used on the face or in the flexures.

Steroid and antifungal preparations are needed for flexural psoriasis, e. g. between or under the breasts. Exposure to sunlight is helpful. Psoriasis of the scalp can be helped by a tar shampoo, tar pomade, calcipotriol scalp application and steroid scalp applications, eg. betamethasone. Genital or perineal psoriasis may be helped by an emollient preparation with occasional short courses of a local weak steroid preparation.

Pustular psoriasis, consisting of sheets of small pustules over most parts of the body, as distinct from the pustular dermatosis of palms and soles, is potentially fatal and requires urgent referral to a dermatology department.

Further information on The Psoriasis Association may be obtained from The National Secretary, Milton House, 7, Milton street, Northampton. NN2 7GJ. Tel:01604 711129.

Sleep Walking (Somnambulism)

This condition, often associated with talking in sleep (somniloquy) and performing purposeful acts in addition to walking, is known in children and adults. In the former it is considered to be part of the normal developmental pattern, in adults it is considered to be a hysterical manifestation, perhaps because of some chronic anxiety.

Though uncommon, the dangers in a school dormitory can be appreciated. If a child does show these tendencies, referral to a psychiatrist specialising in child or adolescent behaviour would be worth while in case there is any underlying anxiety which can be resolved. Practical management would consist of a common-sense assessment of the local situation by all members of staff likely to be involved.

The Testes

Conditions of the testes usually met with in schools include torsion, hydocele, varicocele and trauma to the testis, usually arising from games injuries.

Torsion of the testis
Definition and cause

Rotation if the testis on its horizontal axis leads to a twisting of the spermatic cord and impairment of the blood supply to the testis. Certain anatomical abnormalities, e. g. a horizontal lie of the testis, are thought to be predisposing factors. Torsion occurs most commonly in the prepubescent child and the adolescent. About half the cases occur during sleep, often in the early morning: the remainder during or shortly after severe physical exertion.

Diagnosis

The presenting symptom is acute pain, ranging from mild to excruciating, depending on the degree of torsion. The pain is usually scrotal, but may start in an iliac fossa, later radiating to the scrotum. There are no other early symptoms and signs except vomiting and shock in severe cases. Fever is a later sign. Dysuria is not a feature.

Sudden testicular pain in a school child should alert doctors, sanatorium staff and teachers to the possible diagnosis of testicular torsion. Only when this has been excluded by an experienced person, should alternative diagnoses be considered, the most likely one being that of mumps orchitis. Early diagnosis of torsion is vitally important. Unrelieved torsion of the spermatic cord and consequent impairment of the testicular blood supply lead to death of the testis. Few testes survive a torsion of more than 12 hours.

Treatment

Relief of the condition in its early stages is simple. Manual rotation is effective, and can be performed without analgesia, although occasionally, 10 mg of intravenous diazepam is helpful, as an analgesic and a relaxant. If the pain is very severe, pethidine may be required.

With the patient supine, the doctor, using both hands, gently rotates the testis, Correction of the torsion brings immediate relief: incorrect rotation increases the pain and discomfort, so that the doctor reverses the direction. Twists of less than 180 degrees reduce themselves spontaneously.

Although successful manipulative reduction removes the urgency of the situation, recurrence is likely and in order to prevent this, bilateral orchidopexy is indicated.

Torsion of the appendix testis, (hydatid of Morgagni) occurs less frequently. The pain may be severe. If the diagnosis is definite, the appendix testis will eventually atrophy. If there is any doubt however, then surgical exploration is advisable.

Trauma to the testes

The testes are vulnerable to injury, especially in cricket, contact sports, cadet training etc, for protective 'cages' are not always available or permitted. Traumatic orchitis or a haematoma may result. If severe, a surgical opinion should be sought. Otherwise, continued observation, rest, a suspensory bandage and analgesics would be indicated.

The Undescended Testes

In a full term male infant the testes should be in the scrotum at birth: a testis which has not attained this position is undescended. Scorer reported the incidence of undescended testes at birth to be 4%.[21] Descent continues during the first year of life, and at one year of age the incidence of non-descent is 0.8%. This compares well with the probable incidence in adulthood of 0.7%.

Clinically, there are five groups.

(a) The high scrotal testis: or incomplete descent. The testis never reaches the bottom of the scrotum, and always lies at a higher level than its (larger) normal fellow.

(b) The intracanalicular testis. This is very difficult, if not impossible to palpate. If palpable, it can be manipulated downwards but always resumes its intracanalicular position.

(c) The intra-abdominal testis which is impalpable, and is often very difficult to find at operation. Occasionally a so-called intra-abdominal (missing) testis is diagnosed mistakenly for an unnoticed perinatal torsion with subsequent atrophy of the testis.

(d) The arrested (ectopic) testis. This is not an undescended testis but a maldescended one. The testis passes normally through the inguinal canal, fails to enter the scrotum, usually ascending obliquely and upwards and laterally to lie in the superficial inguinal pouch. The importance of this sub-group is that the spermatic cord is of normal length so that surgical intervention is more successful than in the treatment of the other groups.

(e) There are other very rare sites where the testis is truly ectopic, e. g. perineum.

The retractile testis is most often diagnosed in cases of bilateral non-descent. Only careful and, if necessary, repeated examination eliminates unnecessary surgical intervention. The treatment of the undescended testis is surgical: the correct practice is to operate well before the age of 6 years.

Hydrocele

Primary hydrocele presents as an ovoid, irreducible painless swelling of variable size. It is very common in the perinatal period, and is produced by the dilatation of the lower end of of an incompletely closed processus vaginalis. Natural closure of the processus vaginalis is common in the first year of life. If the hydrocele persists, surgical intervention may be advisable.

Encysted hydrocele of the spermatic cord is less common than a primary hydrocele. It presents as a cystic swelling above the testis. It causes no trouble, but can be removed surgically.

Secondary hydrocele is not seen in childhood, but hydrocele may occur as a complication of mumps.

Varicocele

This is difficult to define. It is a varicose proliferation of the veins of the pampiniform plexus exceeding the 'norm' The left side is almost invariably affected. Right sided varicocele occurs only in the very rare cases of situs inversus totalis. Varicocele occasionally leads to diminution in the size of the homolateral testis, and may debar a candidate from service in the armed forces.

The only effective treatment is surgical, but this should not be undertaken lightly, as testicular atrophy may follow.

Urticaria

Urticaria (the 'Hives' or 'heat lumps,' 'weals' or 'nettle rash') is a common skin condition, usually short lived, which may be of rapid onset and characterised by raised itchy lesions of the skin of any part of the body, which may be discrete or confluent, in which case it is called giant urticaria. Often the urticaria is deeper, involving predominantly the eyelids, tongue and lips in which case the condition is called angio-edema. Urticaria and angio-edema are allergic skin conditions, due to the release of histamine. There are several causes, eg. hot or cold water baths (respectively cholinergic or cold urticaria), exercise, certain drugs, e.g. penicillin products, certain foods or food additives (see under anaphylaxis earlier in this chapter), insect bites or stings. Often extensive investigation will fail to disclose the responsible allergen.

Often, no treatment is required, and local antihistamine preparations are not advised because of the risk of skin sensitisation. If therapy is required, then a low sedating oral antihistamine preparation is probably the best, but consult the manufacturers data sheets for information regarding contraindications and possible interactions with other drugs. Chronic urticaria is unusual in children.

Occasionally, an allergen will produce anaphylactic shock and details of how to manage this dangerous condition are given earlier in this chapter and in Chapter 4.

Vaginal Discharge

This may occur at any age. In the very young it suggests an infection and should be investigated.

Some of the causes could be due to threadworms, foreign bodies or trauma, including sexual abuse. (See Chapters 7 and 8).

Late prepubescent girls often go through a phase of having extra vaginal secretion, sufficient to soil underclothes. This is part of normal development and can be ignored unless it is causing soreness or irritation. Imminently pubescent girls may have a mucoid discharge leaving brown staining, which is occasionally mistaken for blood.

Infective discharges are not uncommon amongst older school girls, the most prevalent being monilia, trichomonas vaginalis and chlamydia, but gonorrhoea should always be remembered. A high vaginal swab should be taken and sent to the laboratory without delay. If a sexually transmitted discharge is suspected, then a prompt referral to an STD clinic is required. Urinalysis should be undertaken, especially in the case of a monilial discharge. The girl may be taking oral contraceptives or have a family history of diabetes. A forgotten tampon has been mentioned in an earlier chapter.

Warts

Warts do seem to occupy a great deal of time and it should be explained that they are caused by various types of the human papilloma virus, which have entered the body via a breach in the skin surface. As immunity to them develops, they will eventually disappear, so that ordinarily, they should be left alone especially if they are asymptomatic. Children with genital warts should be referred to an STD clinic.

Plane warts on fingers may be subjected to repeated trauma and may require treatment because of recurrent pain or discomfort. They are no different histologically from verrucae, or plantar warts, which can again be painful if they are traumatised by the under surfaces of the os calcis or meta tarsal heads. There is no lack of choice of local remedies, usually keratolytic agents, but they must be used with care so as not to damage the surrounding skin. During treatment, it is usual to pare down the wart with an emery board on alternate days. Resistant cases may require, cautery, curettage or even liquid nitrogen.

In 1978, MOSA, reviewed the management of plantar warts and recommended that barefoot activities, including swimming, should be unrestricted. This view still obtains.[22]

References

1. Buxton P. K. (1990) 'Acne and Rosacea ' in *ABC of Dermatology* p 40 ISBN 07279 0220 2 BMA Publications, Tavistock Square, London WC1H 9JR.

2. Warner, J. O., Gotz, M., Landau, L. I., Milner, A. D., Pedersen, S., and Silverman, M. (1989) Management of Asthma: A consensus statement. *Arch. Dis. Child.*, 64. 1065.

3. The British Guidelines on Asthma Management. 1995 Review and Position Statement. (1997) *Thorax*. volume 52. Supplement 1

4. Klein, R. G. (1995) The Role of methyl phenidate in psychiatry. *Arch. Gen. Psychiat.* 52. 429.

5. Gill, G. V., Redmond, S. (1993) Insulin treatment, Time Zones and Air Travel: a survey of current advice from British Diabetic Clinics. *Diabetic Medicine*, 10: 764.

6. Meadow, S. R. (1977) How to use buzzer alarms to cure bedwetting. *Br. Med. J.* 2: 103.

7.   Brooks, D., Mallik, N. ((1982) Urology and Renal Médicine. *Library of General Practice.* Chapter3. Churchill Livingstone . Edinburgh.

8.   Cook, N. (1989) Behaviour problems in childhood in Hart, C., and Bain, J. (eds) Chapter 44. p428. *Child Care in General Practice.* 3rd. Edition. Churchill Livingstone, Edinburgh.

9.   Chadwick, D. (1990) Diagnosis of epilepsy. in Epilepsy: A Lancet Review (Epilepsy Octet.) Vol 336 No 8714. page 15.

10.   Meadow, S. R. (1982) Munchausen syndrome by proxy and pseudo epilepsy. *Arch. Dis. Child.* 57: 811

11.   Jeavons, P. M. (1977) Choice of drug therapy in epilepsy. *The Practitioner*, 219 :542.

12   Betts, T. A. (1990) Pseudoseizures: seizures that are not epilepsy. in Epilepsy: A Lancet Review (Epilepsy Octet.) Vol 336 No 8714. page 8

13.   McMorris S, McWilliam, P. K. A. (1969) Status epilepticus in infants and young children treated with parenteral diazepam. *Arch. Dis. child.* 44: 604.

14   Harding, G., F., A. (1997) Four possible explanations exist (for visual field restriction associated with vigabatrin) Letter. *Br. Med. J.* 314: 1694.

15.   Murphy, J. J., Heptinstall, S., Mitchell, J. R. A. (1988) Randomised double blind placebo controlled trial of feverfew in migraine prevention. *Lancet* 2 :189

16.   David, T. J., Parris, M. R., Poynor, M, Hawnaur, T., Simm, S., Rigg, E. and McCrae, F. (1983) Reasons for late detection of hip dislocation in childhood. *Lancet* 2: 147.

17.   Cleare, A. J., Wessely, S (1996). Chronic Fatigue Syndrome: an update. '*Update*'. 14th August 1996. p 61

18   Fulcher, K. Y., White, P. D. (1997) Randomised controlled trial of graded exercise in patients with the chronic fatigue syndrome. *Br. Med. J.* 314: 1647.

19.   Marcovich, H. (1997) Managing chronic fatigue syndrome in children – Liaise with the family and teachers to keep morale high and minimise disability. Editorial *Br. Med. J.* 314: 1635.

20.   Chronic fatigue syndrome. Report of the joint working group of the Royal Colleges of Physicians, Psychiatrists and General Practitioners. London: RCP. 1996. (CR 54).

21.   Scorer, C. G., (1956) The incidence of incomplete descent of the testicle at birth. *Arch. Dis. child.*, 31, 198.

22.   Medical Officers of Schools Association (1978) Proceedings and Report No 26. (1978-79) London.

Further Reading

Davies, S. C. and Wonke, B. (1991) The Management of Haemoglobinopathies. In Paediatric Haematology . eds. Hann, I. M. and Gibson. B. E. S. *Clinical Haematology.* Vol 4(2) p369 Balliere. Tindall.

Serjeant, G. R. (1992) *Sickle Cell Disease.* 2nd. edn. Oxford University Press.

Oni, L., Dick, M., Smalling, B and Walters, J. (1997) *Caring for Your Child with Sickle Cell Disease: A Parents' Guide.* Publisher. Brent Sickle Cell and Thalassaemia Centre, 122, High Street, Harlesden, London NW10 4SP. Tel: 0181 961 9005

Br. Med. J. (1990) Editorial Allergy to peanuts 300: 1354

ibid Anaphylaxis induced by peanuts. Four cases (two fatal) reported from University College Hospital London. p 1377

ibid Vegetableburger allergy p. 1378

Br. Med. J. (1990) Allergy to peanuts (Letter). 300: 1726.

Br. Med. J. 1990) Allergy to peanuts (Letter). 301: 120.

Br. Med. J. (1995) Treatment of acute anaphylaxis, 311: 731

Br. Med. J. (1996) Managing peanut allergy. 312: 1050

ibid Clinical study of peanut and nut allergy in 62 consecutive patients: new features and associations. . 312: 1074.

Mumford, C. J., Warlow, C., P. (1995) Airline policy relating to passengers with epilepsy. *Arch Neurol.* 52: 1215.

Train, A (1996) ADHD *How to deal with VERY DIFFICULT CHILDREN* ISBN 0 285 63311 2 Souvenir Press (Educational and Academic) Ltd., 43, Great Russell Street, London WC1B 3PA

CHAPTER 7

SCHOOLCHILD ABUSE

Please note that this chapter should be read in conjunction with the next chapter on Child Protection Policies and The Children Act.

The school medical officer is likely to encounter at least one case of serious child abuse. The initial information, which must be taken seriously by the person to whom the information is given, may not necessarily come from the victim. Instead, the allegation of wrong doing may be brought to the doctor's attention by another person, e. g. teacher, parent, fellow pupil or friend. Often there are circumstances or events which a sensitive observer will recognise as being at variance with the child's usual behaviour and demeanour.

Although they may have innocent explanations, the following examples could arouse suspicions of child abuse:

The child who does not want to go home after school.

The child who does not want to return from holidays.

The child who runs away from home.

The child whose school work shows a rapid and inexplicable deterioration.

The child who suddenly suffers from a deterioration of bowel or bladder control.

The child who, uncharacteristically, commences to seek attention or affection, or to display inappropriate behaviour, perhaps of a sexual nature, e.g. exposure, coquettishness or sexually explicit language.

The child who is moody, silent or withdrawn or who starts to indulge in anti-social behaviour, especially if of recent origin.

The child who complains of recurrent abdominal pain or of recurrent headaches.

This list, of course, is necessarily incomplete.

All doctors should read and understand their local Child Protection Procedures. These are based on 'Working Together Under the Children Act 1989'. Doctors should also read the addendum to 'Working Together, Child Protection: Medical Responsibilities.'

Suspected child protection concerns should be discussed with the local Social Services Department immediately. Further advice can be obtained from the local Consultant Paediatrician who is the designated Doctor for Child Protection.

In an emergency, medical examination will be required but usually, discussion with Social Services should precede any examination. If informed consent is needed before any examination is performed, it may be more appropriate for a paediatrician to carry out this examination. A paediatrician and an experienced police surgeon will be involved in cases of suspected sexual abuse. A careful, legible, written record should be made as soon as possible after the examination. Evidence may need to be given in a Family Proceedings Court or a Criminal Court.

Social Services take the lead responsibility for investigation of suspected child abuse. They will advise the head and the school doctor about liaison with the child's parents, etc.

All doctors should read the local Child Protection Committee Procedures carefully and follow them. These will include detailed sections concerning recognition and referral of child abuse, including indicators of the various types of abuse. Special advice will be included concerning abuse within a residential setting and its investigation. The advice of the doctor's Medical Defence Union should be sought in serious cases.

During the past ten years the sexual abuse of children, both inside and outside the family, has been given very wide publicity. Undoubtedly, many more disclosures are being made than ever before. However, it is certain that the physical abuse and the emotional deprivation which accompanies it, is as widespread as ever, but now it is recognised. In schools the virtual abolition of formal corporal punishment has reduced the incidence of physical injury with a consequential steep fall in the litigation brought by parents against teachers for assault and bodily harm. Nevertheless, non-accidental injury to school children remains commonplace. Behind the violent acts may be the illicit use of alcohol and drugs by the perpetrator. The development of child pornography has added a new and dangerous dimension to child sexual abuse. Common bullying and mobbing are unlikely to disappear from schools.

The Long Term and Delayed Effects of Child Abuse

Abusers seldom, if ever, volunteer evidence about their violent or deviant behaviour. As a rule, they take extravagant steps to conceal their crimes and 'cover their tracks'. Abused children may be threatened or bribed by the abusers. Small children will tolerate physical violence or sexual abuse for many months, even years.

The Minnesota studies in the 1970s demonstrated clearly that sexual abuse of children occurred as commonly as physical abuse.[1,2] These important and revealing investigations showed that incest existed at all social levels. Many of those parents were outwardly respectable, professional people and church attenders. The sexually abusive family is united by very strong, though pathological bonds. In 60% of the Minnesota cases, the sexual abuser was the father: 39% were stepfathers or males functioning in the role of father. Sometimes, the wife or the mother colludes.

The possible outcomes for the child later in life are nearly always damaging. Young women may become promiscuous, resort to prostitution or develop a profound aversion to sexual activity. Marital breakdown is common as is drug dependency. Alcoholism and suicide may be other serious consequences of abuse.

Most authorities now accept that many abused children become abusing parents. Violence begets violence. For this reason alone, the earliest detection of child abuse is of paramount importance.

A Family Division Judge spelt out very clearly the guidelines which must be followed during the investigation of the possibility that small children had been abused. He said that the Cleveland Report should be the required reading for all doctors.[6] This advised doctors and barristers to listen to but not to take literally every detail of a child's story. He went on to say that every interviewer 'should be experienced in talking to children.' The school medical officer surely fulfils this judicial criterion.

The Children Act 1989

This Act came into operation in October 1991 and it replaces most of the pre-existing legislation. The Act aims to protect children from harm that may arise from within the family's life. The welfare of the child is paramount and no action must be taken unless that child benefits in a positive sense.

The Children Act (1989) does not diminish police powers to investigate alleged crime. The Act gives local authorities statutory duties to conduct investigations where:

1. A request is made by a court in family proceedings.

2. Where a child is subject to an emergency protection order.

3. Where a child is taken into police protection.

4. Where there is reasonable cause to suspect that a child is suffering (or likely to suffer) significant harm.

5. When directed by the court on the discharge of an education supervision order.

6. When notified by the local education authority that the child, who is the subject of an education supervision order, persistently fails to comply with directions.

Legal orders may be sought by the local authority.

A child of sufficient understanding to make an informed decision may refuse to submit to a medical or a psychiatric examination or other assessment ordered under the Act.

No court may make an order unless making the order would be better for the child than making no order at all. For the purposes of the Children Act, a child is defined as a person under the age of 18 years.

Under the Act, harm is defined as ill-treatment or the impairment of health or development. Development means physical, intellectual, emotional, social or behavioural development. Health includes both physical and mental health and ill-treatment includes sexual abuse and forms of ill-treatment which are not physical.

All doctors should read their local Child Protection Committee procedures carefully and follow them. These will include detailed sections concerning recognition and referral of child abuse including indicators for the various types of abuse.

References

1. Jacobson, V, (1978) *Observations on the long-term effects of incest on the woman.* Minneapolis: University of Minnesota Medical School.

2. James, H. (1975) *Little Victims.* New York. David McKay Company.

3. *Working Together under The Children Act 1989 – A Guide to Arrangements for Inter-Agency Co-operation for the Protection of Children from Abuse.* (HMSO published 1991).

4. *Child Protection: Medical Responsibilities. Addendum to Working Together under the Children Act 1989.* HMSO London.

5. Local Child Protection Committee Procedures. (Social Services).

6. *Report of the Enquiry into Child Abuse in Cleveland 1987.* London: (HMSO 1988). London.

7. *An Introduction to the Children Act 1989.* (HMSO).

8. *The Children Act – An Introductory Guide for the NHS 1989.* (Department of Health).

9. *Child Protection: Clarification of Arrangements Between the NHS and Other Agencies. Addendum to Working Together under the Children Act 1989.* (Department of Health, Welsh Office). HMSO London.

10. Riley, Diana. (Ed.) (1991) Sexual Abuse of Children: Understanding, Intervention and Prevention Radcliffe Medical Press, Oxford.

11. Physical Signs of Sexual Abuse in Children Second Edition (1997). *Report: Royal College of Physicians,* London.

12. Meadow, R. (Ed.) *ABC of Child Abuse* Third Edition. BMA Books. ISBN 07279 11066.

NB. It is important that this chapter should be read in connection with the following chapter on Child Protection and the implementation of The Children Act, with an illustrative example of a specimen school policy on child protection.

CHAPTER 8

CHILD PROTECTION POLICIES INCLUDING THE CHILDREN ACT

Please note. This chapter should be read in conjunction with chapter 7 on Child Abuse.

Introduction

From school bullying to non-accidental injury and proven child abuse, the school medical officer and the school nurse are likely to be involved, often from the initial reporting. Skills are needed in order to recognise abuse when faced with complicity to hide the true facts in a severe case, or in the exaggeration and fantasising which can take place in a young mind.

However, all schools should have bullying policies which identify a trained member of staff to whom reports can freely be made and who can lay down guidelines for dealing with bullying. These are usually based on:

- *education* of the bully and the victim, often in a peer group setting and in Personal and Social Education classes.

- *behaviour modification* for the bully and the victim.

- *support* for the bully and the victim.

All schools should have been inspected under the Children Act (1989) and recommendations implemented.[1]

Most schools have sent identified members of the teaching, medical and boarding house staffs on training courses covering these emotive issues and when a case of abuse is suspected, the Child Protection Handbook for the area gives the guidance needed to:

- identify needs

- observe medical and judicial requirements

for the protection of the child. It should be referred to in all cases. A copy should be available in all schools and surgeries and is usually in loose leaf form so that it can be updated.

Child Protection

'The real numbers of abused children are not known but in 1992, 38,600 children were entered on child protection registers. 59% were between the ages of 5-15 years.

3.7% per 1,000 children aged 0-18 are on child protection registers.

Up to 85% of reported concern is investigated and up to 30% of referred children are registered.[2]

The Children Act (1989)

This Act came into operation in October 1991, replacing much of the preexisting legislation.

A number of important principles are embodied in the act...

- *the welfare of the child* is the *paramount* consideration in court proceedings;

- wherever possible, children should be brought up and cared for *within their own families*;

- children should be safe and *protected* by effective intervention if they are in *danger*;

- when dealing with children, courts should ensure that *delay is avoided*, and may only make an *order* if to do so is *better than* making *no order at all*;

- *children* should be kept informed about what happens to them, and should *participate* when decisions are made about their future;

- parents continue to have *parental responsibility* for their children, even when their children are no longer living with them. They should be kept informed about their children and participate when decisions are made about their future;

- parents with *children in need* should be helped to bring up the children themselves;

- this help should be provided as a service to the child and his family, and should;

+ be provided in *partnership* with the parents;

+ meet each child's *identified* needs;

+ be appropriate to each child's *race, culture, religion and language*;

+ be open to effective independent representations and *complaints procedures*;

and

+ draw upon *effective partnership between the local authority and other agencies*, including voluntary agencies.

Every area of the country has its own.

CHILD PROTECTION HANDBOOK

The guidelines may vary from area to area but have been developed by the Area Child Protection Committee and they set expectations about the way professionals should approach their responsibilities and draw attention to the considerations needed before making judgments.

General Guidelines include;

Definitions
Stages of intervention
Who is involved and what to do
Recognition
Investigation
Child Protection Conferences
Child protection Register
Comprehensive Assessment and Planning
Implementation and Reviews
Case Reviews
Child Protection Committee

Definition of child abuse

Children may be harmed by a parent, a relative, a sibling, a carer, (i. e. persons who, while not parents are looking after a child, such as a foster parent, a staff member in a residential home), an acquaintance or a stranger. The harm may be the result of a direct act or by a failure to act to provide proper care, or both.

Neglect:

The persistent or severe neglect of a child, or the failure to protect a child from exposure to any kind of danger, including cold or starvation, or extreme failure to carry out important aspects of care resulting in the significant impairment of the child's health or development, including non-organic failure to thrive.

Physical injury:

Including actual or likely physical injury to a child, or failure to prevent physical injury (or suffering) to a child including deliberate poisoning, suffocation and Munchausen's syndrome by proxy.

Sexual abuse:

Including actual or likely sexual exploitation of a child or adolescent. The child may be dependent and/or developmentally immature.

Emotional abuse

Including actual or likely severe adverse effects on the emotional and behavioural development of a child caused by persistent or severe emotional ill-treatment or rejection. All abuse involves some emotional ill-treatment. This category should be used where it is the main cause of abuse.

These categories for child protection register purposes do not tie in precisely with the definition of 'significant harm' in section 31 of The Children Act which will be relevant if court proceedings are initiated. For example, with a case of neglect it will be necessary to consider whether it involves actual or likely 'significant harm', and whether it involves 'ill-treatment' or 'impairment of health or development' (in each case as defined by the Act.) The Courts may well provide an interpretation of sexual abuse (which is not defined in the Act) which is different from that used above in particular cases, in which case their definition should be used in relation to those cases.

Recognition

The school, GP and nurses who are monitoring child health have a vital role to play in the protection of children and with any other members of the primary health care team they are well-placed to identify early stage family stress, which can lead to abuse or to recognise significant harm or likelihood of significant harm. They will usually make a vital contribution to child protection conferences and long-term support for the child and family. Child abuse may present in many ways and there is often considerable overlap with other conditions. However, the diagnosis cannot be made unless it is first thought of! The various 'forms' of child abuse are not mutually exclusive and any child thought to be abused should be examined with *all types in mind, and it must be remembered that abuse can take place in any class of society.*

Reporting

When it is suspected that a child may be at risk it is essential that the information is shared with the statutory services responsible for child protection within the time limits laid down by that particular Area Child Protection Committee.

The duty is clear: *if you suspect child abuse, take action but not alone.*

The agencies and independent practitioners concerned with child abuse may include identified members of:

Social Services Departments
District/Area Health Authorities
Health Services
Education Authority and Schools
Police
NSPCC
Other Voluntary Organisations (Where relevant.)
The Armed Forces (Where relevant.)

The Joint Working Party on Medical Confidentiality and Child Protection has stated – 'Professional expertise and judgment are pivotal to decision making in child protection, including the child protection conference, and it is essential that a medical contribution is made at all stages. Multidisciplinary work is essential for the proper protection of children. Doctors have a responsibility to participate fully in all aspects of child protection.'

It is thought that only very rarely will medical confidentiality override the need to protect children.

GUIDELINES

These are given for individual agencies including:

Doctors   )
) SPECIMENS SHOWN
Nurses   )

GENERAL PRACTITIONERS

1. In many cases of suspected child abuse, the child may be seen by a doctor who has not had specialist training in this area. All cases which arouse suspicion need to be considered carefully. Other professionals already involved with the child and family should be asked if they can give additional helpful information, e. g. health visitors, school nurse, social worker, district nurse, teacher. When there is a strong suspicion about child abuse then a referral to Social Services, Police or NSPCC should be made without delay.

2. The doctor's duty is to take a careful medical and social history. Careful consideration should be given to previous incidents including those initially thought to have been accidental. It is essential that *a full general examination is made since injuries may be concealed by clothing*. Depending on the history, and the age and distress of the child, a visual inspection of the genital area may be made. The child and the parents should be aware of the position regarding consent to medical examination. (See below, under 6.)

3. If the child is not known to the GP a check should be made with:-

   (i)   the Child Protection Register

   (ii) the local Social Services office

4. After assessment, referral to a specialist Paediatric Unit for further investigation may be advisable, even though the injuries appear trivial.

5. Any GP who is concerned about the condition of a child due to abuse may ask for a case conference to be arranged.

6. For a full *forensic* examination, such as described above, it is necessary to obtain written informed consent. A child over 16 years can give consent in most cases but consent to the examination of a minor must be given by a parent (or guardian), a teacher when in *loco parentis*, or by a social worker when the child is 'in care'. A chaperon should be present and must be of the same gender as the examinee. When the clinical findings are of crucial visual significance then line drawings and photographs become a valuable aid and may be used as exhibits in Court.

A full medical, social and family history must be taken and recorded. A school medical officer may hold a record on file (or computer) about the victim but this will require updating and revision in the light of the allegations. Careful note-taking and a record of all the positive and negative clinical findings must be made. A full clinical examination is imperative. The restriction of the examination to the site of the injury or to one part of the body, is bound to be misleading. A meticulous examination of the mouth, breasts and ano-genital tracts is essential in all cases of child sexual abuse. All abnormalities discovered, relevant or not must be listed. All wounds, bruises, and marks must be described and measured. When appropriate, X-rays should be included and blood and urine samples taken. A pregnancy test may be required. In sexual offences swabs must be taken from the mouth, the nipples, the penis, the vagina, the perineum and the anus. Head and pubic hair and nail clippings must be collected. The careful and experienced physician may choose to use a hand-lens, a proctoscope, a vaginoscope, or Glaister-Keen illuminated globes to inspect the introitus and hymen, where very tiny lesions can only be seen with some form of magnification and extra illumination.

At the end of the examination the doctor may have reached certain conclusions which can always be revised or modified when the laboratory results or the radiograph reports arrive. In the case of teenage girl victims the prescription of post-coital 'pills' will have to be considered seriously when un protected vagino-receptive coitus has occurred.

Cooperation with other professionals dealing with abuse is *essential*. This includes attendance at initial case conferences which should be given high priority. If this is not possible, then a written report should be submitted for inclusion in the conference.

GPs should acquaint themselves with publications already issued, namely:

(i) Working Together	)	published by
	)	The
(ii) Diagnosis of Child	)	Department of
Sexual Abuse	)	Health.

A further book – The Medical Aspects of Child Abuse – published by the Childrens' Research Fund, may be helpful.

Subsequently, GPs must ensure that they receive minutes of the conference and have a duty to keep themselves updated.

NURSING STAFF

Nurses have a vital role to play in the process of identifying and monitoring vulnerable children and the subsequent support to families. The Social Services Department has the statutory responsibility to investigate all cases of child abuse. The action to be taken by nursing staff will depend on the level of concern.

Where there is clear evidence of abuse:

1. Seek medical attention for any of the child's injuries needing it.

2. Inform /discuss with relevant staff (GP or hospital doctor).

3. Inform /discuss with identified member of school staff.

4. Ensure the Social Services Department is informed. Nurses will normally do this in conjunction with their GP. In evaluating concern it is useful to check the Child Protection Register.

5. If the child is in school or other day care, then the person **in loco parentis** (i.e. headteacher, identified staff member) must be informed of the situation.

6. All referrals to the Social Services must be confirmed in writing within 24 hours.

Where there are suspicions about abuse but no clear evidence:
1. The presenting signs/symptoms must be carefully observed and a history taken in a non-judgmental way.

2. Relevant medical staff (GP or hospital doctor) must be informed of the concerns.

3. The suspicions should be re-evaluated and the Social Services Department consulted unless a well-founded alleviation of concerns leads to no further action or a watching brief being kept.

In All Situations
1. Departmental reports should be written within 24 hours. They should contain a concise, factual account of any action taken, including dates and times. They must be signed.

2. Nurses and doctors should adhere to the following basic principles when listening to a child's account.

i) Listen to the child rather than directly question him or her.

ii) Never stop a child who is freely recalling significant events.

iii) Make a note of the discussion, taking care to record the timing, setting and personnel present, as well as what was said.

iv) Record all subsequent events up to the time of the substantive interview by Social Services or the Police.

3. Provide appropriate assistance to the investigation, e. g. accompanying child during medical examination, working with other agencies and helping the family.

4. Prepare for any subsequent case conference. This will involve a full appraisal of all relevant nursing records and the preparation of a report to distribute to the members of the case conference. Legal advice, if required, will be sought.

The interests of the child are paramount and successful protection of children is dependent on professional staff exchanging relevant information.

Professional codes of confidentiality are important but must not work against the protection of the child.

CONCLUSION

'Most authorities now accept that many abused children become abusing parents. Violence begets violence. For this reason alone the earliest detection of child abuse is of paramount importance'.[4]

The aims of child protection are

• to minimise the emotional and physical disabilities which occur as a result of child abuse and to prevent recurrences.

- to provide a well-trained comprehensive service, available at all times, to respond to emergencies and to take part in an integrated plan for prevention, identification, follow up and management.[3]

'It is well established that good child protection work requires good inter-agency co-operation. It is important for all professionals to combine an open minded attitude to alleged concerns about a child with decisive action when this is clearly indicated. Intervention in a family, particularly if court action is necessary, will have major implications for them, even if the assessment eventually leads to a decision that no further action is required. Public confidence in the child protection system can only be maintained if a proper balance is struck, avoiding unnecessary intrusion in families while protecting children at risk of significant harm.'[5]

References

1. *The Children Act* (1989) HMSO London. ISBN 010544

2. *Health Needs of School Age Children* (1995). P77. British Paediatric Association. Now the Royal College of Paediatrics and Child Health.

3. *Ibid.*

4. *Handbook of School Health* (1992) p103, Trentham Books Ltd. 17th Ed. ISBN: 0 948080 66 3

5. *Working Together* (1991) HMSO London. ISBN 1113214723

6. Lawrenson, F. (1997) Runaway children: whose problem? A history of running away should be taken seriously: it may indicate abuse. *Brit. Med J.* (Editorial), 314. 1064.

CHECK LIST

ALLEGATION/ OBSERVATION	made by?
	when?
	how?
	to whom?
ACTION TAKEN	by whom?
	type of action?
CHILD SEEN	when?
	by whom?
	parents seen?
	have all other children in the household been seen?

CONSULTATION WITH

Medical Authorities:
General Practitioner?
Health Visitor?
Paediatrician?
Child Psychiatrist?
Social Services:
Area Team?
Hospital Team?
Residential /Day Care?
Child Protection Register?
Local Authority Solicitor
NSPCC?
Police
Joint investigation?
Probation?
Education:
Educational Psychologist?
Other (specify)

MEDICAL EXAMINATION	when?
	where
	by whom?
NOTIFICATION	have all relevant agencies been notified?
RECORDING	have all telephone conversations been confirmed in writing?
CASE CONFERENCE	date?

MILLFIELD PREPARATORY SCHOOL GLASTONBURY
POLICY ON CHILD PROTECTION

I. INTRODUCTION:

A   All members of the school staff should be alert to the possible signs of abuse of a pupil. Abuse may take several forms, which are not mutually exclusive.

> *Physical abuse* results from acts or omissions by others which cause injury to the child. Bruises, burns, scalds and abrasions should be of concern to staff.

> *Neglect* involves not providing the basic necessities: food, warmth, shelter, caring, supervision or reasonable cleanliness.

> *Emotional Abuse*, which is harder to detect or define, may result from locking the child away, excessive shouting, teasing or humiliation, the denial of love, affection, interest or friendship, or overprotection so as to deny the child the normal experiences of life.

> *Sexual Abuse* is the involvement of emotionally immature young people in sexual activity with an adult or significantly older person, to which they cannot give informed consent or which breaks social taboos. It is more common than was previously believed and can have serious long-term damaging effects on the victim.

There will be other circumstances, not amounting to abuse, which give cause for serious concern about the welfare of pupils. Questions of the young persons being in moral danger, being uncared for, engaging in anti-social or inappropriate behaviour and so on may be referred on to the Headmaster, and through him to the Social Services Department.

B DESIGNATED MEMBER OF STAFF:

This member of staff liaises with the outside agencies in cases of suspected abuse, and can advise on the appropriate procedures. The Designated Member of Staff for child protection and welfare is currently Mr/Mrs/Miss/ Ms...........................

Staff have an obligation to report all suspicions of abuse either to the Designated Member of Staff, the School Doctor, or to the Headmaster, and to the Houseparent of the pupil concerned.

It then becomes the responsibility of the Designated Member of Staff, working with the Headmaster, to pass these concerns on to the Social Services.

This is an inescapable personal and professional responsibility for the protection of children from harm.

2. PROCEDURES

(i) **Cases where abuse may have been inflicted by parents.**

(a) Suspicion or knowledge of abuse must be reported immediately to either the Head master or the Designated Member of Staff and to the Houseparent of the pupil concerned.

(b) Any adult to whom abuse is reported by a pupil has a duty to listen to the pupil, to provide reassurance, and subsequently record the pupil's statements. S/he must not press the pupil, ask probing questions or suggest answers. The situation will then be discussed with the Headmaster or the Designated Member of Staff. The Somerset Child Protection Handbook must be referred to at all stages.

(c) Expert diagnosis may be required quickly. The Headmaster or the Designated Member of staff will arrange this.

(ii) Cases where abuse may have been inflicted by staff.

If an allegation is made against a member of staff, there is an obvious need to act immediately and with the utmost discretion. The informant should be told that the matter will be referred in confidence to the appropriate people. This must be done, and the written record passed on the same day.

The circumstances should be kept strictly confidential until the Headmaster has been able to judge whether or not an allegation or concern indicates possible abuse. The next step is always to discuss the situation with the appropriate Social Services manager.

If it is decided that an investigation is indicated it is the responsibility of the Social Services manager to arrange a meeting to discuss how the next steps are handled. This would normally involve the police and preferably a member of the governing body of the school and the Headmaster.

The arrangements agreed upon will include informing the parents and seeking their consent for any immediate medical examination.

S/he would normally be informed as soon as possible after the result of the initial investigation is known, or the decision is made to dispense with one, but not invited to make a response. There should be a warning that anything said will be recorded.

If it is established that the allegation is not well founded, either on the basis of medical evidence or further statements, then the person against whom the complaint has been made would normally be informed that the matter is closed.

If the police decide to take the matter further and the allegation is against a member of staff, he or she should normally be suspended or, where the circumstances are considered to warrant it, dismissed. It is reasonable to ask the police to give some indication of the time scale. There have been cases where the period of suspension has been unacceptably long.

January 1996.

NB: This Policy on Child Protection is currently in place at Millfield Preparatory School, Glastonbury, Somerset and is reproduced here, by kind permission of the Headmaster, Mr Simon Cummins.

CHAPTER 9

SPORTS INJURIES AT SCHOOL

Throughout this chapter, where the term 'sportsman' is used, the reference should be understood as being to persons of either sex who play sport. Where physiological differences between the sexes are under discussion, the context will make it clear.

Introduction

The attitude to sport at school has changed in the last few years. Too often, games and PE were competitive, team-based and slanted to those who already had sporting ability. Ridicule and misery were often the lot of the rest. So, the fit got fitter and the fat got fatter.

Now, public appreciation of the benefits of exercise is widespread and the 'Sport for All' movement has convinced many who would never have seen themselves as sportsmen that regular exercise can be enjoyable, relaxing and health-promoting.

Importance of Sport and PE

Training for sport enhances:

> Strength
> Speed
> Endurance
> Flexibility
> Skill

All these can be measured objectively, to some extent. In addition, team sports encourage team working and foster leadership skills.

The National Curriculum

The National Curriculum imposes the following General Requirements for Physical Education for Key Stages 1-4 (Ages 5-16 years).

1. To promote physical activity and healthy lifestyles, pupils should be taught:

    a   to be physically active

    b   to adopt the best possible posture and appropriate use of the body c   to engage in activities that develop cardiovascular health, flexibility, muscular strength and endurance

d   the increasing need for personal hygiene in relation to vigorous physical activity

2.   To develop positive attitudes, pupils should be taught

a   to observe the conventions of fair play, honest competition and good sporting behaviour as individual participants, team members and spectators.

b   how to cope with success and limitations in performance

c   to try hard to consolidate their performances

d   to be mindful of others and the environment.

3.   To ensure safe practice, pupils should be taught

a   to respond readily to instructions

b   to recognise and follow relevant rules, laws, codes, etiquette and safety procedures for different activities or events, in practice and during competition.

c   about the safety risks of wearing inappropriate clothing, footwear and jewellery, and why particular clothing, footwear and protection are worn for different activities.

d   how to lift, carry, place and use equipment safely.

e   to warm up for, and recover from exercise.

Risk of Injury: a necessary consequence

All vigorous exercise involves the risk of overuse or self-injury and most sports carry their own particular risks. It is important that the safety requirements of an activity are explained to new participants and any inherent dangers pointed out to them. Certain sports, for example SCUBA diving, carry risks which necessarily exclude some (in this case some people suffering from asthma, but see later.) who would be quite able to take part in other activities.

Disability and Illness

Great ingenuity has been shown in adapting sporting events so that those with disabilities can take part.

Incidence

Accurate data on the incidence of injury in different sports are hard to come by and difficult to compare. Difficulties arise in deciding what to classify as a significant injury. MOSA Members are collaborating in a cohort study led by Dr. Elizabeth Haworth, Consultant Public Health Physician, Berkshire Health Authority. In that study significant injuries are those requiring treatment in or at hospital, or at least three clinical consultations.

Anecdotal and published figures agree that Rugby Football causes more injuries than any other team sport, though the reported incidence varies from

30 to 200 injuries per 10,000 player-hours. As might be expected, contact sports carry the most serious risk of injury, followed by cricket, cycling, fencing and judo. Combat sports such as boxing and judo have a low incidence of injury, but those that do occur tend to be more serious. The cumulative effect of boxing on the brain makes it a supremely unsuitable sport for schools.

Every sport will have characteristics tending to produce particular types of injury. Some common or important associations are shown in Table 1.

Table 1: Typical Injuries associated with Sporting Activities

Sport	Injury
Running, Athletics	Overuse injury to lower limb, especially knee, ankle. Osgood-Schlatter's disease, compartment syndromes, stress fractures.
Boxing	Metacarpal fractures, head injury (acute and chronic), facial injuries.
Karate	Limb, head, face and trunk injuries.
Rugby Football	Superficial lacerations, cervical spine injury, limb injury, shoulder dislocation, clavicle fracture.
Hockey	Injury to face, eye, leg . Low back pain.
Squash	Eye injury.

Disability and Chronic Illness

Disabled pupils can take part in many sports on equal terms and with few or no adaptations, for example, swimming, riding and target events such as shooting or darts. In other cases, sports can be modified to allow participation, e. g. wheelchair basket ball. There are sports which have been specially developed for disabled people, such as a roll bar for the visually handicapped.

Diabetes Mellitus

Exercise reduces insulin requirements and promotes cardiovascular fitness, reducing the risk of complications such as ischaemic heart disease. Diabetics learn to avoid hypoglycaemia by reducing their insulin dose or taking extra carbohydrate before and during exercise.

Epilepsy

People with epilepsy should not take part in activities where a seizure would put themselves or others in danger. Thus, lone sports such as hang gliding are discouraged. SCUBA diving is forbidden. Caving and climbing, for example, present special risks. Many sports remain open, though, with the proviso that the person with epilepsy is accompanied by someone who will know what to do if they have a seizure.

Intercurrent Illness and Injury

The school doctor is frequently called upon to decide whether or not a pupil is fit enough to participate in games. In the author's experience, malingering is uncommon and it is always safest to start from the premise that one's patient is telling the truth. More often, keen pupils (or their coaches) will be pressing for them to continue playing in spite of illness or injury. In these circumstances, the school doctor must take a wider view. Rarely, if ever, will a pupil's future depend solely on the outcome of Saturday's match, however important it might seem at the time. Likewise, few pupils will eventually earn their livings as professional sportspersons. If there is any risk of long-term sequelae, they must be forbidden to play.

Viral illness is common at school, especially in the Autumn and the Winter terms. It must be borne in mind that heavy exercise in the presence of systemic infection carries a small but real risk of myocarditis or even sudden death on the field. Anyone with a febrile illness should be resting, not taking part in vigorous sport.

Sports Medicine as a speciality. Sports Clinics
Sports Physiotherapists
As a result of the burgeoning interest in exercise and the large amounts of money often involved in professional sport, Sports Medicine is now a sub-speciality in its own right. Many school doctors will find a nearby consultant colleague who professes an interest in treating sports injuries. Physiotherapists, too, often specialise in treating sportsmen. Usually, they practise privately and often attach themselves to a Leisure Centre or a Sports Complex. Links with such practitioners are well worth fostering. It is possible that they may be persuaded to provide a regular clinic at the school, to the benefit of both.

Resource, Courses and Qualifications.
There are many books on Sports Medicine and Sports Injuries, but they are of mixed quality. A selection, which has been found to be useful is listed, with comments, in the bibliography at the end of this chapter. The doctor interested in learning more about the subject will find courses in the medical journals, advertised from time to time.

Qualities of a School Doctor
A prudent school doctor will want to be confident that he has a sound know-ledge of:

- *First Aid and the immediate management of injury.* Even if not present at the time of injury, he will be called upon to advise members of staff who will be there, usually a sanatorium nurse or the sports dept. staff. He will want to know that their ideas on manage-ment agree with his own.

- *Basic Orthopaedics.* chiefly the recognition and management of sprains, fractures and soft tissue injuries.

- *The particular demands and risks of sports practised at his school,* so that he can advise pupils and staff knowledgeably.

In addition he will quickly find that a good working relationship with local consultants and physiotherapists both private and NHS, will pay dividends.

Prevention of Injury
Training, Safety
It is important that the safety requirements of an activity are explained to new participants and any inherent dangers spelled out. In some pursuits, for example climbing, caving and SCUBA diving, safety is the major component of the sport which has to be learnt by the newcomer.

Strength, Skills

Players who are unfit are more likely to be injured. A large part of any sport is learning how to avoid the risk of injury. A skilled horserider is less likely to fall or be thrown than a novice: a rugby team which has had adequate pre-season training is less likely to sustain injury in the scrum. All sportsmen should be taught the importance of warming-up and warming-down, with appropriate stretching exercises.

Protective Equipment

The school doctor should co-operate with trainers and coaches in insisting on the use of appropriate safety equipment. For some sports this is mandatory. Some examples relevant to schools are shown in Table 2.

Table 2: Protective Equipment for Sport

Riding	Hard hat
Rugby	Mouthguard, shin pads, gumshield.
Hockey	Shinpads, mouthguard.
Cycling	Helmet
Squash	Goggles
Cricket	Helmet, Abdominal protector.
Lacrosse	Mouthguard

Supervision, Refereeing, Selection of Teams and Matching

The rules of a game, and the manner in which they are enforced, can influence the injury toll. The Laws of Rugby Football Union have been amended with the aim of reducing the risk of injury in the set scrum and the ruck, and the introduction of different rules for younger players has helped to protect them from harm.

Adolescents of the same age can vary widely in size and strength. There is a danger of teams or individuals being inappropriately matched if they are selected by age rather than by size, skill or strength. The annual Old Boys' fixture presents a special risk in this regard.

Management of Sports Injuries

A distinguished American orthopaedic surgeon with a special interest in knee injuries insisted that personal observation of the mechanism of the injury was vital for accurate diagnosis. For that reason, no doubt, he felt obliged to be present at all of the fixtures of his favourite team, to whom he was honorary specialist. Most schools insist on the doctor's presence at First XV Rugby matches at least, though except in the rare cases of serious cervical spine injury or life-threatening collapse (and assuming in those cases that he is equipped with, and skilled in the use of, resuscitation equipment and neck immobilizers), it is unlikely that his physical presence will add anything vital to the management. Indeed, as has been mentioned before, injuries are more likely on the junior pitches.

Immediate and Early Management

The immediate management of soft tissue injuries, and indeed of suspected fractures, pending X-ray or definitive treatment, is shown in Table 3. The mnemonic RICE is often suggested, though it omits the element of chemical pain relief. ERICA suggests herself as an alternative.

Table 3: Principles of Early Management of Sports Injuries

Elevation	High arm sling for hand injury. Bed rest, leg elevation for leg and foot injury.
Rest	Off games.
	Sling (arm, hand), neighbour strapping (digit), strapping, plastering.
Ice	Cold packs, cold flannels.
	Never apply anything from a freezer or freezer compartment directly to the skin.
Compression	Tubigrip, crepe bandage.
Analgesia	Paracetamol, Co-codamol, NSAID.

This management is appropriate for the first 48-72 hours after trauma. During that time, bleeding, swelling and inflammatory changes occur. The aim of the ERICA manoeuvres is to minimise them. Cold relieves pain and reduces blood supply to the injured part, while compression and elevation oppose haemorrhage and extravasation of fluid.

Later Management – Rehabilitation and Return to Competition
As pain subsides, the priorities are:

- Preventing stiffness in injured joints and muscles.
- Maintaining cardiorespiratory fitness.
- Restoring strength in the injured part.
- Consideration of the cause of the injury, and attention to equipment and technique.
- Staged, gradual return to competition.

Anatomical Survey of Injuries and Common or Important Conditions
Head
Scalp lacerations
The scalp has a very good blood supply and scalp injuries usually heal well. The nerves enter the skin from below – for effective anaesthesia when suturing, the deeper layers of the scalp should be thoroughly infiltrated. The skull and brain are insensitive. A haematoma can mimic a depressed fracture.

For tiny lacerations where the skin edges appose easily, the new cyanoacrylate tissue glues are well worth a trial.

Skull fractures
Casualties who have been knocked out usually get a skull X-ray, but in assessing head injuries, the level of consciousness is more important than the presence or absence of a fracture. Indeed, it is the single most important observation. If the conscious level is deteriorating, urgent transfer to a neurosurgical unit and not to a casualty or an X-ray department is indicated.

Brain Injury
'The brain is a jelly in a steel box'. It can be bruised or lacerated by direct blows or by penetrating injuries. It can bang against the sides of its container, the skull (contre-coup injury). It can be compressed by bleeding or swelling,

even hours or days after the injury. An injured brain is at higher risk from further injury. Repeated injury can cause subtle, long-lasting, disabling damage. Thus, repeated head injuries have a cumulative effect, seen most clearly in the 'punch drunk' boxer. The object of restricting sporting activity after head injury is to avoid further trauma while a player may be less able to avoid it because of inco-ordination or slow reflexes as a result of the first blow.

Head Injury – Immediate Management

A player who falls to the ground after a blow to the head can continue playing if:

- he gets to his feet unaided and immediately, **and**

- he appears fully conscious and orientated.

He must leave the field for the rest of the game, and be admitted to the sanatorium for observation if:

- he is unable to get up for 10 seconds or more, **or**

- he appears confused or disorientated 2 minutes after the blow.

He must be transferred to hospital, preferably with a neurosurgical unit, **if**

- he is unconscious for 60 seconds or more, **or**

- he has retrograde amnesia (cannot remember the blow or the events leading up to it).

This should not be delayed to await the arrival of the doctor, nor to arrange transport: – dial 999 for an ambulance. If he is unconscious on the field, the game must stop and he should not be moved until the arrival of the ambulance personnel.

Late Management of Concussed Patient

Some neurological damage can be suffered even by those who have not lost consciousness. The 'Post-concussion Syndrome', comprising headaches, dizziness, irritability and difficulty in concentrating can persist for weeks or even months. The treatment is:

- Rest (lying down when the symptoms are bad).

- Simple analgesia (paracetamol)

- Reassurance that things will improve.

- Prevention of further injury (see above)

- Someone who has been unconscious for 60 seconds or more, or has post traumatic amnesia of 30 minutes or more, should not play contact sports for 3 weeks – this is the policy for Jockeys and of The Rugby Football Union, and relaxation of the ban would be indefensible if damage resulted.

- Someone who has had two minor episodes of loss of consciousness (10-60 secs) in the same season should not play contact sports for 4 weeks.

- With repeated episodes, however minor, if there has been definite loss of consciousness, or there are any post-concussional features, a complete ban on contact sport should seriously be considered. At this stage, it is best to consult with parents and get a neurological opinion.

Prevention of Head Injury

Representative measures of value in preventing head injury in various sports are listed in Table 4. It should be noted that the value of mouth guards is as much in minimising the effect of injury by reducing transmission of force to the cranial cavity from a blow to the chin as it is in guarding the teeth.

Table 4: Prevention of Sports Injuries

Protective headgear	Cycling, riding, climbing, motorcycling, (boxing)
Mouthguards	Rugby
Design of apparatus and floors	Playgrounds
Spectator control	Golf
Training and ethos	All sports
Rules, refereeing	Team, combat sports.

Face

Most school doctors will be confident to suture simple facial lacerations under local anaesthesia. Teenagers tend to produce rather exuberant scars, and it is worth mentioning this point before the blame for any disfigurement is laid at the doctor's door! Injuries to the inside of the mouth and pharynx heal very well, and rarely, if ever, require suturing. Frequent rinsing with warm water or a mouth wash should be advised.

Dental Injuries

As many as one in four children sustain some sort of injury to their front teeth.[1,2] Many of these injuries are caused by sport, and dental injuries have been reported to account for 40% of injuries sustained in contact sports.[3] Sparks recorded 157 cases of fractured teeth (3 per 10,000 player hours) in his 30 year survey of Rugby injuries.[4] A blow on the face sometimes knocks out an incisor tooth from the root without fracturing it.

Prevention

Fractures of the teeth can largely be prevented by mouth guards if they are properly fitted. This should only be done by a dental surgeon, but it is not available as an expense on the National Health Service. The cost could well be regarded as an insurance premium against the life-long discomfort and expense which may result from a dental fracture. Opinions differ about the cheaper mouthguards fitted by a nurse or a lay person, but it is likely that appliances bought over the counter are often not quite satisfactory. Mouth guards are recommended for all serious rugby and hockey players who are sufficiently well-motivated to wear them. This applies to younger as well as older players, although new guards will have to be fitted as the face grows.

The British Association for the Study of Community Dentistry have kindly advised as follows: 'Properly constructed mouthguards are recommended for those engaged in contact sports where there is a risk of injury to the mouth and teeth. EC regulations may mean that mouthguards may be considered to be personal protective equipment rather than medical devices and bear the CE mark. At the time of writing (February 1997, Ed.) these new arrangements are in transition but pupils and parents are advised to consult their dentist for advice on the most appropriate mouthguard, bearing in mind the developmental stage of their dentition and the frequency of exposure to risk from a sports injury. The use of mouthguards may also be appropriate in certain aspects of Combined Cadet Force training such as assault courses and self defence training.'

Management

All those concerned with contact sports should understand that if a permanent incisor tooth is knocked out completely it may well survive if promptly replaced in the socket. However, reinserting a tooth in this manner is NOT a suitable procedure for a child with a history of cardiac lesion(s) or cardiac surgery, who would normally require antibiotic prophylaxis for dental treatment.

Replanting an avulsed permanent tooth:
First Aid advice at the scene of the accident

If the tooth is clean:
- Push it gently back into the socket
- Seek dental advice

If the tooth is dirty:
- Rinse gently in milk or cold water then push the tooth back into the socket. If reimplantation is not possible:
- Place the tooth in milk, or in saliva (in the pupil's mouth)
- Go to a dentist immediately

DO NOT
- scrape the root
- place in disinfectant
- wrap in dry tissue

Tetanus prophylaxis should be given if the patient has not had an injection of tetanus vaccine in the last ten years. (See 'Immunisation')The patient should be seen by a dental surgeon as soon as possible after the replacement of the tooth. The outlook is usually good if replacement is done within 20 minutes of the injury. Patients with fractured teeth should be seen as soon as possible by a dental surgeon, particularly if the pulp has been exposed.

Neck

Cervical spine injury with paraplegia is the most feared consequence of rugby football and of diving. Head injury often occurs at the same time and can make assessment difficult. The safe rule is to assume that a neck injury is present until proved otherwise. If full and pain free active neck movement returns quickly, and there is no sensory alteration or weakness in the limbs, significant spinal damage can be discounted. Flexion and rotation are most likely to produce spinal cord damage, either at the time of injury or in the subsequent handling of the casualty. To immobilise the neck while awaiting evacuation to hospital, Necloc, two-part collars can be applied on the field by one operator. The neck is held rigid during transport or further evaluation. A range of sizes is supplied in a handy bag which can be carried in the car or kept in the pavilion (Jerome Medical, 309, Fellowship Road, Mount Laurel. NJ 08054). In their absence, neck movement must be prevented by wedging with sandbags or similar improvised means, or by an assistant controlling the head.

Shoulder

Dislocation, usually anterior, results from a fall on the shoulder or external rotation of the abducted humerus. It is worth making a *single, gentle* attempt at reduction if:

- the doctor is there very soon after the injury, and
- he is skilled in the manoeuvre, and
- an associated fracture is unlikely.

Then or later, traction is the secret of success. In the classical manoeuvre, traction is applied through the flexed elbow, while the upper arm is successively abducted and externally rotated, then adducted across the chest while rotating internally. If immediate reduction is unsuccessful, the casualty should lie prone on a couch with the affected arm hanging over the side, applying weight or continuous traction. In combination with sedation and pain relief (not by mouth, lest reduction under general anaesthesia is required later), this alone sometimes achieves a reduction.

Upper Limb
Falls on the outstretched hand

The following list of injuries produced by a fall on the out-stretched hand is in Table 5, presented as an aide-memoire rather than an exhaustive account.

Table 5: Injuries caused by a fall on the outstretched hand

Injury	Important points in Management
Fractured clavicle	'Accurate reduction is neither possible nor essential.' (Apley). Sling, plus progressive mobilisation.
Fractured neck of humerus	Reduction, possibly internal fixation if deformity severe. Usually sling, progressive mobilisation.
Fractured shaft of humerus	'Collar and cuff' sling.
Elbow fractures	Referral to hospital advisable. Immediate and late complications frequent. Accurate reduction needed.
Colles/Smith type fractures (distal radius and ulna) Check elbow if only one bone appears to be fractured – may be a Galleazi or Montéggia fracture – dislocation.	Reduction if significant deformity. Immobilisation in PoP backslab, converted to completed plaster after danger of swelling is past (24 hours).
Scaphoid fracture	May not be seen on early X-ray. Ask for scaphoid views. Repeat X-ray after 2 weeks if pain persists and first X-ray negative. Scaphoid plaster for 6+ weeks.

Metacarpal Fractures

For single metacarpal fractures, accurate reduction is unnecessary and immobilisation futile. A padded crepe is applied for comfort, and mobilisation encouraged. Deformity, due to a 'dropped knuckle' and the lump formed by callus, subsides over 3-5 years. Other finger and thumb fractures are frequent and often demand a hand surgeon's skill in reduction, fixing or splinting.

Ribcage

The possibility of pneumothorax, splenic rupture (possibly with delayed presentation) or associated kidney injury must be borne in mind. In uncomplicated cases, analgesia and pain-relieving measures are all that are needed. Crack fractures, especially of the lateral part of the ribcage, may be elusive on X-ray, but worried parents will need convincing that the investigation does not alter management.

Hip
The 'Irritable Hip'

This useful but non-specific term describes the child with pain and a limp. The pain may be in the hip, groin, thigh or knee. The child should be put to bed, with analgesia. A history of trauma is of little help in establishing a diagnosis; the trauma producing a slipped epiphysis may be so mild it is not recalled, while an injury preceding the onset of juvenile rheumatoid, say, may be a complete red herring.

Table 6 summarises the important clinical features by which the likely or important diagnoses may be distinguished. All except the so – called 'transient synovitis', which rapidly settles with rest in bed, require urgent referral.

Table 6: Diagnosis of the 'Irritable Hip'

	'Transient Synovitis'	Inflammatory Arthritis e. g. Still's disease	Septic Arthritis, or TB Hip	Perthe's Disease	Slipped Epiphysis
Typical Age	Any	Any	Any	5-10 yrs	12yrs (girls) 15yrs (boys)
Fever, Systemic upset	–	+or –	+or++	–	–
Raised ESR	–	+	+	–	–
Abnormal X-ray	–	–	+or–	+	+

Knee

Knee injuries and knee pain are very common in adolescents. Relatively benign causes of anterior knee pain such as Osgood Schlatter's Disease and chondromalacia patellae seem to be, at least in their milder forms, almost variants of the normal. The main problem is convincing anxious parents and zealous coaches that a benign outcome is assured and that the only wise course may be to avoid precipitating activity.

In assessing knee injuries, an accurate account of the mechanism of the injury is most useful. Was the affected knee weight-bearing? Was the body turning, and which way? Most importantly, did the knee swell, and how quickly? A knee which became swollen within an hour or two, almost certainly contains blood, suggesting injury to a vascularised structure such as bone, meniscus or cartilage. If the swelling took several hours or more to appear, the knee more probably contains clear joint fluid.

Details of the subsequent symptoms yield valuable clues. Retropatellar pain is worse on going up, as against going down, stairs. Clicks commonly represent patello-femoral crepitus or tendon snaps but may be produced by loose bodies or meniscal tears. In true locking, the flexed knee cannot be straightened, but **un**locks with a 'clunk' on manipulation by the injured person or another. It is the unlocking that is crucial. The knee that gives way may have ligament (especially anterior cruciate) laxity or a mechanical derangement.

Examining the Injured Knee

Comparison with the uninjured side, as always, can uncover subtle abnormalities. If an effusion is present, intra-articular mischief is almost assured – 'a swollen knee is an unhappy knee!'. The exact location of tenderness will lend a valuable clue. Joint line tenderness suggests a meniscal lesion, while the tenderness of a sprained collateral ligament is more diffuse. Pain or joint laxity (compare the normal side) on valgus, varus or antero-posterior draw stress suggests injury to the medial or lateral collateral, or anterior cruciate, ligaments respectively. Clicks clunks or locking suggest ensnarement of a torn meniscus or loose body in the joint.

In addition to the general principles of ERICA, isometric quadriceps ('Static Quads') exercises are vital from the start, even pending an accurate diagnosis. The thigh muscles will waste at an alarming rate after injury, loss of bulk and tone becoming evident within a few days.

Aspiration of an effusion is justified to improve comfort if the knee is so intensely swollen that flexion is severely limited. Reassessment after few days of resting, when pain, swelling and tenderness have gone, may allow more accurate assessment of ligament injury and internal derangement.

Lower Leg

Athletes often present with a self diagnosis of 'shin splints', describing aching varying in intensity from a nagging ache to an agonising pain, associated with running. Early treatment, whatever the cause, will include ice, elevation of legs and avoidance of precipitating activity. Diagnosis may depend on sophisticated investigations; tibial stress fracture may be revealed only by an isotope bone scan, while objective proof of the raised pressure of anterior tibial compartment syndrome requires pressure recordings from transducers implanted inside the fascial compartment.

Ankle

Most doctors will be confident at assessing and treating the ubiquitous inversion injury of the ankle. Again, treatment strategy depends more on the clinical picture than the X-ray findings, but patients, coaches and distant parents will need careful explanation to go along with this.

Foot

'March' fracture of a metatarsal (classically the second) may cause initial puzzlement, and, again, may require an isotope bone scan for diagnosis. A pupil complaining of a painful foot after an adventure trek or early season training, gives the clue.

Insurance

Every year a small number of school children are permanently disabled by sports injuries. While injuries due to road traffic accidents are generously compensated in the courts, and many adults carry sports insurance, the school child accidentally injured in the course of a game at school will receive no compensation unless insurance cover has been arranged. It is not sufficient to expect the parents to take the initiative for individual accident insurance and it is now recognised, at least in independent schools, that insurance against accidental injury is a responsibility which must be accepted by the school, irrespective of who finally pays the premium. A number of schemes have been drawn up by the insurance companies, and school authorities are very strongly advised to participate. The best policies cover all sport and adventure activities officially organised by the school, and require registration of every pupil in the scheme. Death benefit is limited in the case of a minor, but the most important provision is for adequate cover for the lifelong cost of permanent total disablement. £1,000,000 should be regarded as a minimum, and some schemes now insure for £2,000,000. The premiums for group insurance schemes are much lower than for individual accident policies. Details can be obtained from the Hon. Secretary, MOSA and from the Independent Schools Joint council.

References

1. Blinkhorn, A. S., and Mackie, I. C. (1996) My child's just knocked out a front tooth – Urgent treatment can save the tooth and the smile. *Br. Med. J.* 312, 526

2. O'Brien M. *Childrens' dental health in the United kingdom 1993.* London; Office of Population Censuses and Surveys, 1994.

3. Page. J (1996). *Personal communication.*

4. Sparks, J. P. (1981) Half a million hours of rugby football. Br. J. Sports Med., 15, 30.

Reading and Further Study

Mackie. I. C. and Worthington, H. V. (1992) An investigation of replantation of traumatically avulsed incisor teeth. *Br. Dent. J.* 172 17

Many organisations connected with particular sports publish leaflets about safety, injury prevention, first-aid and rehabilitation after injury. Of particular interest may be those from the Rugby Football Union. In the excellent series of monographs, 'Practical Problems' and free on request to doctors from the Arthritis and Rheumatism Council, No.12, 'The Management of Acute Soft Tissue Injures in Sport', deserves special mention. The same organisation produces leaflets for patients in quantity on request, for the cost of the postage.

Books

There are many books on Sports Medicine and Sports Injuries, but they are of very mixed quality. Two which the author has found useful are:

'*Sports Injuries – A Self-Help Guide*' by Vivian Grisogono (John Murray ISBN 0-7195-4111-5). A most excellent book, written in a lucid, logical and accurate style. The lay sportsman will understand it and every doctor will learn something useful from it. Once a copy is seen by the Games Department staff, they will order several copies and a large part of the doctor's mystique will disappear! However, as a result, surgeries will be smaller!

'*ABC of Sports Medicine*' (BMJ Publishing ISBN 0-7279-0844-8). This is another book in the authoritative but digestible series from Tavistock Square. It contains the essentials of a truly comprehensive range of topics, with useful details where appropriate (for example, telephone numbers of Diving Emergency Centres). If the Bursar will run to only one book on Sports Medicine, let it be this one.

Training. The doctor interested in learning more about the subject will find courses advertised from time to time, in the medical journals. Structured and comprehensive schemes are run by:

British Association of Sport and Medicine c/o. The National Sports Institute, St. Bartholomew's Medical College, Charterhouse Square, London EC1M 6BQ. It organises academic meetings, publishes *The British Journal of Sports Medicine*, and organises a structured Education Programme comprising a series of five-day courses and a week-long Practical Sports Medicine Course.

University of Bath Centre for Continuing Education Claverton Down, BATH. BA2 7AY offers a modular course consisting of Distance Learning modules and clinical week-ends.

CHAPTER 10

SAFETY AT SCHOOL

Introduction

Safety at School covers a very wide field and schools are subject to the Health and Safety at Work Act 1974.

Health and Safety at Work Act (HASAWA) 1974.

This is an enabling piece of legislation setting down broad duties analogous with common law. It is applicable to all work places and allows for the introduction of more specific regulations and Approved Codes of Practice in the future. There are many sections ie:

Employers' Duties

These are to ensure the health, safety and welfare of employees at work, providing them with safe plant and equipment and to maintain the work place/environment in a safe condition.

Employees Duties

Employees must now be responsible for the health and safety of themselves and others. They must co-operate with the employer to enable the employer to comply with statutory duties.

Approved Codes of Practice (ACOPS)

These suggest the means by which a regulation may be implemented practically. Those which accompany Health and Safety legislation do not constitute statutory duties and are not enforceable in law. However, failure of individuals to comply with the provisions may result in the presumption that they were in breach of the statutory requirements applicable. This is laid down in Section 17 of HASAWA and applies only to criminal proceedings instigated as the result of a breach of a statutory duty.

Section 17 states that during criminal proceedings for contravention of requirements made under HASAWA (or any other Health and Safety legislation still in place), if there is an ACOP with which the accused has not complied, then proof of that breach equals evidence of guilt. It is therefore, the duty of the accused to satisfy the court that he was meeting the statutory requirements in a way other than that stated in the ACOP.

Types of Statutory duty

Statutory duties are identified legal requirements falling into three main categories:

Absolute – Where the risk of injury or ill-health is inevitable and it is possible to follow Health and Safety precautions, then the duty to implement those precautions is absolute.

Practicable – A requirement which must be carried out 'as far as is practicable'. In other words, if in the light of current information and technology it is feasible to do so, then it must be done.

Reasonably Practicable – This involves the weighing of the risk involved against the time, trouble and cost of implementing any action required to meet the duty. These are open to interpretation.

Personal Protective Equipment – If personal protective equipment (PPE) is issued as a means of controlling exposure to hazardous substances /operations, it is subject to risk assessment under the Personal Equipment Regulations, 1992. The PPE should be suitable for the use intended and all staff issued with PPE should receive information, instruction and training on the correct selection, use, maintenance and storage of the equipment.

Legislation Issued Under the HASAWA (Section 16)

The Control of Substances Hazardous to Health (COSHH) Regulations 1989, updated 1994.

COSHH is concerned with any hazardous substance and how it will be used. Also certain substances may have additional requirements to those of COSHH, eg. asbestos, cyanide.

There are three ACOPS issued under COSHH. These are:

i   COSHH Regulations

ii   Biological Agents (Issued as a result of an EC directive on the protection of workers from risks related to exposure to biological agents at work).

iii Carcinogens (This ACOP was updated in 1994 to reflect the current state of knowledge.)

Every employer is required to undertake a suitable and sufficient assessment of the risks to the Health and Safety of their employees arising from their work with hazardous substances.

Such assessments must be reviewed at regular intervals or if circumstances change. Each assessment will include:

Assessment of the risks to health

Means of prevention of exposure to such substances

Measures to use substances safely where it is impossible to avoid exposure, ie suitable control measures.

Employers must then give information (including all hazards and their associated risks) instruction and training in the control of such substances to any staff involved in their handling.

Hence, these regulations place obligations on school authorities to assess the toxic, corrosive or irritant qualities (if any) of substances used in school and to prevent exposure to them if necessary. Staff and pupils are not exposed to hazardous substances to the same degree as industrial and other workers, yet problems can arise and the COSHH regulations compel the use of proper systems of management at work. These should protect not only pupils and staff but also visitors, outside contractors and members of the public.

Schools should appoint a member of staff to be responsible for implementing COSHH, even if this is delegated to an outside consultant. Briefly COSHH involves assessing any substances in use in the school which could possibly be harmful, including micro-organisms and substantial dust of any kind. The use of any personal protective equipment (PPE) (e.g. respiratory protection equipment) and general control measures (e.g. fume cupboards), should be subject to regular inspection, testing and maintenance, which is recorded, signed and dated.

COSHH and its ACOP can be relevant to schools as in the following examples:

Craft Design and Technology departments – wood dust, welding fumes, solvents, paints, glues and related substances.

Art departments – clay, glazes, glues, paints, dyes.

Home Economics departments – bleaches, cleaning fluids, dyes.

Clerical staff – photocopier toner, correction fluid, thinners.

Science staff – a large number of potentially hazardous substances are used and produced in school laboratories. Science teachers' own professional organisations have already produced suitable guidance for most schools and so appreciable expertise is already likely to be focussed on the production of chlorine gas (toxic) which is acceptable on a small scale in a well-ventilated classroom.

Cleaning and Domestic staff – cleansing fluids, bleaches, polishes, wooden floor sealers.

Caretaking and maintenance staff – especially if they are associated with the upkeep of swimming pools and shower areas. For example, a swimming pool of even modest dimensions may have the capacity to produce a major gassing accident due to chlorine gas. Pool chlorine donors and acid used for pH correction will produce chlorine gas if accidentally mixed and should always be bunded separately. Also, staff responsible for the upkeep of shower areas will be affected by the ACOP for biological agents, in that this work may place them in contact with Legionella bacteria especially at the start of a new term when shower heads have not been in regular use for some time.

Medical/sanatorium/First Aid staff – will also be affected by this ACOP in relation to possible contact with biological agents, including possibly HIV and Hepatitis B viruses.

NB. The member of staff responsible for COSHH should assess any areas where potentially hazardous substances are stored as well as used.

The Reporting of Injuries, Diseases and Dangerous Occurrences Regulations – RIDDOR 1995

The purpose of RIDDOR is to establish a set format for the generation of written reports (within 24 hours) to the Health and Safety Executive (HSE), or relevant parties in the event of:

An accident which results in death or inability to carry out normal work for three days or more.

An injury requiring a minimum stay in hospital of 24 hours.

A dangerous occurrence or contraction of a specific disease.

The individual responsible for reporting such events is called the 'responsible person' and further explanation of this is given in the guidance notes for implementing RIDDOR.

The Noise at Work Regulations 1989

These regulations state the duties of employers in controlling noise in the working environment. If noise levels in the work area are thought to be in excess of 85 decibels (stated as 85dB (A) in the regulations), then the appropriate assessment of noise levels must be carried out by a competent person. Should noise levels be thus identified as reaching this level, then employers must provide suitable effective ear protection. At levels of 90 dB(A) and above, the wearing of such protective devices becomes mandatory and must be enforced by the employer. As a rough guide, if someone standing two metres away from another person finds it necessary to shout to be heard, the level is likely to be above 85 dB (A).

The Management of Health and safety at Work Regulations (1992)

These regulations were introduced as the UK means of compliance with specific EC directives on Health and Safety and set out explicitly what are implicit within HASAWA. The regulations require an employer to make suitable and sufficient assessments of the Health and Safety risks to which employees may be exposed during the course of their work. These assessments must be recorded and reviewed on a regular basis. An employer must introduce appropriate measures to eliminate or reduce any identified risks. Employers must then give information (including information regarding all hazards and their associated risks), to their employees.

The Manual Handling Operations Regulations 1992

Employers have basic duties under these regulations:

- To avoid handling hazardous material where reasonably practical.

- To carry out suitable risk assessment where manual handling cannot be avoided.

- To reduce the risk of injury by implementing suitable control measures.

- To train/instruct all relevant staff accordingly.

Employees also have a duty to inform their employer about any injury, regardless of its age or how it was sustained, which may compromise their working abilities.

The Health and Safety – Display Screen Equipment (DSE) Regulations 1992

These regulations apply to display screens where *users* habitually use the display screen equipment as a significant part of their normal work.

Employers must undertake suitable and sufficient assessments of DSE work stations and introduce appropriate measures to reduce any identified risks.

Employers must ensure that work stations satisfy the minimum requirements set out in the regulations for display screen, keyboard, desk and chair, working environment, task, design and software.

DSE work should be planned to include regular work breaks/changes of activity.

Employers must also give information (including all hazards and associated risks), instruction and training to any relevant staff.

DSE users are entitled to specific eye examinations and eyesight tests carried out by a doctor or optician, with the cost of these tests, together with any indicated spectacles or contact lenses being met by the employer.

A DSE user is someone who habitually uses DSE as a significant part of their normal work. It is unlikely that they will be able to do their job satisfactorily without using DSE.

NB. These regulations could be of relevance in school Information Technology Departments

Contractors

Now that schools are increasingly employing outside contractors to do a variety of tasks which were hitherto done by school maintenance departments, the HSE has issued a booklet of information for headteachers, school governors and bursars.[4]

Publications

Publications relevant to regulations referred to above, may be obtained from: HSE Books.

See the references at the end of this Chapter.

Swimming Pool Safety

Adequate supervision by a life-saver trained in the use of mouth to mouth artificial respiration is essential at all times because of the possibility of drowning, which may follow trivial mishaps, as well as vasovagal attacks and fits. The preservation of good pool discipline also prevents other accidents such as skidding on slippery pool surrounds and collisions between swimmers. Swimming pools should be out of bounds after dances and parties where alcohol has been consumed.

School authorities should carefully adhere to the safety guidelines contained in the recent publication by the Health and Safety Executive, especially if the school pool is used by staff and families and hired out to outside organisations.

Diving Accidents

In recent years there has been a greater awareness of the risks of diving and very large sums of money have been awarded by the courts following spinal injuries from this cause. A Code of Practice has been agreed between a number of interested national organisations. Swimming should not be allowed near diving installations which are in use and there should be separation of swimmers and divers in these circumstances.

It should be noted that vertical diving should never be taught or allowed except in deep water especially reserved for diving. There should be no diving into less than 1.5 m of water and starting blocks should only be used by swimmers who are proven to be skilled in their use and under careful supervision.

If the public, parents or staff are allowed to use the pool a notice should be prominently displayed stating 'No Vertical Diving'.

Accident Prevention

The following aspects of safety in school are dealt with in more detail in the DFEE publications. See under 'References'at the end of this Chapter

Fire Precautions.

The design of buildings plays an important part in fire prevention and periodical inspections should be made by the Chief Fire Officer. Fire drills to practice evacuation of buildings should be carried out regularly and fire extinguishers should be regularly inspected, maintained and recharged according to the manufacturer's instructions.

Precautions in the Use of Electrical Equipment.

All mains electrical apparatus must be properly wired to an appropriate plug. Particular care is required over electrical musical instruments, as fatalities have been caused by the failure of the earth or the transformer. Electric guitars and sound reproduction apparatus should be forbidden until they have been inspected and approved by a qualified electrician. Automatic circuit breakers are increasingly used in boarding house establishments.

Physical Education

Sports injuries are dealt with in Chapter 9. The rules of the Amateur Athletic Association on Safety are reproduced in the DFEE publication 'Safety in Physical Education'. These rules are particularly important in throwing events. See under 'References' at the end of this Chapter.

School Premises

Wherever possible reinforced or shatter-proof glass should be used in partitions and swing doors. Roller towels should be avoided as they have caused occasional fatal strangulation accidents in young children.

Science Laboratories

All teachers should be aware that the splashing of hot acid or alkali into the eyes is fairly common and that immediate first aid treatment by prompt flooding of the eyes with copious amounts of cold water is the best way of preventing permanent damage. Hospital referral afterwards should be mandatory. The DFEE booklet 'Safety in Science Laboratories' provides information about other accidents. See at the end of this Chapter.

First Aid in Schools.

The HMSO booklet entitled 'First Aid in Educational Establishments', which is commended to all schools has a 'Statement of first-aid policy' as follows: 'It is recommended that every educational establishment should prepare a written statement of its policy on first aid, covering both employees and non-employees. Where appropriate, this could form part of the written statement of policy on health and safety required by section 2 (3) of the Health and Safety at Work Act. This statement should be brought to the attention of all concerned within the establishment and should include such information as the names and locations of all first-aid personnel and the locations of equipment (this is also relevant to para 34 of the Approved Code), special arrangements for dealing with accidents away from the establishment or outside normal hours, and arrangements for liaison with ambulance services. Employers may find it useful to contact their local HSE Employment medical Advisory Service (EMAS) office for advice on drawing up their policy'.[3]

Perhaps it may be helpful to quote the 'Recommended scales of provision'. viz. 'The 1981 regulations and the Approved Code of Practice are framed to allow employers considerable scope in deciding how to tailor first-aid provision to the particular circumstances of their establishments. General advice on the criteria to be used by employers in deciding the appropriate level of provision for their employees is given in paras 6 to 22 of the Approved Code. The most important questions to be considered relate to the number (and type) of first-aid personnel to be employed and whether a first aid room should be provided. The main criteria which apply to these questions are on the number and location of staff, the nature of the hazards to which they are exposed and the accessibility of NHS emergency facilities. These principles should apply equally to facilities provided for pupils, students and other non-employees. In primary and secondary schools, which may be regarded as establishments with relatively low hazards, the Approved Code suggests that a first-aider would be required only where there are150 or more employees and a first-aid room where there are 400 or more. Consequently most schools will not need a first-aid room for employees (although many already have medical rooms or rest rooms) and few will need qualified first-aiders. However, this does not prevent trained first-aiders being appointed in primary and secondary schools where this is considered appropriate. Where the total number of employees is below 150, employers may consider the total number of people on site in assessing first-aid needs.

Where no first aiders are provided, the regulations require 'appointed persons' to be available to look after first-aid equipment and to take charge of a situation if an accident occurs. No training is specified for appointed people, although HSE recommends the value of instruction in emergency first-aid (resuscitation, control of bleeding and treatment of unconsciousness) for such people. Such instruction would be especially valuable where the appointed person(s) may be responsible for children.

In further and higher educational establishments, hazards will vary greatly from department to department. Libraries, offices, teaching rooms and lecture rooms may be regarded as areas with relatively low hazards attracting a commensurate level of first-aid provision. Research or teaching laboratories and workshops may be classified as areas with more hazards requiring a higher level of first-aid provision, such as more first-aiders. In establishments where special or unusual hazards exist, both occupational first-aiders and a first-aid room may be necessary, irrespective of the number of employees.'

Guidance is then given on the content and locations of first-aid boxes, the purpose, location and facilities of first-aid rooms, the selection, duties and training of first-aid personnel, arrangements for 'out of hours working' first-aid cover and the importance of preparatory arrangements with the ambulance service and nearby hospital A and E departments.

There is a special paragraph on 'Sports injuries and field trips' This is: 'Pupils and students often suffer sports injuries and arrangements should take account of them. In particular, those in charge of sporting activities may need special training in dealing with such injuries. A number of organisations run courses in this area (information available from the Central Council for Physical Recreation, London). First-aid requirements (e.g. travelling first-aid kits) should be considered when planning field trips or expeditions. Special training may be needed for those accompanying expeditions to locations remote from emergency services or where activities involve specialised hazards (e.g. pot-holing, mountaineering or diving).

N.B. References at the end of the Chapter.

First-aid Instruction for Staff and Pupils

Emergency first-aid as previously indicated, ie resuscitation, arrest of bleeding and management of unconsciousness, should really be within the capability of all members of staff and senior pupils. If the school doctor has an aptitude and the requisite enthusiasm for teaching first-aid, then he can make a very worth-while contribution to the school. It would be helpful if schools possessed 'Resusci-Andy' or 'Resusci-Annie' manikins for teaching mouth to mouth resuscitation and afterwards, it would be very worth-while to demonstrate the Heimlich manoeuvre to relieve choking, as matters of priority. Some senior pupils need to learn first-aid as part of their Duke of Edinburgh's Award scheme training.

Alternatively, it might be possible for first-aid instructors from the St John Ambulance Brigade, or The British Red Cross Society to visit the school and give first-aid instruction (at the school's expense) and perhaps arrange for keen first-aiders to take their proficiency certificates in due course.

Road Safety

Road safety is an important part of nursery and primary school teaching. Bicycle training and testing are organised by the Royal Society for the Prevention of Accidents. All cyclists should know the Highway Code and wear safety helmets of an approved design and reflective clothing. Also, consideration should be given to encouraging the taking of cycling proficiency tests. Bicycles should be maintained in good order, reinforced by inspection if necessary. Motor vehicle instruction should be given only by qualified instructors and pupils under instruction should have the written consent of their parents.

It is reassuring to note that the safety of children in motor cars is receiving the attention of the Child Health Monitoring unit, at the Institute of Child Health, London WC1N 1EH, who claim that 'child restraints should be built in safety features, not optional extras' and 'that if children must be condemned to motorised monotony then cars should be designed with them in mind'.[1]

Safety in School Vehicles

1. All school passenger carrying vehicles (PCV's) should be in a roadworthy and clean condition, regularly serviced and maintained according to the manufacturer's schedule and checked for faults before each day's journeys. Any faults should be recorded, reported and rectified before any children are carried in the vehicle.

2. Distinctive (preferably) illuminated signs of official design, indicating that children are being carried should be fixed to the front and the rear of the vehicle.

3. Each passenger must occupy an individual seat and wear a correctly installed and fitting seat belt of approved design, whenever the vehicle is in motion.

4. Drivers of school PCVs should be competent drivers, trained to work with children and receive regular instruction and examination in first-aid, resuscitation and vehicle evacuation. Verbal or preferably, written instructions (as in passenger aircraft) should precede each departure.

5. Drivers of school PCVs should drive for no more than nine hours out of the 24 and must not drive for more than four and a half hours, either cumulatively or continuously, without a minimum break of 45 minutes, which may be taken as a passenger in the same vehicle.

6. Preferably, school PCV drivers should be between 25 and 65 years of age, have at least five years driving experience, be appropriately licensed and have no conviction for a serious driving offence. They should be in good health, with no history or evidence of any condition likely to impair their conscious level, cognitive function, neuromuscular coordination or power. They should be free from the untoward effects of illegal, prescribed or OTC drugs and, of course, alcohol, including the effects of the 'carry over' from the previous day. Ideally, pending further legislation, school PCV drivers should meet the recently revised standards of medical fitness required for the holders of Group 2 licences. (Drivers who drive

for hire or reward, Large Goods Vehicles (LGV) over 7.5 tonnes or Passenger Carrying Vehicles (PCV) of nine seats or over.)

7. Adult supervision, in addition to the driver, should be present whenever children are being carried to enforce safety procedures, ensure acceptable behaviour, supervise boarding and alighting and to deal with any emergencies.

8. All school PCVs must be equipped with a first-aid kit and a fire extinguisher, conforming (at least) to the statutory requirements of Appendix E of the PCV booklet No. 385, together with a neck collar and an assortment of splints, all of which should be regularly checked, repaired and replenished as necessary. Also, it is strongly recommended that a correctly functioning mobile telephone or a two-way radio should be carried on all journeys.

9. No smoking or consumption of alcohol by driver, escort or passengers, immediately before or during journeys. (See 6 above)

10. Any luggage must be stored intelligently and securely, both on the roof and inside the vehicle, thus ensuring that entry to and exit from the vehicle are unimpeded. If a trailer is towed,* it must be securely loaded (not overloaded) with proper regard to the condition and pressures of the tyres, the tightness of the wheel nuts and correctly functioning lights and, if fitted, brakes. All passengers should have ready access to an inside door and the vehicle must not be refuelled whilst children are on board.

N.B. The above apply equally to private school vehicles, or to 'self-drive hire' vehicles hired from commercial firms and to passenger carrying vehicles hired from a local education authority. The above relate to individual schools and are enforceable by them. The absence of appropriate legislation and dedicated school buses preclude the enforcement of national distinctively coloured school bus stop signs and the compulsory stopping of all traffic in the vicinity of stationary school buses whilst discharging or taking on passengers, although MOSA would generally support these measures. (Incorporating MOSA Policy Guidelines on School Vehicle Safety February 1996)

* Implementation of the second EC Directive on the Driving Licence (91/439/ /EEC) means that the new regulations changing the entitlement to tow trailers came into force on 1st July 1996. These regulations will affect a few existing drivers. A fact sheet, INF30, is available from Vehicle registration Offices or DVLA's Customer Enquiry Office, 01792 772 151 (lines open 0815-1630 hours, Monday to Friday.)

ADVENTURE TRAINING AND OUTDOOR ACTIVITIES AT SCHOOL

Outdoor education covers many different activities aimed at broadening the scope of pupils' interest and abilities. As a result of recent widely publicised enquiries into accidents at sea or on the mountains, there has been an increased stress on the concept of risk assessment and on the training and qualification of staff leading all such parties. The problems common to most training, such as leadership and the management of extreme conditions, will be considered before referring to the individual activities. A list of contact addresses is given.

Leadership and Planning

Whatever the activity, the leader must be known to be both competent technically and to possess the maturity to lead, control and encourage parties of young people. Certificates should not be the main basis by which a teacher's capability is judged, but local authorities and governors now lay down required standards for various outdoor activities, and schools in the independent sector must generally match these standards. A list of addresses of governing bodies of relevant sports and useful institutions is provided for those seeking further details about particular activities including training and certification.

There is a fine line between a well-planned adventure which extends children towards their physical and mental limits, and the event or chain of events which, by pushing them beyond those limits, risks injury or death. The modern concept of systematic risk assessment allows the leader to note down the possible risks, and to analyse the hazards and strategies for countering those hazards under the headings of 'people', 'equipment' and 'environment'. After considering the standards and guidelines applicable and the staff skills required, he can then choose to accept or reject the planned activity. It encourages a preliminary assessment combining experience, local knowledge and gathered information on the weather, capacity and fitness of members of the party, available equipment, etc., in an area where control and prevention are all important. A useful review of leadership requirements for all outdoor activities is 'Outdoor Pursuits: Guidelines for Educators' published by The Ministry of Education, Wellington. N.Z.

Exposure (Hypothermia)

This is generalised cold injury secondary to body chilling. It is caused primarily by any combination of the factors cold, wetting and wind. Extremes of cold are not necessary to produce hypothermia; the wet and wind common in the British hills, even in summer, can be as dangerous as the dry cold of the Himalaya.

Prevention is all important; teachers should be aware that the risk of it is raised by fatigue, fear and thinness, and should look out for these early symptoms, any one of which should alert them to the possibility of hypothermia:

Odd behaviour and judgment.
Lethargy, lack of response to orders, etc.
Repeated stumbling.
Irrational outbursts of energy, irritability.
Slurred speech, grumbling.
Uncontrollable shivering.
Dimness of vision and hallucinations.

Treatment; the vital principle is to prevent further heat loss.

1. Stop and shelter at once, using buildings, a tent (e.g. an emergency group shelter), a snow hole or at least some wind break.

2. Conserve heat using a sleeping bag, down jacket, polythene bag or 'space blanket'; insulate from the ground; the body heat of companions may be life saving.

3. Give hot drinks and sugar by mouth.

4. Be prepared to start resuscitation if respiration or pulse stops.

5. DO NOT encourage the patient to try and walk on even after he has apparently recovered.

6. DO NOT try to warm him by giving him alcohol, rubbing the skin or using hot water bottles.

7. Get transport as near to the patient as possible. A stretcher should be used for the shortest possible distances.

One person showing signs of exposure in a party means that others, perhaps even the leader, may be close to being affected; a decision on whether or not to turn back or seek shelter should be made *in good time*. It is recommended that clear, brief instructions on the recognition and treatment (on waterproof cards) are carried by leaders and their deputies.

Heat Exhaustion

Under hot conditions, the sweating brought on by physical exertion can cause heat exhaustion. This is due to the associated loss of salt (sweat contains approx 0.25% sodium chloride). Heat exhaustion causes giddiness and nausea, followed by typical 'fainting' (cold, pale, clammy skin, dilated pupils and a rapid, weak pulse; the temperature is initially subnormal and the blood pressure low). Muscle cramps are a warning symptom.

Prevention is by ensuring that the drinking water carried in hot conditions has enough salt added to make a 0.1% solution. This will replace the chloride loss.

Treatment involves resting and shading the patient, and giving 0.1% saline solution by mouth. Severely affected people may require active cooling and intravenous fluids.

Mountain Activities

These activities include hill-walking, orienteering, mountain cycling, fell-running, rock climbing and snow and ice climbing. The need for pre-activity fitness training for staff and pupils is stressed. The range of risk and skill requirements is wide, and the leader should be operating well within his or her competence, with a routine of written risk assessment before any venture, and a readiness to recognise early when the situation requires retreat. LEAs and independent schools should now require the leader to hold the appropriate certificates and awards of the UK Mountain Training Board or their local equivalent; these include the Mountain Instructor's Certificate for all-season mountaineering, the Single Pitch Supervisor's Award for rock climbing Instruction and the Summer Mountain Leader Award for non-technical summer hill-walking.

The standards of mountain clothing and equipment have improved and the leader should ensure that the party is adequately protected against cold, wind and rain, and that boots are suitable for the projected activity; there can be no compromise on the standards of equipment such as helmets, ropes and harnesses.

Emergency Kit needs vary according to the potential risks;some summer trips might need little more than a first-aid kit, but for remoter mountain areas, particularly in cold or unstable conditions, the following emergency kit for each group of 8 climbers should be considered:

Two survival bags or a group emergency shelter tent.

One sleeping bag or duvet jacket (in a dry bag.)

Emergency rations and a flask of hot drink (or a small stove with fuel and lighter to heat fluids).

Two torches with spare batteries and bulbs.

First Aid Kit.

20 metre length of rope.

A miniflare pack (for more serious expeditions).

Extra clothing.

Waterborne Activities

Advice on the leader qualifications and training appropriate to these activities can be obtained from the Royal Yacht Association, National Schools Sailing Association, British Canoe Union and British Sub-Aqua Club.

As with all such activities the leader should make a full risk assessment with special reference to wind, tide, temperature, and local hazards, ensuring that craft and equipment are adequate for the conditions, that rescue provision and communication are arranged and that most pupils are confident in the water, have enough buoyancy, and are clothed to survive the chilling effect of most British waters. Wet suits are usually worn for wind-surfing and sub-aqua diving, but may also be useful for sailing, especially in the colder months.

Canoeists run a real risk of hypothermia on British rivers in winter and should be able to recognise its early signs. Proper attention to insulation, particularly of the hands, is vital, and neoprene gloves and insulation of alloy-shafted paddles are recommended. Since sudden immersion in cold water can cause headaches and blackouts, leaders should be watchful and assist a canoeist off the water if necessary. For white water rafting, canoeing and surfing, wet suits and helmets should generally be worn.

Sub-aqua diving is increasingly popular, but the medical risks are somewhat higher than with most outdoor activities. Existing ear and sinus problems can be worsened by the effect of water pressure. Trainees must be medically examined before they take their first open water dives, and the British Sub Aqua Club provides doctors with details of the examination and the standards required; a chest X-ray is no longer routinely required but only when clinically indicated; children with asthma are not necessarily barred from diving, but should be assessed individually. No school diving club can operate without a qualified diving instructor, and all equipment including compressors must be maintained to a high standard. Snorkelling is encouraged at many schools; advice on medical examinations is required and safety standards can be obtained from any British Sub-Aqua club.

Anyone whose occupation or recreation takes them into fresh water should bear in mind the risks of leptospirosis (Weil's disease). This disease occurs when the organism (leptospira) gains access to the bloodstream through cuts and abrasions or via the surface membranes of the eyes or nose. This condition and ways of reducing its risk, are considered in greater detail in the Chapter on Communicable Diseases.

Underground Activities
Caving, pot-holing and mines-exploration involve common risks and skills, though some caves may be more liable to flooding, and some mines to instability and pollution. Dry caves may require only the simplest of equipment (boots, overalls, helmet with lamp); longer wetter caves may require wet suits and a safety kit containing first-aid equipment, survival bag, candles, waterproof matches, spare torches batteries and bulbs and an emergency ration pack. Simple accidents can produce major problems underground; safety ropes should be used for all ladder work and abseiling, and free diving sumps should have a hand-line and an adult at each end. The leader should know the strength of his party and be aware of the problems of hypothermia. These days, he will be expected to hold the appropriate certificate of the National Caving Association or its local equivalent.

Skiing
School ski parties can reduce the chance of injury by making sure that boots, skis and bindings are correctly fitted, and by encouraging all members of the party to get as fit as possible by pre-ski exercises and visits to dry ski slopes.

Clothing should allow for changes in conditions, with a wind-proof outer layer and several light inner layers which can be worn or carried. Hats and goggles should always be available, though sun-glasses are suitable for good conditions. Sun creams and lip salves are essential in nearly all conditions and should be applied twice daily to prevent sunburn.

Air Sports
Hang-gliding, paragliding and parachuting are not yet common school activities, but training in paragliding for pupils over 16 may well become less unusual in the future. Paragliding training schools will provide instruction and

will hire or sell paragliding equipment and helmets; they are monitored by the British HangGlider and Paraglider Association which also closely controls the training standards. Injury levels are low.

Overseas Expeditions

Increasingly doctors may be asked to advise school parties planning overseas trips to remote areas. They should offer an appropriate immunisation programme and make sure that all members of the party are confident in simple first-aid, the prevention of sunburn and the sterilisation of water. The risks of all outdoor activities are increased by remoteness and the increased scale of the challenge, and the leader should take account of all this in making his risk assessment. (Also, see the risks regarding HIV and Hepatitis B infections in the chapters on Communicable Diseases and Immunisation.).

References and Useful Addresses

1. Roberts, I., DiGuiseppi, C. (1997) Children in cars. Editorial *Br. Med. J.* 314: 392.

2. A booklet, 'Code of Practice for Youth Expeditions' gives good planning and is available from the Young Explorer's Trust.

3. First Aid in Educational Establishments (1986) *Education Service Advisory Committee.* ISBN 0 11 883837 7 HMSO London.

4. Contractors in Schools. Information for head teachers, school governors and bursars (with useful references). (1996) Health and Safety Executive. C250 IAC (L) 98 2/96.

5. List of organisations approved for first-aid training and qualifications. Leaflet IND (G) 5L, free from HSE Area Offices or public enquiry points. i. e.

   St Hugh's House, Trinity Road, Bootle. Merseyside. L20 3QY. Tel: 051 951 4381

   Baynard's House, 1, Chepstow Place, Westbourne Grove, London W2 4TF
   Tels: 0171 221 0416/0171 221 0870

   Broad Lane, Sheffield. S3 7HQ Tel 0742 752539

   DFEE Publications
   Safety in Science Laboratories. ISBN 0 11 270473 5*

   Safety in Physical Education. ISBN 0 11 270320 8*

   Safety at School: General Advice. ISBN 0 11 270305 4*

   Safety in Practical Studies. ISBN 0 11 270305 4*

   * Available from HMSO.

   First Aid (Basic advice on first aid at work) HSE booklet. ISBN 0 7176 1070 5.

   First aid at work. Your questions answered. HSE booklet ISBN 0 7176 1074 8

   First aid at work: Approved Code of Practice Health and Safety Commission 1 74 1997 ISBN 0 7176 1050 0

   HES priced and free publications available from HSE books, Box 199, Sudbury, Suffolk. CO10 6FS. Tel: 01787 881165 Fax: 01787 313995, and from good booksellers.

   For other enquiries, ring the HSE infoline Tel: 0541 545500 or write to the HSE Information Centre, Broad Lane, Sheffield. S3 7HQ.

British Mountaineering Council and UK Mountain Training Board,
177-179 Burton Road, West Didsbury, Manchester. M20 2BB. Tel: 01641 454747.

British Canoe Union, Adbolton Lane, West Bridgeford, Nottingham, NG5 5AS.
. Tel: 01159 821100.

National Caving Association. White Lion House, Ynys Uchaf, Ysradgynlais, Swansea. SA9 1RW. Tel:01369 849519.

Royal Yachting Association, RYA House, Romsey Road, Eastleigh, Hants. SO50 9YA.
Tel: 01703 627400.

British Sub-Aqua Club. Telfords Quay, Ellesmere Port, South Wirral. L65 4FY
Tel: 01513 571951.

British Orienteering Federation, Riversdale, Dale Rd North, Darley Dale, Matlock. Derbys.
DE4 2HX Tel: 01629 734042.

British Hang-Gliding and Paragliding Association. Old School Room, Loughborough Road,
Leicester. LE4 5PT. Tel: 01162 612362.

Central Council of Physical Recreation, Francis House, Francis Street, London, SW1P 1DE.
Tel: 0171 388 3163.

Sports Council, 16 Upper Woburn Place, London WC1H OQP Tel: 0171 388 1277.

Youth Hostels Association. Trevelyan House, 8, St. Stephens Hill, St. Albans. Herts. AL1 2DY.
Tel: 01727 855215.

Young Explorers' Trust, c/o Royal Geographical Society, 1 Kensington Gore, London SW7
2AR. Tel: 01623 861027.

British Schools Exploring Society, c/o Royal Geographical Society, 1 Kensington Gore,
London. SW7 2AR. Tel: 0171 584 0710.

CHAPTER 11

COMMUNICABLE DISEASES

The Common Cold

The common cold is an acute respiratory illness in which the infection falls on the mucous membrane of the upper respiratory tract, leading to rhinorrhoea, nasal obstruction, sneezing and a dry cough. The duration of any of these conditions is usually a few days, up to a week. The majority of common colds are caused by rhinoviruses, of which there are over 100 distinct serotypes. Other viruses, concerned to a lesser extent in the causation of colds are coronaviruses, enteroviruses, respiratory syncitial viruses and parainfluenza viruses.

Diagnosis

Diagnosis is on clinical grounds. (The virus is isolated from nasal washings with difficulty, and experimentally, it has been surprisingly difficult to transmit the infection between persons.)

Communicability and Immunity

Colds are most commonly communicated in the active stage, by physical contact and also by droplet inhalation, but may be transmitted up to eight days from the onset of symptoms. Immunity is type specific and prolonged but there is no cross immunity among strains of rhinovirus.

Prevention

There is no method of preventing common colds. Contrary to popular belief, large doses of vitamin C do not prevent, or cure colds.

Treatment

Treatment is purely symptomatic. Antibiotics are not indicated.

Return to School

Children with a heavy nasal discharge or complications should be kept at home or in the sanatorium until free from infection. Swimming, especially if there is a history of otitis media, should be restricted and strenuous physical exercise should not be undertaken until after full recovery, with the resting pulse rate having returned to normal, because of the risk of viral myocarditis.

Streptococcal Pharyngitis and Tonsillitis

Sore throats can be caused by a variety of viruses and bacteria, especially, by the haemolytic streptococcus. Diphtheria (qv) is fortunately now quite rare, and in some cases of glandular fever (qv), there is gross tonsillar enlargement with the tonsils covered by a white exudate.

Human streptococcal throat infection is nearly always caused by strains of the Lancefield Group A streptococci and although other groups may be isolated from throat swabs, they are seldom pathogenic. The symptoms of streptococcal pharyngitis or tonsillitis are severe sore throat coupled with pain on swallowing and usually a constitutional illness with high fever. The tonsillar lymph nodes are usually enlarged and tender. An erythrogenic strain of this organism produces a scarlatiniform rash and a characteristic 'strawberry tongue'. On this basis, scarlet fever, still a notifiable disease, may be diagnosed. Occasionally, a peritonsillar abscess (quinsy), develops, which merits urgent ENT referral. Some epidemic strains of streptococci may cause acute glomerulonephritis. Rheumatic fever, and rheumatic chorea, are other sequelae of streptococcal infection, which are now almost never seen in the UK.

Diagnosis

The final diagnosis is made on the clinical appearance of the redness of the throat in the case of pharyngitis and enlargement of the tonsils with a purulent, cheesy material oozing from the tonsils (follicular tonsillitis). In the case of tonsillitis, however, it is by no means uncommon to make a clinical diagnosis of pharyngitis on one day and to note the undeniable appearances of follicular tonsillitis 24 hours later, supported by the isolation of a group A streptococcus form the throat swab. The isolation of the type of streptococcus will show whether the strain is one associated with rash, rheumatic fever or nephritis.

Infection and Transmission

Transmission is by droplet infection and may be from symptomless carriers. Nasal and salivary carriers are more infectious than faecal carriers. Streptococcal infection, occasionally, has been transmitted by unpasteurised milk.

Incubation Period

The incubation period is short, usually two to three, but may be from one to six days.

Period of Communicability

Adequate antibiotic treatment, usually with penicillin V, will render patients virtually non-infectious within 48 hours. However, a carrier state may persist.

Prevention of Streptococcal Infections

Streptococcal infections may be prevented by long-term dosage of oral penicillin or erythromycin (250 mgm. b. d.) in those for whom such infections would constitute a special risk . In practice, this means those who have had an attack of rheumatic fever. The risk of milk-borne streptococcal infection is eliminated by pasteurisation.

Methods of control

The patient with a suspected streptococcal infection should be kept from school and isolated for the first 48 hours of antibiotic treatment. An extensive outbreak in a school, very unusual nowadays, but with the implied risk of rare but serious sequelae, may continue for longer than an outbreak of Influenza. Throat and nasal swabs are the most effective means of detecting sufferers and carriers. These then should be treated with penicillin or erythromycin to eliminate the infection. (The local Consultant in Communicable Diseases may arrange for laboratory co-operation for mass swabbing.)

Treatment

The streptococcus almost invariably responds dramatically to penicillin. No other antibiotic is indicated except erythromycin for those who are genuinely allergic to penicillin. As the majority of sore throats are self-limiting virus infections, the doctor has to exercise judgment in deciding whether or not to use antibiotics. Ideally, throat swabs should be taken, then a decision on whether or not to treat should be made on clinical grounds while the swabs are being cultured. There is general agreement that all cases of steptococcal throat infections should be treated with antibiotic therapy. There is less agreement however, about what to do in the cases of sore throats. Most would agree that if there is constitutional upset, an acutely red pharynx, tonsillitis, cervical lymphadenopathy, otitis media or a scarlatiniform rash, treatment should begin at once. Oral penicillin V in a dosage of 250 mgm. q.d.s. before meals is usually sufficient, but intramuscular penicillin can be used to initiate therapy in those who are acutely ill or in those where vomiting precludes oral medication. (Erythomycin for those with genuine penicillin allergy.)

If the throat swab is negative, the antibiotic therapy can be discontinued, but if it is positive, it is important to continue for ten days, as relapse is common. On no account should ampicillin or amoxycillin be given, because of the risk of provoking a very unpleasant rash, should the infection turn out to be infectious mononucleosis. (Glandular fever qv).

Return to School

The patient can return to school on recovery, ideally with a negative throat swab.

Adenovirus Infections

There are many types of adenovirus, which may cause different clinical syndromes:

(a) *Pharyngitis* An acute febrile illness with enlargement of the regional lymph nodes. The throat is red and oedematous and there may be a follicular exudate. The nose is often affected and produces a thick mucopurulent discharge. In spite of the fever, constitutional symptoms are not severe and convalescence is rapid.

(b) *Pharyngoconjunctival Fever* – Epidemics occur in schools from time to time. The characteristics are fever, sore throat, swelling of the cervical lymph nodes, and corzya-like symptoms. These are followed by conjunctivitis with purulent discharge and photophobia. The conjunctivitis may be unilateral and may occur in the absence of other symptoms. Pharyngoconjunctival fever is more common in summer than in winter.

(c) *Acute Respiratory Disease.* The throat is again involved but the glandular enlargement is not so marked while the lower respiratory tract may be invaded. Sometimes pneumonia develops.

(d) *Epidemic Kerato-conjunctivitis.* This is a general and chronic condition which affects the eyes only and occurs in minor epidemics. Transmisssion may be by dust with consequent corneal damage or by contamination with ophthalmic instruments or eye droppers.

The transmission of adenovirus infections is largely by droplet. The diagnoses can be made by isolation of the virus from throat and eye swabs, and the incubation period is about a week. The immunity is type-specific and probably prolonged. Isolation is unnecessay and there is no specific treatment.

Croup

Croup is the name given to a condition, largely confined to children, characterised by a typical forceful expiratory noise replacing a typical sounding cough, but sometimes referred to as a 'tracheal cough', which is usually the result of some degree of upper airway obstruction, due to upper respiratory infection. This maybe associated with inspiratory and expiratory stridor. It is most commonly due to laryngo-tracheo-bronchitis, often caused by para-influenza or respiratory syncitial virus, (RSV), and less commonly bacterial tracheitis and acute epiglottitis.

There may have been mild coryza for a day or so with only minimal symptoms and signs. Characteristically in the small hours, the child suddenly awakes from sleep with fright, a painful 'tracheal cough', inspiratory and expiratory stridor, tachypnoea, maybe a fever and some degree of suprasternal and intercostal recession. The child must be carefully observed for restlessness due to air hunger, increasing cyanosis, progressive intercostal and suprasternal recession. If these signs of compromised respiration are noted, then urgent transfer to hospital, by ambulance, equipped with oxygen is indicated. In such cases, the child should be minimally disturbed and examination of the throat must wait until the child is in hospital where facilities for endo-tracheal intubation are at hand, because of the risk of fatal respiratory obstruction.

The likely diagnoses are bacterial tracheitis or, especially, if the child (usually in the three to six year age group) looks gravely ill with drooling of saliva, acute epiglottitis. The latter, often fatal condition is now very much less common, following the introduction of Haemophilus influenzae Type b (Hib) vaccine.

In addition to causing epiglottitis, Haemophilus influenzae caused meningitis, which was prone to relapse and to have neurological sequelae, septicaemia, pneumonia and other significant infections. The fatality rate was of the order of 4-5%.[1]

The majority of children presenting with croup and stridor, however, will be suffering from viral laryngo-tracheo-bronchitis, usually in a lower age group, and once observation has indicated sinister progression of obstructive respiratory signs to be unlikely, symptomatic remedies can be employed. Traditionally, inhalations of steam in a warm bathroom or kitchen are thought to be helpful although latterly, inhalations of corticosteroids (usually nebulised budesonide, 1 mg, repeated after four hours) have been used.[2] There is no place for sedatives.

Otitis Media

Probably only a quarter of cases of otitis media are bacterial in origin. In children under the age of four years H. Influenzae is, or was, involved. Over that age, pneumococci are the commonest pathogens. The complications of otitis media include chronic discharging otitis media, (otorrhoea), deafness of varying degrees and more rarely, mastoiditis and meningitis. The use of antibiotics therefore, has some justification.

Ampicillin is effective against H. influenzae, penicillin and erythromycin against pneumococci and cephalexin is usually effective against both organisms. Now that an effective vaccine against H. influenzae is available, there should be a reduction in upper and lower respiratory infections due to H. influenzae.

Secretory or serous otitis media (Glue Ear) may follow incomplete resolution of otitis media or blockage of the eustachian tubes. Immobility of the tympanic membrane may result, causing some impairment of hearing. Persistence of these signs and symptoms after decongestants have failed, will require ENT referral. Myringotomy and grommet insertion, to ventilate the middle ear and restore hearing, may be indicated.

Bronchitis and Bronchiolitis

Bronchitis may be defined as an infection of the lower respiratory tract with adventitious sounds, but no clinical and radiological evidence of consolidation. It is usually of viral aetiology, the principal symptoms and signs being cough and fever. In children with recurrent attacks of respiratory infection, the diagnoses of asthma or even cystic fibrosis should be considered. Acute bronchiolitis, caused by the respiratory syncitical virus (RSV), affects babies and very young children. There is lower respiratory obstruction and damage to lung tissue. Hospital treatment is urgently necessary.

Pneumonia

Pneumonia is an acute infection of the lungs, usually with radiological and clinical signs of consolidation. Lobar pneumonia is uncommon and can cause diagnostic difficulties due to the high fever, diarrhoea, and prostration. Elevation of the pulse and respiratory rates accompany the fever. Before the appearance of the physical signs in the lungs, there may be a toxic confusional state. Strep. pneumoniae is the commonest cause and penicillin is, therefore, the drug of choice. Bronchopneumonia, with its more profuse and patchy consolidation, may be caused by bacterial or viral infection with approximately equal frequency. It may occur as a secondary infection following an attack of influenza, or, especially in children, complicate attacks of measles or whooping cough. The other bacteria most commonly involved are Mycoplasma pneumoniae, and Staphylococci. Viruses include RSV, para-influenza, adeno-virus and influenza.

Mycoplasma Pneumoniae

Infection with mycoplasma has an insidious onset, with fever, malaise and cough, which may initally be unaccompanied by adventitious sounds in the lungs. Radiological changes, usually consisting of miliary mottling, are often more widespread than would be suggested by the physical signs. Bullous myringitis may accompany the chest infection.

This organism, for which poultry and other birds may be the vector, may be grown from throat swabs or sputum. The diagnosis can also be made serologically from paired sera. Immunity is probably prolonged. Erythro-mycin is the drug of choice in M. pneumoniae infections but it requires to be given for several days after the elevated temperature has subsided.

Staphylococcal Pneumonia

Staphylococci are an uncommon cause of pneumonia in the schoolchild, but may be seen due to secondary invaders in influenza. The infection may then be a fulminating one and will require hospital treatment, initially with intra-venous flucloxacillin or fusidic acid. Lung abscesses are a feature of staphylococcal pneumonia, with the risk of rupture of abscesses at the periphery of the lung and the production of spontaneous pneumothoraces.

Respiratory Syncitial Virus

RSV causes acute bronchiolitis and pneumonia in infants and young children (see previous page). The infection also occurs in older children and adults, who may have mild upper respiratory infections. More severe illnesses with constitutional signs and lower respiratory tract involvement can occur in these groups, occasionally in small winter epidemics.

Para-Influenza Infections

These infections are more severe than rhinovirus infections, but generally they are not as severe as influenzal infections. The signs and symptoms range from common colds and laryngitis to severe laryngo-tracheo-bronchitis and pneumonia. In most cases, fever does not exceed 38 deg. C. and lasts only two to three days; nasal discharge, cough and hoarseness are prominent. In more severe cases the signs of obstructive laryngitis or lower respiratory tract infection predominate. Diagnosis is by isolation of the virus from throat or nasal swabs or by demonstration of a rise in titre in paired sera.

Q Fever

Q fever is caused by Coxiella burneti and is carried by many insects, ticks and animals.[3] In the U.K the main sources of infection are probably cattle or sheep, airborne or direct contact and possibly via unpasteurised milk. The com-monest clinical presentation is of pyrexia of undetermined origin (PUO), which may be accompanied by a bewildering array of symptoms. These include atypical pneumonia and endocarditis. Treatment is with tetracyclines.

Ornithosis and Psittacosis

Ornithosis is an infection caused by chlamydia B organisms, which are transmitted by birds. Psittacosis is the term used for disease transmitted by the parrot and the budgerigar families of birds. Clinically, there is an atypical pneumonia or milder respiratory infection. Treatment is with tetracycline.

Legionnaire's Disease

Legionnaire's disease is a bacterial pneumonia caused by Legionella pneumoniae, which responds to clarithromycin and to a lesser extent, erythromycin. Defective water cooling apparatus and shower heads, especially after not having been used for long periods of time, as in the school holidays, have been seen as reservoirs of this infection.

Influenza

Influenza is an acute viral respiratory infection, affecting all ages, caused usually, by the influenza viruses A or B. Influenza C is rarely isolated from ill patients, probably causing inapparent infection, and serological studies have demonstrated that asymptomatic infections, involving A and B viruses also occur.

For example, at Christ's Hospital school in the H1N1 influenza epidemic of 1978, the clinical attack rate was 50%, but serological studies at the same time demonstrated that the true attack rate was 90%.[4] Influenza A also affects many animals and birds, but Influenza B appears to affect only humans.

Influenza is highly infectious. The incubation period is short, (one to three days) and the disease spreads rapidly in closed communities, such as residential schools, colleges, barracks etc. Influenza viruses are unique in their capacity for antigenic variation. They have two surface antigens, haemagglutinin (H) and Neuraminidase (N), both of which can induce antibody formation in humans. Influenza A, and to a lesser extent influenza B viruses, are subject to minor changes of the surface antigens (antigenic drift), and less frequently, influenza A viruses undergo major alterations (antigenic shift). The sub-types of influenza A are classified according to the surface antigens. H1N1 for example, is the name given to the strain which first appeared in 1947 and reappeared in 1978. The massive epidemics of 1957 occurred after changes in both haemagglutinin and neuraminidase. The virus was named H2N2. The next shift in 1968 involved haemagglutinin alone, so the strain was called H3N2.

Symptoms

Clinically Influenza A and B are indistinguishable, being acute febrile illnesses, generally with sudden onset and considerable constitutional symptoms including prostration and misery. The conjunctivae and fauces show an early non-oedematous flushing. The respiratory tract, especially the trachea, is soon involved. The nose may also be inflamed and excoriated. Epistaxes may occur. There may be a complaint of a sore throat, but inflammation is slight. Headaches, muscle pains and a dry cough are almost invariable. Occasionally the illness is biphasic and in the average case the fever may rise to 40 degrees C and last for two to four days.

Complications

Although the complication rate is low amongst school children, there are nevertheless some potentially serious complications, especially pneumonia. The dangerous fulminating type, which is rapidly fatal within a few hours may be a primary viral infection with the influenza virus, or it may be due to secondary staphylococcal infection. Secondary bronchopneumonia due to Step. pneumoniae occurs more commonly and H Influenzae and haemolytic streptococci are secondary invaders.

Reye's syndrome is a rare complication of influenza and other virus infections. Encephalopathy and fatty liver degeneration produce a very high mortality rate. Because of the association between aspirin in young febrile children and Reye's syndrome, it is urged that paracetamol be used instead of aspirin.

Diagnosis

The virus can be isolated from throat swabs or by special techniques using nasal aspirate which can provide evidence of the infecting virus in three hours. Retrospective diagnoses can be made by serological tests on acute and convalescent sera.

Incubation Period

Two to three days.

Period of Communicablity

Influenza is transmitted to those who are susceptible to the epidemic strain. Communicability is thought to be maximal in the prodromal phase, lasting no more than three days from the outset.

Immunity

Immunity is type specific but is bedevilled by antigenic changes in the virus. (See above). Infection with one sub-type of influenza (e.g. H3 N2) or with Influenza B provides lasting immunity against the infecting strain and minor degrees of antigenic drift. When the surface antigens have been significantly different from the parent strain, the patient may be more susceptible to the new virus. Reinfection with the H1N1 strain appears to occur more readily in school children than with the other strains.

Prevalence

Influenza usually occurs in epidemics, especially in closed communities in which a high proportion of the susceptible community are infected within two or three weeks of the first case. Epidemics are caused more by influenza A than by influenza B viruses. Epidemics of the latter are confined to schools and other institutions, where they tend to occur in cycles of three to five years. Usually, outbreaks occur between the months of April and December.

Prevention

The place of influenza vaccination in schools remains controversial. (See 'Influenza Vaccination') . In residential schools, previously identified helpers can be called in to help nurse uncomplicated cases in converted dormitories, leaving the sanatorium available for severe cases.

Amantadine is effective in the prevention of influenza A, but not influenza B, and although rather costly, has sometimes been used to advantage in school populations. (See 'Influenza Vaccination'.)[5]

Treatment

There is no specific treatment. General symptomatic measures, such as copious fluids, rest, paracetamol, and a mixture of honey, lemon and glycerin for the troublesome coughs are helpful but secondary bacterial infections require to be treated with an appropriate antibiotic.

Return to school

In a boarding school epidemic with pressure on sanatorium accommodation, it is often necessary for pupils to return to school after the fever has settled. This causes no harm, so long as it is recognised that there is likely to be some debility in the convalescent period and no strenuous activity should be permitted, especially until after the resting pulse rate has returned to normal.

The Exanthemata

Measles

Measles is an acute infectious disease caused by a paramyxovirus, transmitted by droplet spread and characterised by fever, respiratory symptoms, (principally cough), conjunctivitis, misery and a dusky red, blotchy, macular rash. The incubation period is approximately ten days. This is a notifiable disease, which before the introduction of the MMR vaccine, was one of the commonest infectious diseases of children.

Symptoms

A particularly troublesome dry cough develops associated with coryza and a considerable degree of fever. The conjunctivae are injected, as is the buccal mucosa and on the latter, Koplik's spots, likened to grains of salt on red velvet, appear about 48 hours before the start of the skin eruption. This usually first appears on the forehead, behind the ears and down the sides of the neck. More spots then occur and become widespread over the body, trunk and the limbs, changing from discrete macules to become confluent. There may be a few scattered petechiae. During this eruptive phase the child is intensely miserable, febrile and nothing will relieve the cough. After about four days, the fever settles, the cough improves, the misery disappears and the widespread blotchy rash takes on a brownish coloured staining as it subsides. (This brown staining and the Koplik's spots are pathognomonic of measles.)

Measles has a mortality (highest in children under one year of age and lowest from one to nine years), which was at an average rate of 13 deaths per year from 1970 until 1988 when immunisation against measles was introduced. Since then the death rate from the disease has fallen significantly.[6]

Complications are thought to occur in about 7% of notified cases and include otitis media, broncho-pneumonia, purulent conjunctivitis and rarely, measles encephalitis. This latter condition occurs in about one in 5000 cases with a mortality of 15% and up to just under a half of those surviving having some degree of residual neurological handicap. For this reason alone, it is vitally important that all children should be immunised against measles, but especially those who are already debilitated from another condition (e.g. cystic fibrosis, Down's syndrome or congenital heart disease).

Immunosuppressed children, especially those suffering from leukaemia, are at risk of severe illness and death, from measles.

There is an even rarer, late, neurological complication of measles, which is invariably eventually fatal, known as SSPE, or subacute sclerosing panencephalitis, against which protection is afforded by measles immunisation.

Diagnosis

In the preimmunisation days, the diagnosis was often delayed in the initial catarrhal stage, especially if there were no other cases nearby, unless the buccal mucosa was routinely and carefully examined. Often the rash was confused with rubella or scarlet fever and perhaps the maculo-papular rashes due to the entero viruses (Echo and Coxsackie). In roseola infantum, thought to be caused by the herpes virus, the sick child's condition improves dramatically and the temperature falls, with the appearance of the rash, which lasts less than a day: quite unlike measles. Erythema infectiosum (fifth disease) is a mild non-febrile erythematous eruption occurring in epidemics in children and causing a characteristic 'slapped cheek' appearance. The parvavirus is thought to be responsible and a reticulate eruption on the trunk follows the 'slapped cheek' sign. There are minimal constitutional signs.[7] Also, it must be remembered that drug eruptions may cause difficulties in the diagnosis of measles, notably those due to ampicillin and co-trimoxazole.

One must remember the possibility of early meningococcal disease, for an erythematous rash may precede the onset of the petechial rash, and also Kawasaki disease, in young children, which presents with an erythematous rash, fever and desquamation. (qv). Finally, in adolescents, especially in menstruating girls using tampons, the 'toxic shock syndrome' (qv) must be borne in mind.

Laboratory diagnosis

Examination of saliva samples for specific IgM preferably taken within three day of the onset of the rash are very accurate and replace the earlier serological tests. Ideally saliva tests should be performed on all notified measles cases.[8] Advice on this procedure can be obtained from the local Consultant in Communicable Disease Control, or Public Health Laboratory or Consultant in Public Health Medicine (CPHM), or in Scotland, Communicable Disease and Environmental Health (CD and EH).

Incubation Period

The incubation period is 10-15 days, usually 10 days from exposure to the onset of the illness, and 14 days to the development of the rash.

Period of Communicability

This is from the day before the development of symptoms until the disappearance of the rash.

Immunity

The attack normally confers permanent immunity.

Prevention

Measles vaccine, ideally offered along with protection for rubella and mumps (MMR) between the ages of 12 and 15 months, and again (since October 1996) with their pre-school boosters, prevents the disease in approximately 95% of those vaccinated. When occurring in a vaccinated child, the disease is usually mild. During an outbreak, measles vaccine given to susceptible contacts, early in the incubation period, is effective (See 'Immunisation'). As in other countries, and in young people from abroad attending school and further education in the UK, measles is now being seen in much older children and even young adults. Be prepared for more in the way of complications from measles in these patients, compared to young children.

Treatment

There is no specific treatment for measles. Antibiotics are used to treat secondary infection, which may be used prophylactically in those children who are widely susceptible to any of the common complications., e.g. otitis media, lower respiratory infections, etc.

Return to school

Pupils may return to school on recovery, provided this is not earlier than seven days.

Rubella (German Measles).

Rubella is a notifiable viral infectious disease. A very mild infection, it is characterised by a generalised pink macular rash, with enlargement of the suboccipital and post auricular lymph nodes. The importance of this disease of course, is the risk to the foetus in early pregnancy, with the baby being born suffering from the Congenital Rubella Syndrome. (CRS).

Symptoms and signs

These are malaise with low fever and minimal respiratory signs which develop simultaneously with the rash. This is a very discrete macular rash which spreads down the trunk and on to the thighs. Occasionally, petechial spots on the soft palate are noted. Joint pains and swellings occur in young adults. The rash fades in about four days and there is minimal constitutional disturbance. Subclinical attacks are known to occur, which can still nevertheless cause the Congenital Rubella Syndrome (CRS). This devastating condition affects some infants born to mothers who contract rubella during the first four months of their pregnancy. Foetal defects in CRS include mental retardation, deafness, cataracts, congenital heart lesions and encephalitis, together with failure to gain weight, enlargement of liver and spleen and thrombocytopenic purpura. Some infected infants may appear normal at birth, but perceptive deafness may become apparent later.

Termination of pregnancy should be considered where laboratory proven infection has occcured.

Diagnosis

Clinical diagnosis is entirely unreliable as the rash is easily confused with many of the rashes considered in the differential diagnosis of the measles rash.

(qv) Little or no credence should be placed on a clinical diagnosis alone. To be absolutely sure of the diagnosis, as for example, in early pregnancy, rubella specific IgM should be sought in a saliva sample taken within three days of the onset of the rash. For details regarding this procedure, see under measles.

Infection and Transmission
This is by droplet spread.

Incubation Period
14-21 days. Usually 18.

Period of Communicability
This is a few days before the onset of the symptoms and for 4 days after the appearance of the rash.

Immunity
The attack usually confers life-long immunity. The common history of alleged recurrent attacks simply emphasises the difficulty of accurate clinical diagnosis of this condition.

Prevention
Rubella can be prevented by a live vaccine, which is a component of the measles mumps and rubella (MMR) vaccine offered to children, ideally between the ages of 12 and 15 months of age, and again, (since October 1996) with their pre-school boosters. Single rubella vaccine is available for those not having the MMR vaccine. The schoolgirl rubella immunisation programme has now been discontinued.

Treatment
There is no specific treatment.

Return to School
Pupils can return to school as soon as they are well. If the school insists on exclusion the period should be four days after the appearance of the rash.

Chickenpox (Varicella)
Chickenpox is an acute highly contagious infectious disease with fever, constitutional symptoms and a vesicular itching rash, due to the varicella-zoster virus.

Symptoms
The rash is distributed centripetally (the opposite of smallpox) and the flexures are involved. Sparse rashes are common. The symptoms tend to be more severe in older patients. Maculopapules last a few hours before becoming vesicles (like dew drops), lasting about four days and then producing scabs. Successive crops of lesions following this sequence usually appear, giving a pleomorphic rash. Because of the intense itching secondary infection is transmitted to the lesions from scratching finger nails, thereby producing pustules. Sparse vesico-ulcerative lesions appear in the mouth early in the course of the disease. Varicella pneumonia, encephalitis and haemorrhagic chicken pox are rare but serious complications. Older children and adults tend

to get numerous lesions, together with fever and constitutional (influenza-like) symptoms appearing just before the rash. (These early symptoms are mild in young children).

Diagnosis
The diagnosis of chicken pox seldom presents any difficulty, as the vesicles are quite characteristic. In a young child, the lesions may be so sparse as to require a search. In older children and adults, they may cover most of the body.

Infection and Transmission
The spread is mainly by droplet spread, but skin lesions are also a source of contact infection. Contact with herpes zoster may cause chicken pox in susceptible children, but the infectivity is not great. However, immuno-compromised children, e.g. those undergoing treatment for leukaemia or those who are on, or have recently been on steroid therapy, may have devastating complications from an attack of chicken pox, eg. encephalitis, pneumonia or hepatitis. Such children, who are chickenpox or herpes zoster contacts and have no previous history of chicken pox or who are already known to be varicella negative, should be given Human Varicella-Zoster Immunoglobulin (VZIG) This preparation is in short supply, so that the Joint Committee on Vaccination and Immunisation of the Department of Health, the Welsh Office, the Scottish Department of Health and DHSS (Northern Ireland) recommend VZIG prophylaxis for all individuals who fulfil all of the following three criteria:

(i) A clinical condition which increases the risk of severe varicella; this includes immunosuppressed patients, (see later), neonates and pregnant women. (There exists a congenital (foetal) varicella syndrome, which features microcephaly, cataracts, growth retardation and varicella near or soon after delivery, which can be fatal for the neonate.)

(ii) No antibodies to varicella zoster (VZ) virus (see later)

(iii) Significant exposure to chickenpox or herpes zoster.

Immunosuppressed patients include the following:

(a) Patients currently being treated with chemotherapy or generalised radiotherapy, or within six months of terminating such treatment.

(b) Patients who have received an organ transplant and are currently on immunosuppressive treatment;

(c) Patients who within the previous six months have received a bone marrow translant.

(d) Children who, within the previous three months have received prednisolone, orally or rectally, at a daily dose (or its equivalent) of 2mg /Kg/day for at least one week, or 1mg/Kg/day for one month. For adults, an equivalent dose is harder to define but immuno-suppression should be considered in those who have received a dose of around 40mg prednisolone per day for more than one week in the previous three months.

(e) Patients on lower doses of steroids, given in combination with cytotoxic drugs (including anti-thymic globulin or other immuno-suppressants);

(f) Patients with evidence of impaired cell-mediated immunity, for example severe combined immune deficiency syndromes, Di George syndrome and other combined immunodeficiency syndromes.

(g) Patients with symptomatic HIV infection. VZIG is not indicated for asymptomatic HIV positive patients with normal CD4 counts as there is no evidence of increased risk of severe varicella in these individuals.

(h) Patients with gammaglobulin deficiencies who are receiving replacement therapy with intravenous normal immunoglobulin, do not require VZIG.

Supplies of VZIG (issued free of charge to patients who meet the above criteria) are available from Public Health Laboratories and the Communicable Disease Surveillance Centre (CDSC) Tel: 0181 200 6868).

Northern Ireland: the Public Health Laboratories, Belfast City Hospital, Lisburn Road, Belfast. Tel: 01232 329241.

Scotland; Available from Regional Transfusion Centres.

Please Note: Immunosuppressed patients with bleeding disorders in whom intramuscular injections are contraindicated should be given intravenous normal immunoglobulin at a dose of 0.2g per kg body weight (ie 4 ml/kg for a 5% solution) instead. This will produce serum levels equivalent to those achieved with VZIG.

Needless to say, consultant advice should be sought in dealing with the above types of patient.

Incubation Period

Between 11 and 21 days, most commonly about 16 days. The incidence of chickenpox is seasonal and reaches a peak from March to May.

Period of Communicability

Chickenpox is probably most infectious from several days before the rash until the last crust has separated. This is of relevance in the immunocompromised children discussed above.

Immunity

One attack confers permanent immunity against chickenpox, but it confers no immunity against herpes zoster, which occurs with the reactivation of the varicella-zoster virus in a dorsal root sensory ganglion.

Prevention

Live attenuated varicella vaccine has recently been licensed in some countries, but as yet, no such vaccine has been licensed for use in the UK.

Treatment

Local treatment consists of the application of calamine lotion or even sodium bicarbonate paste, to reduce the itching and therefore the scratching. Dirty fingernails result in secondary infection which makes the residiual scarring (which occurs in any case) worse. Oral antihistamines may be helpful. There is no evidence that VZIG is effective in the treatment of severe disease.

Return to School
Children may return to school six days after the appearance of the rash, unless heavily scabbed.

Herpes Zoster (Shingles)
Herpes zoster is usually due to reactivation of the varicella-zoster virus which has lain dormant in a dorsal root ganglion resulting from an attack of chicken pox several years previously. More rarely, it results from direct exposure to chickenpox or herpes zoster. It is characterised by a unilateral eruption of grouped vesicles on an erythematous base, confined to the territory of the corresponding sensory nerve.

Symptoms
Adults are affected more frequently than children. The eruption is preceded by pain, often severe, in the same area for a few days and this can cause diagnostic difficulties, especially if the site is the chest, abdomen or head. Patches of erythema develop in which the characteristic vesicles soon appear. These dry up and scab over in about a week to ten days. After separation of the scabs, there may be considerable residual scarring. The intercostal nerves are most frequently involved, but the eruption may occur anywhere on the body. If the naso-labial branch of the first division of the trigeminal nerve is involved, then keratitis and iridocyclitis may follow. This requires prompt ophthalmic referral.

Pain and paraesthesiae may persist in the affected area for months after the disappearance of the eruption, particularly in the elderly. (Post-herpetic neuralgia). Rarely, motor nuclei close to the affected sensory ganglia are involved, causing local pareses. Herpes of the external auditory meatus and palate associated with facial paralysis constitute the Ramsay Hunt syndrome.

Incubation Period
The incubation period when there is direct infection is three to seven days.

Period of Communicability
Herpes zoster is not very infectious, but child contacts may develop chicken pox, and there is some evidence of case to case spread of herpes zoster. The period of communicability is likely to be similar to chickenpox ie until six days after the appearance of the rash.

Immunity
One attack usually confers permanent immunity.

Treatment
Specific treatment with idoxuridine paint four times daily commenced as soon as possible after the appearance of the vesicles reduces the duration of symptoms and the incidence of post-herpetic neuralgia. Aciclovir and famciclovir are other anti-viral agents which may be taken by mouth if the

lesions are extensive or if there is constitutional distress. The former is available in a cream for local application for troublesome herpes simplex labialis lesions. (See below). Pain can be treated with analgesic drugs, or, in accordance with recent work, low doses of tricyclic anti-depressant drugs.[9]

Return to school
The disease is often mild in children and they need not necessarliy be excluded from school in view of the low infectivity of herpes, especially if the lesions are on the thoraco lumbar aspects of the body, normally covered by clothing. Perhaps it would be wise to keep them off games until recovery. In more severe cases, they may return to school on clinical recovery.

Herpes Simplex
There are two serotypes of viruses causing this commmon condition, HSV1 and HSV2, featuring a vesicular eruption on the skin or mucous membrane, preceded by an itching or a burning sensation. HSV1 causes muco-cutaneous and eye lesions and occasionally encephalitis, whilst HSV2 causes genital herpes and occasionally neonatal herpes from contact with the mother's genitalia during birth. The commonest presentation in children is ulcerative gingivo-stomatitis, which in older children can be quite severe with fever, lethargy, halitosis, coated tongue and gingivitis. Vesicles appear on the lips and in the mouth which then ulcerate.

There is often quite marked cervical adenopathy. Other skin lesions appear, largely by direct transmission from the mouth by the fingers and herpetic whitlows occur in this manner. Sometimes the vesicles on the skin may mimic herpes zoster, but they are pain free and often bilateral. 'Scrumpox', thought to be herpes simplex infection of the skin transmitted via rugby football scrums, and often more troublesome than bacterial impetigo, is less common now. Children who are already suffering from eczema are at special risk from HSV1 infections, especially if their eczema is being treated with topical steroids. Consultant advice is indicated. Similarly, children suffering from eczema should not be allowed to come into contact with other children suffering from any kind of herpes

Children with HSV1 eye lesions have corneal involvement and perhaps dendritic ulcers. Vesicles may be noted on the eyelids. Steroid eye preparations must not be used and consultant ophthalmic advice should be sought without delay.

Recurrent herpes simplex infection is the most common cause of 'cold sores', or herpes labialis. The virus lies dormant following a primary infection and when reactivated, produces a vesicular eruption around the lips. Such herpetic eruptions are associated with the common cold, influenza and pneumonia. Also, they can occur after trauma, exposure to cold or to sunlight and during menstruation and emotional upsets. In eczematous subjects, infection may cause eczema herpeticum (Kaposi's varicelliform eruption.)

Systemic infections with HSV1 can occur. These are fortunately rare: the two best known being hepatitis and encephalitis. The latter has a characteristic EEG tracing, is very often fatal and there is a high rate of residual neurological damage in survivors.

Patients, usually adolescents, with genital herpes, HSV2 infections should be referred to a clinic for sexually transmitted diseases.

Diagnosis

Diagnosis is on clinical grounds. It can be confirmed on electron microscopy of fluid from vesicles and by culturing the virus. A serological response can be demonstrated.

Incubation period

Four to five days

Period of Communicability

Seven to ten days.

Prevention

As for bacterial impetigo. Keep away from school until skin lesions have healed. Beware of the risk to other children who suffer from eczema coming into contact with herpes sufferers.

Treatment

Antiviral agents such as idoxuridine, aciclovir and famciclovir are effective against herpes simplex and can be used in severe cases. One recent study showed that all clinical symptoms and viral shedding were shorter in children receiving aciclovir than in those receiving placebo.[10] These preparations are expensive however, and simple antiseptic preparations such as Eusol or povidine-iodine are usually all that is necessary for cold sores. Antiseptic mouthwashes usually suffice for minor degrees of stomatitis.

Other Virus Infections

Mumps

Mumps is an acute, viral infectious disease caused by the Myxovirus and is characterised by salivary gland swellings (usually the parotid). Young children are usually infected, but the disease can occur in older children, adolescents and adults. It is a droplet infection and it is a notifiable disease.

Symptoms

Fever and headache develop in association with swelling of one or more of the salivary glands, lasting about a week, the parotids being the most commonly affected. Orchitis is perhaps the best known complication of mumps, which may occur at any age and may be unilateral or bilateral. This can be very painful in the older male and although some degree of testicular atrophy follows, impotence and infertility are thought to be rare. Oophoritis and pancreatitis are other complications. Neurological complications include meningitis and encephalitis which may occur at any time during or after the disease. Permanent, often total, deafness may occur at any age. Rarely, any of the above complications may occur without any salivary gland involvement, the diagnosis then being made by serological means.

Diagnosis

Parotid swellings fill up the depression behind the angle of the mandible and may cause the ear lobe to rise. Less often, submandibular, or rarely sublingual mumps may occur. The affected salivary glands are not usually tender on palpation, although parotid mumps may occasionally cause trismus. In the acute stage of mumps, there is sometimes a subcutaneous, gelatinous infiltration over the affected salivary gland, which may extend down towards the thyroid or the clavicle. Sharp percussion of this swelling produces a rapid shaking of the tissues, known as the 'jelly sign' which is pathognomonic of mumps. Also, the openings of Stensen's and Wharton's ducts may be red and oedematous.[11]

The first attack of isolated or recurrent bacterial (suppurative) parotitis, is frequently mistaken for mumps, and of course lymphadenitis due to tonsillitis or infectious mononucleosis must be differentiated from the salivary gland swellings of mumps. Occasionally dental abscesses are mistaken for mumps.

Alteration of consciousness, signs of meningeal irritation, fever and vomiting, require consultant advice, if not hospital admission. Mumps meningo-encephalitis is a rare complication of mumps convalescence, with a high mortality rate.

Torsion of the testis must always be remembered and excluded before diagnosing orchitis. The serum amylase is elevated in over 90% of cases with clinical mumps and if necessary, mumps specific IgM can be detected in saliva samples taken within three days of the onset of the salivary gland swellings.

Mumps has been a notifable disease in the UK since October 1988.

Incubation Period

Outside limits of 12-26 days are usually quoted, but commonly, the incubation period is from 16 to 18 days.

Period of Communicability

Mumps, which has a low infective state, is communicable from a few days before the onset of symptoms and signs until about four days after the onset of salivary gland swelling.

Immunity

One attack confers life-long immunity. The mumps virus can cause inapparent or subclinical illness, and laboratory studies show that at least 90% of the population are immune by the age of 14.

Prevention

Spread of the disease may be prevented by the isolation of cases during the acute illnness. MMR vaccine offered to schoolchildren between the ages of 12 and 15 months of age and, since October 1996, with their pre-school booster injections, offers protection against mumps.

Treatment

There is no specific treatment for mumps. If, as is usual in young children, there is no discomfort, then no treatment is required. If the salivary gland swellings are troublesome, then simple analgesics like paracetamol, taking fluids via a straw and local warmth to the neck have been found to be helpful. The acute pain of orchitis will be helped by the use of a suspensory bandage and oral prednisolone, 10 to15 mg four times daily.

Return to School

Pupils may return to school on recovery.

Viral Hepatitis

There are now at least five types of hepatitis virus, designated A to E.[12]

Hepatitis A

This is common, notifiable and cyclical in the UK and is transmitted by the faecal-oral route, either by person to person contact or from consuming contaminated food, e.g. shellfish. Epidemics may occur in closed communities, especially those catering for children with learning difficulties, but usually the cases are sporadic. Only one serotype of hepatitis A virus (HAV) is recognised throughout the world. The disease is generally mild, although the severity does tend to increase with age. The prodromal stage commences with fever, anorexia and malaise, followed by nausea and vomiting. There may be some pain in the right hypochondrium and about this time, bile may appear in the urine followed by bradycardia and pruritus. The liver may be enlarged and tender. In an outbreak or an epidemic, mild cases may fail to develop any jaundice – the anicteric state. In most cases the disease is mild and resolves spontaneously in three to six weeks. Occasional cases of fulminating hepatitis may occur but there is no chronic carrier state and little likelihood of chronic liver damage.[13]

The highest risk areas are the Indian sub-continent, the Far East and Eastern Europe.[13]

Diagnosis

Hepatitis A can be diagnosed accurately by serological immunoassay from a single blood specimen (Refer to Microbiologist for special precautions re. taking blood.)The differential diagnosis is large, bearing in mind that many other viruses cause hepatitis with jaundice, e. g. cytomagalovirus, E. B. virus, yellow fever and herpes simplex. Toxoplasmosis and Weil's disease are non-viral conditions which can produce hepatitis and jaundice.

Incubation Period

The incubation period varies from 15 to 40 days.

Period of Communicability

This is from before the onset of clinical signs for at least three to four weeks.

Immunity

Relapses occur in about 30% to 40% of patients within about two months of the original illness. Second attacks later than this are rare.

Prevention

Infective hepatitis is a notifiable disease and patients should be isolated at home or in the school sanatorium. Since the spring of 1992, Hepatitis A vaccine, a formaldehyde inactivated vaccine has been available, prepared from one of two strains of hepatitis A virus (HAV) grown in human diploid cells. (See 'Immunisation' for further details)

Travellers

Protection against hepatitis A is recommended for travellers to areas where the disease is endemic or where sanitation and general hygiene are poor, especially where a camping or 'backpacking' holiday is envisaged. Immunisation with hepatitis A vaccine is recommended, especially if the stay is over three months, or frequent visits are planned for such areas. Immunisation is considered not necessary for visitors to Northern and Western Europe (including Spain, Portugal and Italy) or to North America, Australia or New Zealand. (See 'Immunisation.')

Patients with chronic liver disease

Infective hepatitis A can produce a very serious illness in people with chronic liver disease and it is recommended that such patients should be immunised with hepatitis A vaccine. This will include intravenous drug misusers with chronic liver disease. (See 'Immunisation.')

Haemophiliacs

Immunisation against hepatitis A is recommended for haemophiliac patients who are receiving Factor VIII and Factor IX concentrates, in the preparation of which, the hepatitis A virus may not have been destoyed.

Sufferers form haemophilia may be infected with the viruses of hepatitis B and C and may even have established liver disease. In these cases, superimposed hepatitis A infection would result in severe illness. (See 'Immunisation'.)

Human normal immunoglobulin (HNIG)

This preparation offers protection for up to four months to people who by reason of recreation or employment may be temporarily at risk of contracting infection with hepatitis A. Such people might be close family contacts of an infected person or short term travellers. HNIG is of value in conferring protection against HAV on members of staff working in establishments dealing with young children e.g. nursery schools, or in closed communities with poor standards of personal hygiene. For further information (See' Immunisation.')

Treatment

There is no specific treatment for HAV. General measures like adequate rest and optimum hydration are important. Potentially hepatotoxic drugs like paracetamol must not be administered.

Return to School

Pupils may return to school on recovery. However, liver function tests may not revert to normal for several months and convalescence may be prolonged with some restriction on sporting activities.

Hepatitis B

Hepatitis B is caused by a more complex virus than hepatitis A and its aftermath is generally much more serious. All ages are affected and the disease is transmitted parenterally by infected blood or blood products from a sufferer or a carrier, or by sexual contact with an infected person. Vertical transmission is known to occur from mother to baby, as the virus is present in many body secretions. A particular risk occurs with injecting drug abusers and infection can be transmitted by such procedures as tattooing, acupuncture and ear piercing. Biology lessons, which until a short time ago required children to prick their fingers in order to obtain blood for microscopic examination, are not now permitted. Particular care is required in taking blood specimens, after needle-stick injuries and in dealing with children who are bleeding as the result of an accident. Rarely, transmission has also followed bites from an infected person.[14]

Transfusion associated infection is now rare in the UK, following the adequate treatment of blood products.

Clinically, hepatitis B sufferers usually have jaundice, but may have an anicteric form as was described in the case of hepatitis A. Usually the onset of the illness is mild, comprising nausea, anorexia, malaise, headache and maybe fever, but with the added features of arthropathy and urticarial rashes. Initially, hepatitis B may be clinically indistinguishable from hepatitis A, although Hepatitis B is usually more prolonged. The severity of the disease ranges from inapparent infections, which can be detected only by liver function tests or serological markers of acute hepatitis B infection, to cases of fulminating acute hepatic necrosis. Among cases admitted to hospital, the fatality rate is about 1%.

Diagnosis

Hepatitis B can be diagnosed serologically and the carriers identified in this way. The complete virus particle of HBV has an outer surface antigen (HBsAg) and an internal core antigen (HBcAg). A subunit of the core antigen is called the 'e antigen' (HBeAg), which is easy to detect in the serum of carriers and serves as a useful marker in indicating hepatitis B virus activity and therefore, infectivity. For example, the presence of the 'e antigen' (HBeAg), without the corresponding antibody (anti-HBe) indicates that a sufferer will be very infectious. Those with antibody to HBeAg (anti-HBe) are generally of low infectivity.

Of those infected as adults, 2-10% become chronic carriers of the hepatitis B virus, with surface antigen (HBsAg) persisting for longer than six months. Chronic carriage is more frequent in those infected as children and rises to 90% in those infected perinatally.

20-25% of hepatitis B carriers world-wide develop progressive liver disease with an active hepatitis leading in some patients, to cirrhosis. The prognosis of such people is uncertain, for chronic hepatitis B carriers are at increased risk of developing hepato-cellular carcinoma.

Known cases of Hepatitis B should be monitored serologically, together with liver function tests for many months after the onset of the infection, and remain under constant supervision. The number of overt cases in the UK has fallen in recent years and as of June 30th 1996, there were 612 reports in 1995.

About two thirds of infections are asymptomatic and therefore may not be diagnosed.[14]

Incubation Period

This is long: the range being 40 – 160 days.

Period of Communicability

This depends on serological assessments, i. e. the persistence of HBeAg and HBeAb.

Immunity and Prevention

Prevention depends on risk avoidance (i.e. drug misuse with shared needles and unprotected sexual contact with partners of unknown hepatitis B status.) Hepatitis B is the only sexually transmitted infection which may be prevented by immunisation.

For people, who by reason of their occupation are likely to encounter blood from infected patients, e. g. doctors, dentists. nurses, midwives, policemen, active immunisation is available, to which the immune response is good, but tends to fall off in those over 40 years of age. (See 'Immunisation').

Similar precautions as exist for the prevention of HIV infection should be followed after potential infection, accidentally acquired, as with a needlestick injury, specific immunoglobulin should be administered as soon as possible and in any case, within 48 hours. There must be adequate cleansing of the wound, with proper precautions (See 'Immunisation') with reporting to the doctor, who may wish to take consultant advice.

Treatment

There is no specific treatment for acute hepatitis B but chronic hepatitis B has been treated with anti-viral agents, e. g. alfa-interferon, with some success. As with hepatitis A, mild cases can be treated in the home or in the school sanatorium with due precautions in the handling of body fluids. Menstrual blood from an infected girl will contain the virus and soiled sanitary towels should be handled by nurses wearing disposable gloves and both gloves and towels incinerated afterwards.

Hepatitis C

Hepatitis C (HCV) used to be called Hepatitis, Non-A, Non-B. The condition is found in people accidentally infected with blood products (e. g. Factor VIII) and in people who are injecting drug users. Choo, Weiner, et al consider this infection to be responsible for most cases of transfusion hepatitis in America, Europe and Japan.)[15] Also, there are now eight recognised HCV genotypes, all with different isolates into subtypes, allowing each individual patient to be infected with several different strains. This variation is thought to permit the virus to escape recognition on serological testing, thus permitting persistence of infection and resistance to treatment.[16]

The detection of antibodies to hepatitis C, does not distinguish between an active infection or a previous exposure to the virus, unlike the case of Hepatitis B, with surface and 'e antigens'. The acute illness is usually mild and may be anicteric. However, fulminating hepatitis may occur. Groups at high risk: haemophiliacs (80%), current, or previous, intravenous drug users (50-70%), haemodialysis patients (2-5%), infected patients from high risk countries and multiple transfusion recipients. There is a low risk to health care workers eg

5-15% risk of infection from needle stick injuries. Generally, there is thought to be a low risk of death or complications from HCV, although in about 20% of cases, chronic HCV infection will progress to cirrhosis. However, fewer than 10% of chronic carriers will die, even after 20-40 years. Biopsy and long-term follow up required for assessment of prognosis. Consultant advice should be sought.

Diagnosis
Serological testing is required to make the diagnosis, but some of the difficulties are outlined above.

Incubation Period
The range is thought to be from 15 to 160 days.

Period of Communicability
This is likely to be long. Prolonged serological testing is indicated.

Immunity
No vaccine is yet available.

Prevention
Effective screening of blood and blood products, otherwise as for Hepatitis B, with regard to intravenous drug abuse and casual unprotected sex, although some authors think that the risk of sexual transmission of HCV is not as great as with HBV. Care should be taken in dealing with spilt blood and there should be no sharing of razors and tooth brushes.

Treatment
Alfa-interferons have been used and possibly, ribavirin, but this must be under consultant supervision.

Hepatitis D
This is caused by a viral agent which is exclusively associated with the virus which causes hepatitis B. Thus hepatitis D is a parenteral infection which is diagnosed serologically.

Prevention
Since this virus (sometimes called the delta agent) is intimately associated with the hepatitis B virus, the methods of prevention are those for hepatitis B.

Hepatitis E
Initially, it was thought that all cases of hepatitis acquired by the faecal-oral route were due to the A virus. However, recent serological work has identified another enteral virus which is distinct from hepatitis A. This virus, Hepatitis E, has been isolated from cases of hepatitis, largely from Asia and the tropics, where for many years, large numbers of acute viral hepatitis cases had been recognised for which neither hepatitis A viruses nor hepatitis B viruses were responsible.

It seems likely that hepatitis E was the responsible virus for these cases. Usually, this is a self-limiting condition which does not progress to chronic hepatitis. However, Pregnant women seem to be particularly at risk, with a high fatality rate (of the order of 20%) due to disseminated intravascular coagulation.[17]

Diagnosis

This diagnosis should be considered in all cases of Non-A, Non-B hepatitis, especially if there is a history of recent foreign travel in developing countries in the tropics and in Asia.

Incubation Period

The range is though to be 14-60 days.

Prevention

There is no active immunisation and there is no protection from hepatitis A immunoglobulin. High standards of public sanitation and sewage disposal are important factors in controlling the spread of this infection, and this needs to be adressed in developing countries.

Treatment

There is no specific treatment.

The Acquired Immune Deficiency Syndrome (AIDS)

This is the most significant new disease entity to be recognised in the UK (and elsewhere) in the last decade and a half. It first appeared in the UK in the early 1980s and according to figures issued by H. M Government, in the UK, 27,730 cases of AIDS, of whom 4,202 were women, had been reported by the end of September 1996.[18] The disease is a secondary immunodeficiency state caused by a virus occurring in individuals without any previous history of immunologial abnormality. This severe degree of immunodeficiency results in infectious, malignant and neurological disorders. The causal virus is a retro-virus, which is called the Human Immunodeficiency Virus. (HIV).

Retroviruses affecting humans have an affinity for lymphocytes, parti-cularly the T4 lymphocytes. The loss of function of the T4 helper lymphocytes caused by this virus, can explain the AIDS spectrum of immunological malfunction, including the opportunistic infections which have been recorded. (vide infra.)

HIV is not transmitted by casual contact, for example, such close non-sexual contact which normally occurs at school, home or work. Transmission of body fluids containing infected cells, e. g . blood, plasma, semen and breast milk, is required for spread to another person. Infected cells can reach target cells directly through the blood stream or via mucus membranes. Trans-mission through the latter is easier in inflamed or damaged tissue, explaining the higher risk of infection in the presence of other sexually transmitted diseases. Children may also be infected by HIV in utero and during delivery, by contaminated blood products, by dirty needles, and by sexual abuse.

The World Health Organisation divides the world into two categories according to the means of spread of HIV. In Pattern 1 countries (North America, Western Europe, Australasia and parts of South America) spread is principally through homo/bisexual males and I.V. drug use, with a male to female ratio of 10:1. In Pattern 2 countries (sub-Saharan Africa, Caribbean and part of South America and Asia) spread is principally heterosexual with male to female ratio of 1:1. Much of sub-Saharan Africa, where around 20 % of the adult population is HIV positive, is experiencing devastating demographic effects from high mortality among wage-earners and an exploding population of orphaned children.[19]

There is wide variability in the length of time between exposure and the development of the AIDS process, and a small number of people are still well 15 years after being found to be HIV positive. In children there is a very wide spectrum of disease with HIV infection. Approximately one third will have the early onset of opportunistic infection or severe encephalopathy, while approximately two thirds follow the adult pattern of symptoms. Statistically, more HIV infected children are reaching school age and such children may present in one of several ways; with another family member being ill, their mother being diagnosed as HIV positive in pregnancy, or an incidental finding on routine examination. In the management of these children, there were some similarities with infected adults, but also some important differences. The main features were:

> bacterial infections
> growth failure
> developmental delay
> encephalopathy
> LIP (lymphocytic interstitial pneumonitis.)
> malignancy is rare

Chicken pox could be very severe in immunocompromised children and if a suseptible child is exposed to the infection, they should be given varicella zoster immunoglobulin, preferably within 48 hours, but certainly not later than 96 hours, after exposure. The effect of the imunoglobulin is to prolong the incubation period to 28 days and if a second exposure to chicken pox occurs three weeks after the immunoglobulin has been given, a further dose is required. Lastly, intravenous aciclovir could be administered. A similar situation pertains to measles, where human immunoglobulin may be given within six days of exposure. (See under 'Immunisation' for details of the immunisation of HIV infected children).

Ideally, HIV infected children should be seen in hospital outpatients at three monthly intervals for blood tests to be taken for the monitoring of immune function and general review by a multi disciplinary team, with regard to diet and control of intercurrent infection. 'Septrin' is used for antibiotic prophylaxis and this has been found to have fewer side effects than in adults. Anti-HIV drugs are prescribed as appropriate.

With regard to school attendance, it is important to appreciate that the risk of non HIV infected children being infected from HIV infected children is extremely small indeed, only one well documented case of horizontal transmission having been recorded. The risk to the HIV infected child from attending school is that of infection, particularly from measles and chicken pox, but since children require the companionship and competition of other children for their all round development, the benefits of attending school and enjoying the normal social relationships, far outweigh the risk of the child acquiring a harmful infection, especially if the above procedures are followed.

It must be appreciated that many parents are reluctant to disclose the diagnosis of their child's condition, even to members of their own families. There is the risk of children becoming stigmatised and it is important that schools address matters of staff training, confidentiality, standard good hygiene practices for all children and adequate sex education including, in particular, the prevention of HIV infection.[20]

As far back as 1988, MOSA produced policy guidelines for Headteachers when approached regarding the admission of a child known to be HIV positive or to be a hepatitis B carrier . The revised versions (1994), are as follows:

(i) Accept the child.

(ii) Explain to the parents the policy of confidentiality in the school and the need for the School Medical Officer and Nurse to be aware of the situation.

(iii) Ensure that all first-aid equipment and practices are updated regularly in accordance with the Department of Health guideliines.

(iv) Ensure that counselling is provided.

(v) Ensure that the Head Teacher, House Master, medical and nursing staff have ready access to Department for Education and Employment publications on AIDS and Hepatitis B in school children.

Confidential testing for HIV antibodies may be arranged for any person requesting such a test but only in association with pre and post test counselling by a suitably qualified person. The long term implications for job prospects, eligibility for insurance and the social life of the individual concerned require very careful evaluation. Although no regulations exist for the statutory notification of HIV infection, there is a voluntary system for the anonymous reporting of such cases to the Communicable Diseases Surveillance Centre in England and Wales or to the Communicable Diseases (Scotland) Unit, so that the national scale of this infection may be monitored.[19]

See under 'References' for details of DFEE publications on AIDS and Hepatitis B which are recommended to all schools.

Surfaces contaminated with blood or other body fluids should be cleaned carefully by experienced staff wearing disposable gloves and aprons which then should be disposed of according to the locally agreed scheme of management. The immunodeficiency virus is readily inactivated by heat and commonly used disinfecting agents. A 1 in 10 household bleach solution diluted in cold water should be used for cleaning contaminated (or potentially contaminated) surfaces.

For sports injuries where there is bleeding, the traditional bucket and sponge should be replaced by individually pre-packed sterile sponges or pieces of gauze, with sterile water from sealed bottles. The person administering the First Aid should wear disposable gloves. As in the case of Hepatitis B, there should be no finger pricking to obtain blood for biology lessons, neither should there be any blood mixing by means of which certain children demonstrate their mutual affection. Ear piercing and tattooing should be actively discouraged.

With the increase in foreign travel associated with various school groups for sporting and cultural activities the school doctor is likely to be asked for guidance on matters of hygiene in the context of AIDS, whilst the group is abroad. By far the greatest risk in Pattern 2 countries is heterosexual intercourse. Commercial sex workers can be very seductive and many supposedly sensible visitors succumb to their blandishments under the influence of alcohol. Those in charge of school groups therefore have a heavy and unenviable responsibility for the welfare of their charges.[19]

Packages are now available which contain disposable sterile sponges, needles, surgical gloves, suture material and dressings so that responsible teaching staff, with suitable training, will be able to carry out first aid.

Poliomyelitis

Poliomyelitis is an acute viral illness following invasion of the gastro-intestinal tract by polio viruses. About half the patients have a minor prodromal illness. The major illness which may follow a few days later, ranges from aseptic meningitis without paralysis (Non-paralytic .poliomyelitis), to flaccid paralysis of all degrees of severity, in any part of the body. Other symptoms include head and neck ache, fever, stiff back and neck. The causal organism is an enterovirus, of which there are three main types, (1, 2 and 3), each of which having a special affinity for nervous system tissue. They are known to replicate in anterior horn cells and motor neurones.

The infection rate in households with young families is very high, depending on the infecting virus and the prevailing social conditions. In many of the developing countries, poliomyelitis is endemic and cases may occur sporadically or in epidemics.

Mode of spread.

Transmission is via contact with the faeces or by the oropharyngeal secretions of an infected person.

Incubation period

Three to 21 days. It is thought that cases are maximally infective from a week to ten days before the onset of symptoms and it is believed that the virus may be shed in the faeces for at least up to six weeks afterwards.

Fortunately, the disease is now very rare in the UK, but travellers abroad must ensure that their polio vaccination status is intact. (See 'Immunisation').

Other Enterovirus Infections (Coxsackie and Echo)

In addition to the three main polio viruses, other enteroviruses consist of many different sero-types of Coxsackie A, Coxsackie B and Echo viruses. (Coxsackie, an island off the coast of America. Echo, an acronym of Enteric cytopathic human orphan.)

They are spread by the faecal-oral route to infect the pharynx and the alimentary tract. They may then cause a viraemia with further spread to other organs and especially, the central nervous system. All of them can cause acute febrile illnesses with a variety of signs and symptoms including meningism, myalgia, respiratory tract infection, glandular enlargement, mild diarrhoea, vomiting and different kinds of skin eruptions and rashes. There are certain specific syndromes associated with different viruses and subtypes, some of which are:

(a) *Epidemic Myalgia.* (Bornholm Disease, so called after a small island in the Baltic sea). Coxsackie B viruses cause this febrile illness with severe stitch-like pains in thoracic, abdominal and limb muscles. Fever is present to 39 degrees C and a biphasic course is common. Complications include pleurisy, pericarditis and orchitis. Myocarditis may occur and infected infants may die from this. Differential diagnoses from intrathoracic and abdominal disese is crucial, yet often very difficult.

(b) *Lymphocytic Meningitis.* Most of the enteroviruses and the mumps virus (see earlier) can cause lymphoyctic meningitis. The onset is usually sudden with headache, photophobia, vomiting and drowsiness. Neck stiffnesss is usually present. The main illness may follow a minor illness due to the same virus. The CSF shows an increased cell count with a preponderance of lymphocytes but without visible organisms. (At the onset, there may be an excess of neutrophils.) The course of the illness is usually mild and short. Many transient mild cases occur, with little more than meningism. Epidemics may occur in the community.

(c) *Hand, Foot and Mouth Disease.* Small discrete vesicles about 0.5mm in diameter with surrounding erythema occur on the hands and the feet, both on the soles and the palms and also on the sides of the fingers and toes. Also, they occur on the buccal mucous membrane and tongue and cause soreness. The patient may be febrile or have pharyngitis with fever. The illness is especially associated with Coxsackie virus A 16 and is usually mild and short. No treatment is indicated.

(d) *Herpangina.* This too, is caused by Coxsackie A virus. It has an abrupt onset, with fever up to 40 degrees C., sore throat and enlarged cervical glands. Small vesicles, 1-2mm in diameter on an erythematous base develop on the soft palate and fauces, and these are followed by shallow ulcers. The lesions do not extend to the anterior part of the mouth. The illness lasts up to 4 days.

Diagnosis
Enterovirus infections can be diagnosed by isolation of the virus from the throat, faeces or CSF.

Incubation Period
The incubation period for enterovirus infections is betweeen two and five days.

Period of Communicability
These illnesses are probably communicable during the acute phase of the illness, and possibly longer when the virus is excreted in the faeces.

Immunity
Immunity is type specific and long lasting.

Prevention
Little that is effective can be done to prevent the spread of enterovirus infections, but cases of meningitis should be isolated during the acute phase of the illness, and care should be taken over the disposal of excreta.

Treatment and Return to School
There is no specific treatment and pupils may return to school on recovery.

Infectious Mononucleosis (Glandular Fever)
Infectious mononucleosis is caused by the Epstein Barr virus (E-B virus). In young children infections are often mild and unrecognised, but those in the 15-25 year age-group usually develop a more severe illness.

Symptoms
The onset is often gradual and ill-defined, with headache, malaise and fever. Sore throat follows immediately, or within two days of the onset, and is often severe. Within a few days, the patient may be very uncomfortable, with prostration, a fever as high as 40 degrees C., grossly enlarged tonsils and a confluent white exudate covering the tonsillar area. Often, petechiae are seen on the palate. The naso-pharynx may be congested, with some oedema of the eyelids. Swallowing and respiration may be embarrassed. The cervical lymph nodes, especially those in the posterior triangles, are enlarged and cause discomfort but they are not very tender. (This is sometimes called the 'anginose' type of glandular fever.) Other lymph nodes, the liver and the spleen may be enlarged. Illness and fever fluctuate for seven to ten days (exceptionally up to three weeks) and then the symptoms and signs gradually resolve. Convalescence may be slow and the patient may tire very easily after only minimal effort. Prolonged debility occasionally occurs. After the acute stage, relapses do not usually occur. Second attacks after a few years, are not unknown.

A variant, ('the febrile type') includes fever and lymph node enlargement, with some enlargement of liver and spleen, but without throat involvement. Jaundice is uncommon in glandular fever, usually not more than 10% of cases, although in most cases it is possible to demonstrate minor abnormalities of liver function tests; usually slight elevations of the serum bilirubin and the transaminases. These revert to normal on recovery.

Very occasionally, and usually in adults, glandular fever may present as a pyrexia of undetermined origin, (PUO), or even as acute abdominal pain.

Complications
Complications are rare, but include a rash which is usually faint and transient. However, a florid morbiliform rash may occur in up to 90% of cases treated with ampicillin and the rash is directly due to the use of this drug. For this reason, ampicillin and amoxycillin are contra-indicated whenever there is a possibility of infectious mononucleosis.

The spleen is very friable and may rupture during the acute or the convalescent stages of the disease, and should be examined very carefully. Such an event, would of course require prompt surgical referral. Rarely, neurological complications may occur in the form of meningoencephalitis.

Diagnosis

There is a lymphocytosis, usually with an atypical lymphocytosis visible on a blood film. Heterophile antibodies are characteristic of glandular fever and these will agglutinate washed sheep or horse red blood cells (after absorption with guinea pig kidney). This is the Paul-Bunnell test, which requires to be done in the laboratory and is positive in all cases of glandular fever, usually by the end of the second week of the illness. Other tests, which can be performed in the school or in the surgery, are the fast slide agglutination tests, the 'Monospot' being one of them.

If initially, the Paul-Bunnell or the Monospot tests are negative, it is advisable, if glandular fever seems likely on clinical grounds, to repeat the test in 10 to 14 days. Similarly, with requests seeking atypical lymphocytes in the blood film. The Paul Bunnell test remains positive for a variable length of time in the convalescent period, but there is no correlation with this period of antibody reponse and the nature or severity of the clinical state.

Streptococcal and other, viral or parasitic infections mimic the clinical picture of glandular fever and require to be differentiated from it and most school doctors will have met the situation of a patient with signs and symptoms of glandular fever and persistently negative Paul Bunnell and Monospot tests. In these cases, cytomegalovirus and toxoplasma gondii infections, described below, require to be considered.

Incubation Period

The incubation period is unknown, but maybe up to several weeks.

Period of Communicability.

There is some evidence that contact has to be close for its transmission. The period of communicability is probably confined to the acute phase.

Immunity

Immunity is thought to be permanent after an attack but individuals may be immune because of sub-clinical or mild infections early in life.

Treatment

There is no specific treatment but symptomatic treatment may be required during the acute phase. When threatened with pharyngeal or respiratory obstruction, then steroids are needed. As mentioned before, amoxycillin and ampicillin are strongly contraindicated. In fact antibiotics are of no benefit in glandular fever. However, the condition may coexist with a streptococcal throat infection. In this situation and the commoner situation of a child being ill with an infected throat requiring treatment pending the arrival of the results of laboratory tests, then penicillin 'V' (or erythromycin in the case of genuine penicillin allergy) may be used.

Return to School

Pupils should return to school after clinical recovery and a period of convalescence.

Cytomegalovirus Infection

Infection with cytomegaloviruses is world wide and antibodies to the infection are present in a large proportion of the adult population. Although most infections are inapparent, the organism is important as it may cause severe damage or death to the foetus or to the neonate. In school children, it causes a glandular fever like illness with atypical monocytes and abnormal liver function tests. The Paul-Bunnell and Monospot tests are negative. Lymph gland enlargement and throat infection are not as common as in glandular fever. Pneumonia and liver disease have been described in children and adults due to CMV infection. The diagnosis is made from serological tests, particularly a raised IgM or an antibody rise in paired sera.

Toxoplasmosis

Although a protozoal and not a viral disease, toxoplasmosis is best considered here because its commonest manifestation at school age is a glandular fever like syndrome with negative Paul-Bunnell and monospot tests. The cervical lymph nodes are most often involved but the spleen and liver are not usually enlarged. Sore throat is not consistently present but the fever is generally slight and long-lastiing so that the illness may pursue a protracted course for several months. More severe manifestations include choroidoretinitis, an acute encephalitis and pneumonia. Like CMV infections, toxoplasmosis can cause severe damage to the foetus and to the neonate. Diagnosis is usually serological, although since it is a parasitic condition, there may be an eosinophilia. The source of the infection is raw or undercooked meats or vegetables contaminated by the faeces of domestic animals, such as dogs and especially, cats. Great care should be exercised in disposing of cat litter (feline pets in school boarding houses!) and in the preparation of raw vegetables and seeing that all meat dishes are adequately cooked. Pregnant women are particularly at risk from these two diseases, especially the latter.

For normally healthy schoolchildren, the infection is usually not very significant and in uncomplicated glandular toxoplasmosis, specific treatment is not indicated. If however the patient is ill yet without evidence of any serious complication, e.g. encephalitis, a combination of pyrimethamine and sulphadiazine may be given, but since the former can depress the bone marrow, it would be prudent to obtain consultant advice about this.

Bacterial Infections
Strepococcal Infections

Streptococci are amongst the most important bacteria causing illness in school children. They are dealt with in the sections on skin and respiratory infections.

Staphylococcal infections

Numerous infections are caused by staphylococci; the usual pathogenic staphylococcus being the coagulase positive variety of which there are many phage types. It is the organism most likely to develop antibiotic resistance.

Most manifestations of staphylococcal infection are dealt with in the sections on skin, respiratory and intestinal infections. The very important remaining infection caused by this organism is osteomyelitis.

Osteomyelitis occurs as a complication of septicaemia or local spread of sepsis, usually, but not always due to staphylococci. The usual source is skin sepsis. The cardinal symptom is bone pain, which can be very severe, at the site of infection, which is generally in the metaphysis of a long bone. The child is usually febrile with a leucocytosis. Often, marked tenderness over the diseased bone can be elicited. The leucocytosis is usually polymorphonuclear and often the leucocytes show toxic granulation. Indeed, in the early stages of the disease, this may be the only significant diagnostic sign. Early diagnosis is important and is best made by blood culture, since X-ray changes do not develop for a week or more. Nowadays however, bone scans are useful in the early stages as 'hot spots' reveal where the infection is long before there are X-ray changes. There may be a recent history of trauma to the affected bone and a septic focus must be sought. (e.g. dental abscess). Once the blood cultures have been taken and the diagnosis made, the prompt use of antibiotics like flucloxacillin or fusidic acid, may make surgical drainage unnecessary, but early consultation with an orthopaedic surgeon is strongly advised. If prompt treatment is not instituted, chronic infection may develop, with the ultimate need for operation to remove bony sequestra. Septic arthritis may develop in an adjacent joint.

Acute Bacterial Meningitis

The common cause of acute bacterial meningitis, which is a notifiable disease, is the meningococcus, Neisseria meningitidis, of which there are several different types, followed by the pneumococcus and Haemophilus influenzae, although, fortunately, infections due to the last named organism are now very much less common since the introduction of the Hib vaccine in 1993. (See under 'Immunisation'.)

Numerous other organisms may be responsible for acute bacterial meningitis such as streptococci and staphylococci, which, together with pneumococci, are usually secondary to infections of the middle ear and the para-nasal sinuses. Other pyogenic forms of meningitis, due to E. coli and salmonellae are more common in infants, or may be secondary to infections in other organs. Tuberculosis was an important cause of meningitis in children until about the early to mid 1960s. During the last three years there have been small year on year increases in the notification of new cases in the UK and also, it should be remembered that HIV infection is also a risk factor for tuberculosis.

The majority of meningococccal infections in the UK are due to the Group B strains (approx 2/3rds) whilst Group C strains account for most of the rest of the cases. Group A strains account for less than 2% of cases in the UK, but they are the epidemic strains in other countries.[21]

The meningococcus may be responsible for an acute fulminating septicaemia, with adrenal haemorrhage and failure, with or without signs of meningitis. A petechial or purpuric rash is one which does not fade on pressure, is diagnostic of septicaemia, and may precede, accompany or replace, the signs of meningitis, and this rash may be preceded by a non-specific erythematous rash.

A rapidly developing purpuric rash is a grave sign and a patient suffering thus, must immediately be transferred to hospital, ideally, to one with an intensive care unit. Deaths are caused by the septicaemia rather than the meningitis, and the septicaemic form is seen in about 25% of cases of meningococcal infection. Although the meningococcus is very sensitive to penicillin, the pathogenesis of the disease involves the release of toxins and inflammatory substances which cause septic shock, and these substances continue to be released after the antibiotics have killed the causative bacteria.

The septic shock involves increased vascular permeability, intravascular thrombosis, vasoconstriction and then vasodilatation and heart failure because of decreased stroke volume. The lungs are affected and artificial ventilation is required.

Acute bacterial meningitis is ushered in by fever, headache, vomiting, rapidly developing confusion, delirium, coma, twitching and convulsions. While the patient is conscious, meningismus, photophobia and Kernig's sign (spasm of the hamstrings on extending the lower leg when flexed at 90 degrees to the upper leg, whilst the latter is flexed at the hip by 90 degrees, and the patient supine), may be present. If a child exhibits these signs, especially if there are signs of markedly increased intracranial pressure (fixed non-reactive pupils), then, again, urgent transfer to hospital, preferably with an intensive care unit, is mandatory. The diagnostic lumbar puncture will be performed in hospital, once the child is in a stable condition, because of the risk of coning.[22]

Pending the arrival of the ambulance, a patient with the signs and symptoms of meningitis and /or septicaemia should be given an intramuscular injection of benzylpenicillin in accordance with the following schedule:

1200 mg for adults and children over 10 years or more,
600 mg for children aged one to nine years
300 mg for those less than a year.

(Assuming of course, that there is no history of anaphylactic shock following an earlier dose of penicillin.)

Although the above may appear contrary to the hitherto accepted practice of witholding antibiotics until the identity of the infecting organism has been established, particularly since the meningococcus is so very sensitive to penicillin, this procedure is now considered to be beneficial to the patient. New techniques are now becoming available which facilitate the diagnosis of meningococcal disease even after antibiotics have been administered, as indicated above.[23]

Infection and Transmission

Infection is usually by direct contact or droplet spread from the nasopharynx of an infected person or a carrier. The carriage rate for all meningococci in the normal population is about 10%, depending on age. About 25% of young adults may be carriers at any one time.[23]

Incubation Period

For meningococcal meningitis, this is from three to five days.

Prevention

Outbreaks of meningococcal infection most often occur in overcrowded conditions such as army barracks and maybe the 'old type' school dormitories. Sleeping 'head to toe' was designed to reduce the spread of infection.

Close contacts of cases of meningococcal infection are at greatly increased risk of developing the disease, despite chemoprophylaxis. Even so, it is helpful for close contacts to receive chemoprophylaxis and rifampicin is the drug of choice. The duration of the treatment is two days and adults should receive 600mg 12 hourly. Children over one year of age should receive 10mg/Kg and children less than one year should receive half this dose. Warn contact lens wearers of irritation and staining and advise extra contraception where appropriate, because of the liver enzyme induction from the rifampicin.

Immediate family or close contacts of Group A or Group C meningitis should be given meningococcal vaccine in addition to the chemoprophylaxis. The drugs should be given first and the appropriate vaccine should be given when the results of typing of the organism are available. At present, there is no effective vaccine against Group B organisms and the A and C vaccines should not be given to the contacts of Group B cases.[24]

Local outbreaks

In addition to sporadic cases, outbreaks of meningococcal infections with Group C organisms tend to occur in closed or semi-closed communities such as schools and military establishments. Immunisation has been shown to be effective in controlling epidemics, reducing infection rates but not carriage rates.

As well as the local Community Paediatrician, the Consultant in Infectious Diseases and the Consultant in Public Health, advice on the use of meningococcal vaccines is available from:

PHLS Communicable Disease Surveillance Centre.
(0181 200 6868)

Public Health Laboratory Service

Meningococcal Reference Laboratory
(0161 445 2416)

Scottish Centre for Infection and Environmental Health
(0141 946 7120)

Scottish Meningococcal and Pneumococcal Reference Laboratory
(0141 201 3836)

For further information regarding vaccines for meningococcal infection, see 'Immunisation'

Diphtheria

Diphtheria is a serious, notifiable acute infectious disease of the naso-pharynx caused by Corynebacterium diphtheriae. The characteristic lesion is an inflammatory exudate, which forms a grey coloured membrane in the upper respiratory tract, not confined to the tonsils, which threatens obstruction to respiration, often requiring tracheotomy . The diphtheria bacillus produces a toxin with a particular affinity for heart muscle, the CNS and the adrenal glands and is capable of causing myocarditis, palatal palsies and adrenal shock. This disease used to be a common and much feared cause of death in children (and adults). It is now fortunately extremely rare in the UK, due to the national immunisation programme introduced in the latter 1930s and since there is virtually no remaining natural immunity in the country, it is vital that every child should be fully immunised. Nevertheless, should a case be suspected then urgent admission to an Infectious Diseases Hospital should be arranged. Modern air travel increases the risk of carriers of the disease introducing the infection into the UK, especially if they are coming from Russia or the Newly Independent States of the USSR, from where diphtheria epidemics have been reported recently.

Infection and Transmission

Spread is by droplet infection and by contact with articles contaminated by an infected person, (fomites). In countries with a poor standard of hygiene, a cutaneous form of the disease exists and this is a significant source of infection.

Incubation Period

The incubation period is short (2 to 5 days) but patients suffering from the disease can be infectious for up to a month and carriers, for much longer. Since the UK has been free from the disease for many years, there is negligible natural immunity in the country. Thus, in order to guard against infection imported from abroad, the immunisation rate must be maintained. People travelling abroad to endemic or epidemic areas should have primary or booster doses as appropriate. See 'Immunisation'.

Tetanus

Tetanus is an acute, notifiable disease carrying a high mortality. The cause is a spore forming anaerobic bacillus, Clostridium tetani, which lives in soil and animal faeces, especially from the horse. The bacillus or its spores, enter the skin through puncture wounds of all degrees of severity, and burns. Some of the wounds may be so small as to be unnoticed. Multiplication of the bacilli and the consequent production of the powerful neurotoxin are facilitated by the presence of devitalised tissue. The first symptoms are usually muscle spasms superimposed on generalised rigidity, producing agonising contractions. Typically, the masseter muscles are first affected, hence the synonym 'lockjaw' and the description of the facial appearance, 'risus sardonicus'.

Neonatal tetanus, due to infection of the infant's umbilical stump, is an important cause of death in many developing countries.

Incubation Period

This varies from 2 days to 3 weeks, and it is thought that the longer the incubation period, the better the prognosis.

Prevention

Tetanus can be prevented by active immunisation. (See 'Immunisation'). At the time of an injury, the use of tetanus toxoid or anti-tetanus immunoglobulin where indicated, must be accompanied by thorough cleaning and débridement of the wound. (See 'Immunisation.')

Tetanus can never be eradicated and it is not spread from person to person.

Treatment

Urgent hospital admission is mandatory, for tracheal intubation, assisted ventilation and parenteral fluids, in addition to treatment with antitoxin and antibiotics.

Whooping cough (Pertussis)

This notifiable and highly infectious disease, is caused by the bacteria Bordetella pertusis. Commencing with a catarrhal stage lasting about a week, it progresses over the next two weeks or so, to a clinical picture of distressing, repeated, prolonged, paroxysms of coughing often ending in vomiting. The pitch of the cough rises during a paroxysm (the 'crescendo' cough) and the child may not be able to breathe until it is over, when the first inspiratory breath causes the characteristic 'whoop'. The 'whoop' is often absent in infants and young children and periods of apnoea may follow the paroxysms. The duration of the symptoms can often be several months, and recovery gradually occurs as the paroxysms of coughing become less frequent and less severe.

Commonly, children develop conjunctival and petechial haemorrhages on the neck and forehead as a result of the coughing. Cerebral petechiae are thought to occur because of the coughing and, together with cerebral hypoxia from associated periods of apnoea, account for the risk of brain damage. Other complications include bronchopneumonia, basal lung collapse, bronchiectasis and encephalitis, although these, with death, tend to occur in young children and infants. Repeated attacks of vomiting result in failure to gain weight and even weight loss. Adolescents and even adults can suffer from pertussis and this was not uncommon in the pre-war days of extended families. Mild pertussis, often without the whoop, can occur, occasionally, in children who have received pertussis vaccine.

Diagnosis

The clinical suspicion may be confirmed, if necessary, but not without difficulty, by bacteriological examination of pernasal or supra-laryngeal swabs. The taking of these swabs requires some patient cooperation (in both senses of the word) and, since the Bordetella pertussis is a difficult organism to culture, the laboratory usually require advance notice before the swabs are sent, so that they may be anticipated and cultured without delay.

Incubation Period

Usually 7 to 10 days.

Period of Communicability

A case of pertussis is infectious from seven days after exposure to about a month after the appearance of the coughing paroxysms, and the youngest siblings or class-mates of the patient are those most at risk of serious illness.

Immunity

An attack confers life-long immunity.

Prevention

Pertussis immunisation (See 'Immunisation') is the most effective means of prevention. Petussis continues to be a dangerous infection, especially to infants, so special efforts must be made to protect them. Parents should always be notified of cases occurring in a school and advised to take appropriate precautions. The period of communicability can be reduced by giving erythromycin and the main reason for giving the drug is to reduce the rate of transmission to infant contacts.

Treatment

Pertussis is an unpleasant and prolonged illness where good nursing is important. The place of antibiotics is controversial, but if they are used, then erythromycin has replaced chloramphenicol as the drug of choice.

Return to school

A pupil should not return to school until at least three weeks has elapsed after the onset of the paroxsmal cough and then only if clinically recovered.

Tuberculosis

This infectious disease can occur in animals and birds in addition to the human species. Human tuberculosis is caused by infection with Mycobacterium tuberculosis. Since the latter 1980s, there have been slight increases in the annual notifications of the disease in the UK, the provisional totals for 1994 and 1995, being 6, 229 and 6, 249 respectively.[25] As discussed earlier, HIV infection is an additional risk factor for tuberculosis, although this is thought not to have contributed significantly to the recent increases in the UK.[25] Tuberculosis, as in previous years, is a disease associated with overcrowding and substandard nutrition and generally is found in crowded urban areas amongst people originating from areas of the world where the disease is widespread.

Primary tuberculosis of the lungs is usually self-limiting and symptomless but detectable on X-ray examination and subsequent conversion of the skin reaction to tuberculin protein in the form of the Mantoux and Heaf tests. (See 'Immunisation'). In complicated cases, pleural effusions, segmental collapse of lobes of lungs, gland rupture, tuberculous bronchopneumonia and miliary tuberculosis may occur. This occasionally leads to tuberculous meningitis, in which the symptoms can develop slowly, but then proceed inexorably until treatment is instituted. Tuberculous bone and joint disease and tuberculous lymphatic disease are now very rare.

Post primary or adult infection of the lungs leads to variable degrees of chronic inflammation and destruction of lung tissue and these patients are the usual source of infection by droplet infection. The school doctor should bear in mind the possibility of tuberculosis in adults or children who have recently returned from certain developing countries and also, those with a chronic cough, with or without fever, haemoptysis or if there has been evidence of an earlier chest problem.

Tuberculosis is a notifiable disease and when an open case occurs, then contact-tracing and isolation of contacts are important public health measures. (See 'Immunisation' for BCG vaccination.)

Conjunctivitis

Infective conjunctivitis may be caused by a wide variety of bacterial and viral agents and may be difficult to distinguish from allergic conjunctivitis, which is especially common in the hay fever season. Mucopurulent conjunctivitis is important in schools as it can spread rapidly through direct contact and the use of communal towels. There is catarrhal inflammation of one or both eyes, with conjunctival injection and a variable amount of discharge. The discharge is thin and slight at first, later becoming mucopurulent and occasionally purulent.

Exclusion from school is only necesssary for younger children and in very severe cases. Improved personal hygiene and the use of individual, or, better still, disposable towels, all help to reduce the level of infection. Culture is seldom informative and treatment with chloramphenicol or soframycin eye ointment is usually satisfactory.

Brucellosis

Brucellosis is an infectious disease caused by Brucella abortus, suis, or melitensis, exhibiting a febrile stage without specific clinical features ('PUO') and a chronic stage characterised by relapses of fever, malaise, sweating attacks, lassitude and headache. A form of arthritis can occur. This is a milk-borne infection and is now very rare in the UK following its virtual elimination from dairy herds and the wide-spread pasteurisation of milk.

Leptospirosis

In the UK several pathogenic leptospires have been isolated from wild and domestic animals which, whilst remaining well, excrete large numbers of leptospires into the environment. Humans become infected through contact with the urine or tissues of infected animals or through contact with water – harbouring leptospires. The organisms enter through skin cuts and abrasions or through the mucous membranes of the eyes or nasopharynx. Leptospirosis is a notifiable disease.

Leptospirosis presents in many ways, from inapparent or trivial, to fulminating and fatal infection. About 90% of the infected patients present with a mild influenza like illness which usually resolves uneventfully in two or three weeks. Occasionally, patients present with lymphocytic meningitis. Only a small proportion develop haemorrhagic complications and severe kidney and liver failure (Weil's disease) and only 20% of these patients die. (Two or three people annually in the UK.)

Farmers and agricultural workers are now the main occupational groups at risk but people in contact with rats or natural inland waters are potentially at risk. No human vaccine is available in the UK but the following precautions, which may be put on rainproof cards may further reduce the risk.

Reducing the risk of Leptospirosis

Eliminate rats and don't touch them with unprotected hands.

Cover all cuts with waterproof plasters and wear protective clothing.

Avoid immersion in natural waters.

Wear footwear.

Shower after canoeing, windsurfing, water-skiing or swimming.[26]

In England and Wales, the Public Health Laboratory service will provide advice and serological tests.

Intestinal Infections
Food Poisoning

Food poisoning is a disease which must be notified on suspicion whatever the cause. An acute inflammation of the lining of the stomach and intestine results from the ingestion of infected or contaminated food. The causal agents may be:

(a) bacterial e. g. salmonella, Clostridium welchii, B. cereus and atypical Escherichia coli.

(b) bacterial toxins, e.g. staphyloccoccal enterotoxin, botulinum toxin.

(c) non-bacterial, e.g. fungal, chemical (including pesticides), which usually cause neurological symptoms, as well.

Diagnosis is by isolation of the causal agent from the food, faeces or vomitus.

Mass outbreaks in schools or parties are suggestive of food poisoning due to bacteria or to bacterial toxins. In such cases, the outbreak may be explosive, occurring within a few hours of the ingestion of the contaminated food. Food may be contaminated by handlers with infected wounds, naso-pharyngeal discharges or enteric infections. Bacterial contamination may occur in raw, inadequately cooked and/or re-heated food. The staphylococcus produces a heat stable enterotoxin which may resist cooking. (See also Chapter 2 for details of kitchen hygiene)

In B. cereus food poisoning the source is rice which either has been boiled in bulk and stored under warm conditions before reheating, or fried for a short time with freshly beaten egg. Nausea and vomiting are the predominant symptoms.

Incubation Periods

These vary according to the degree of contamination. Staphylococcal food poisoning due to an enterotoxin has a more rapid onset than types due to bacterial infection.

The following periods are a rough guide.

Staphylococcus	one half to 6 hours	(usually 1 to 2 hours.)
B. cereus	one half to 11 hours	(usually 1 to 4 hours)
Salmonella	6 to 48 hours	(usually 12 to 24 hours).
Cl. welchii	8 to 24 hours	(usually 10 to 12 hours).

Prevention

Food poisoning is best prevented by attention to the principles of hygiene described in Chapter 2. Outbreaks should be fully investigated by the local Environmental Health Department or The Public Health Laboratory Service.

Treatment

The most important, and often the only treatment for most forms of gastro enteritis is fluid replacement. A suitable solution can be made up of a pinch of salt and a teaspoonful of sugar in 250ml of water. More sophisticated solutions are sodium chloride and glucose oral powder compound, and similar preparations listed in the British National Formulary. Kaolin or codeine preparations may relieve the diarrhoea. The anti-emetic, metoclopramide, should not be given to children because of the risk of dystonic reactions. Antibiotics are of no help and are specifically contra-indicated as they may prolong the carrier state and actually aggravate the diarrhoea by specifically altering the bacterial flora of the gut. The use of anti-motility drugs against diarrhoea may prolong the illness by preventing the excretion of toxins.

A contrary view, as far as adults are concerned, has been put forward by Gorbach, who advocates bismuth subsalicylate for mild to moderate diarrhoea, noting the black tongue and stool, with loperamide for more severe diarrhoea, (up to four loose motions per day), maybe combined with a quinolone antibiotic. He counsels caution in applying the recommendations to children, largely because of the potential toxicity of quinolones, although he observes that they are used in children with life threatening diarrhoea in developing countries. Also, he advises that anti-motility drugs should not be given to any patient with diagnosed shigellosis or with dysentery (bloody, mucoid stools and fever), which is commonly seen in developing countries or in returning travellers. He cites other studies along these lines.[27]

Return to school

Patients may return to school on clinical recovery. In cases of salmonellosis a negative stool should ideally be obtained before return to the community. This rule may have to be relaxed for prolonged (symptom-less) excretors who must, nevertheless, be excluded from all forms of food handling until three successive negative stools, taken at intervals of not less than two days, have been obtained.

Bacillary Dysentery

Bacillary dysentery is a notifiable disease caused by the Shigella group of organisms. In the UK, S. sonnei accounts for over 90% of cases and S. flexneri for most of the rest. Usually it is characterised by diarrhoea of acute onset with fever, blood and mucus in the stools, abdominal colic and tenesmus. Many infections, however, are mild and some are symptomless. Young children are particularly susceptible and outbreaks can be particularly troublesome in nursery schools and in residential childrens' homes. The diagnosis is made by stool culture or by examination of rectal swabs.

The source of infection is from excreta of patients or carriers, the route being faecal-oral directly or through contaminated food, toilets, eating utensils and, rarely, water. Flies may act as vectors.

Incubation period
This is usually 2-4 days but may be 1-7 days.

Period of communicability
Dysentery may be transmitted as long as the organisms persist in the faeces. This is usually days or weeks, but a carrier state may persist for several months.

Prevention
Prevention is by attention to hygiene. Contacts should be instructed on strict hand washing and scrupulous personal hygiene.

Treatment
Severe cases in infants require hospitalisation for correction of dehydration and electrolyte imbalance. Ordinary acute cases require rest, fluids and symptomatic treatment.

Return to school
Pupils may return to school after two successive negative stool cultures. However, the return to school of the persistent carrier calls for special consideration and consultation with the local Environmental Health Department. Symptomless carriers however, are not highly infectious and play little part in the spread of an outbreak, unless they are engaged in food handling.

Management of an Outbreak
'It is a golden rule in the management of any infection never to take any swabs, unless one has decided what to do with the positives.' Christie discusses the problems of managing an outbreak in an institution and the reader is referred to his book.[28]

Amoebic Dysentery
This is not an indigenous infection in the UK. It is caused by the Entamoeba histolytica and usually presents as a colitis with bloody mucoid stools, but late forms such as amoebic hepatitis may occur. Diagnosis and treatment are difficult and should be carried out whenever possible, by a hospital for the treatment of tropical diseases.

Gastroenteritis
A large number of organisms cause diarrhoea and vomiting which may occur in epidemic form in schools. Dysentery and food poisoning including salmonella infection, have been dealt with above. Other causes of intestinal infection are as follows:-

Campylobacter jejuni

Campylobacter organisms, only recognised as human pathogens since 1977, are now thought to cause as many cases of diarrhoea as salmonella organisms. The sources are most commonly inadequately cooked poultry and un-pasteurised or contaminated milk. The organism is readily destroyed by heat. Cases occur sporadically and also in large outbreaks. Outbreaks in schools have been traced to unpasteurised milk and in one case, to a contaminated water supply. The incubation period is usually from three to five days. Severe, often prolonged abdominal pain, and fever often precede the diarrhoea and these may mimic an acute abdomen. There is often blood in the stools. Vomiting is uncommon but diarrhoea may persist for several days. Diagnosis is by isolation of the organism from the stools. Spread from person to person rarely occurs except in very young children.

Erythromcin is effective, but is often unnecessary because the disease is self-limiting. Although the disease is not statutorily notifiable, the nature of the signs and symptoms make it advisable to inform the local Environmental Health Department.

Yersinia enterocolitica

Y. enterocolitica is another organism which has only come to our attention in recent years and has been involved in school outbreaks of abdominal pain and diarrhoea. The effect of the infection is to cause mesenteric adenitis with abdominal pain and fever. Diarrhoea is more common in young children than in adolescents. Transmission is by the faecal-oral route and an important feature may be that these organisms can survive and even proliferate in con-taminated food at temperatures as low as 4 degrees C.

See under thalassaemia major in Chapter 6.

E. coli

Enterotoxic strains of E. coli cause infantile gastroenteritis and travellers' diarrhoea. The outbreak in the months of November and December 1996 in Scotland, traced to contaminated meat, was particularly severe, causing several deaths.

Viruses

A number of viruses is responsible for gastrointestinal infections, and these may be identified by electron microscopy. Enteroviruses cause minor gastro-intestinal symptoms. Rotaviruses cause extensive outbreaks, most commonly in young children. Winter vomiting disease occurs in explosive outbreaks in boarding schools and appears to be caused by parvoviruses, of which the Norwalk agent is one.

Giardia lamblia

Giardia lamblia is a protozoan infection which causes persistent travellers' diarrhoea. The diagnosis is made by microscopy of the stools and metro-nidazole is effective treatment; 2g per day for 3 days, or 400 mg t. d. s. for 7 days. Chronic giardiasis can lead to malabsorption.

Typhoid and Paratyphoid Fever

Typhoid and paratyphoid are caused by salmonella typhi, A, B and C. Typhoid is found throughout both temperate and tropical zones, particularly in areas with poor sanitation and hygiene. While local residents may exhibit a high degree of immunity, the unprotected traveller is at special risk. Most cases in the UK in recent years have been in persons infected on holiday abroad: indigenous infection in the UK is rare.

Typhoid is a systemic illness of insidious onset characterised by a slowly rising fever, bradycardia, rose spots on the abdomen and the back, splenomegaly and an apathetic mental state. Constipation is common in the early stages and may be followed by diarrhoea. In the later stages of an untreated case, bowel haemorrhage, perforation and peritonitis may occur and require prompt treatment. Blood culture is the most important early diagnostic measure. Culture of the faeces and urine, and the Widal agglutination test may also be helpful. Sources of the organism are the faeces or urine of a patient or a carrier. Food and milk contaminated by an infected handler, water from a contaminated source, fly borne infection, or inadequately sterilised canned food may be responsible for outbreaks of typhoid.

The epidemiology of paratyphoid is similar to that of typhoid fever except that it is nearly always food borne.

Incubation Period
Usually 10-14 days.

Period of Communicability
Patients after clinical recovery, may excrete S, typhi in the urine and faeces for many years. Therefore, any patient is a potential source of infection for as long as the organism can be cultured from the urine or faeces.

Prevention
Typhoid and paratyphoid are notifiable diseases. Prevention is by good hygiene and the avoidance of raw food and water in endemic areas. Travellers to these areas should have typhoid vaccines. (See 'Immunisation').

Treatment
Chloramphenicol is the most effective antibiotic, but in view of its potential toxicity, (blood dyscrasia), some practitioners prefer to use ciprofloxacin, or, if the patient has no penicillin allergy, amoxycillin.

Return to School
Patients may return to school when clinically fit and after three succcessive negative faecal and urine cultures at 2 or 3 day intervals

Tropical and Imported Diseases
Malaria

Malaria is a notifiable disease caused by a parasite protozoon of the genus Plasmodium. The early development of the parasite takes place in the gut of the Anopheles mosquito from where it passes through the salivary apparatus and is injected into the blood stream of the human host when the female mosquito feeds. The distribution of malaria follows that of the Anopheles mosquito and is mainly confined to tropical and subtropical regions throughout the world. Since the mosquito requires water for the completion of its life-cycle, malaria may show a seasonal variation in incidence in regions which have a wet and a dry season. Two to three decades ago, there was a chance that malaria might be eradicated, but now the situation is much worse, with more areas of the world being involved and the emergence of drug resistant strains of parasite to both first and second line drugs.[29] Today, malaria is a public health problem in more than 90 countries, inhabited by 40% of the world's population, and is responsible for up to 500 million clinical episodes and 2.7 million deaths a year, predominantly in young children in sub-Saharan Africa.[30]

Doctors looking after schools attended by children from overseas must be alert constantly, to the problem of malaria. Children from areas where the disease is endemic may be pupils at school and travel home for holidays, and children normally resident in the UK may visit malarious areas on holiday. A few years ago it was recommended that even if a person was planning to visit a non-malarious area it was worth considering giving malaria prophylaxis if there was the likelihood of a scheduled (or the risk of an unscheduled) stop for refuelling etc. in a malarious area. 'Runway malaria' was described where travellers have been bitten by mosquitoes at such stops. However more effective methods of spraying the interior of aircraft on such stops are thought to have reduced the risk of this mode of infection.[31]

Malignant tertian malaria is caused by P. falciparum, benign tertian by P. vivax or P. ovale, and benign quartan by P. malariae. The symptoms of all types of malaria are an abrupt onset of fever with headache, joint pains, rigors, anorexia and vomiting. A pattern of remitting and then recurring fever develops later, but the diagnosis should be made before this is established. There are many grave complications of malignant tertian malaria, perhaps the most dangerous one being the usually fatal, cerebral malaria. Approximately, 2,000 cases of imported malaria annually, are notified in the UK, and whilst this figure has been roughly constant for the last few years, the proportion due to P. falciparum has steadily increased, and the proportion of the benign P. vivax infections has fallen. In the decade 1979-1989, there was an increase of 51% of reported cases of malaria in the UK, in which period of time, the proportion of the dangerous falciparum cases had risen from 20% to 56%.[32]

From a practical point of view, each child or adult, returning from a malarious area, whether they are UK residents returning from holiday, ethnic minority travellers visiting the UK, or pupils (or staff) returning to school in the UK from their homes abroad, should be observed carefully. They should be urged to seek advice as soon as they are unwell, even during an epidemic of another disease, e. g., influenza, and assumed to be suffering from malaria until urgent blood investigations prove otherwise. Malaria very often presents as an influenzal like illness several weeks after the person has been bitten by an infected mosquito.

Adults and children returning from extended holidays in malarious areas, especially of the back-packing variety, are particularly at risk and should be observed accordingly. Protection against malaria can never be 100% complete, but observation of the following four types of measures will help:

Be aware of the risk

All travellers to malarious areas must be aware of the malaria risk, act to reduce the risk, and urgently seek medical advice if they get a fever.

Avoid being bitten by mosquitoes

Sleep in screened rooms. Use knock down sprays in rooms in the evenings. Sleep in intact mosquito nets impregnated with pyrethroids. Burn mosquito coils. Wear long sleeved clothing and long trousers if out of doors after sunset. Use mosquito repellents on the skin and impregnate clothing with them. eg. diethyltoluamide.

Take Chemoprophylaxis as appropriate

Observe the following four principles.

(i) Compliance is essential.

(ii) Continue to take chemoprophylaxis for four weeks after returning to UK from a malarious area.

(iii) Start chemoprophylaxis one week before departure for a malarious area.

(iv) Take antimalarial drugs after meals to minimise side effects.

Seek early diagnosis and treatment

Medical advice should be sought promptly for any febrile or flu-like illness occurring within a year, and especially within three months, of returning from an endemic area even if all recommended precautions have been taken.[32]

Updated advice in the frequently changing sphere of malaria prophylaxis is available via the Dept. of Health 'Health Information for Overseas Travel' and in other medical journals. Up to date authoritative advice is now available at a number of centres, detailed below.

School doctors should be aware of the adverse drug reactions of the anti-malarial drugs, so that they can select the drug in accordance with the medical history of the patient and risks assessed.

Specialist advice regarding antimalarial therapy may be necessary for patients suffering from epilepsy, renal failure or for splenectomised or pregnant patients.[32] Antimalarial drugs can no longer be prescribed on Forms FP 10. See also Chapter 6 for advice for patients suffering from haemo-globinopathies

Centres for Advice on Malaria Prophylaxis

Ross Institute of Tropical Hygiene 0171 636 8636
School of Tropical Medicine Liverpool 0151 708 9393
East Birmingham Hosp 021 772 4311
Ruchill Hospital, Glasgow 041 946 7120.

Viral Haemorrhagic Fever

Viral haemorrhagic fevers, Lassa fever, Marburg disease and Ebola fever are diseases of West Africa and the Sudan which have occasionally been imported into Europe with attendant publicity, on account of their considerable mortality rates. These fevers should be thought of, in addition to malaria, in cases of pyrexia of undetermined origin in travellers who have arrived from these areas within the three weeks preceding the onset of their illness. If suspected, the Medical Officer for Environmental Health should be notified imediately.

Rabies

The few occurences of rabies in the UK are in patients who have contracted the disease overseas, for not since 1902 has a case of indigenous rabies been reported in the UK, apart from a rabid bat on the south coast during the summer of 1996. Rabies is an acute viral infection, resulting in encephalomyelitis. It is acquired from the bite or lick of a rabid animal, and is almost invariably fatal once neurological symptoms have developed. The cause of death is usually respiratory paralysis. After a prodromal illness of headache, fever and malaise there follows a progression of signs consisting of cerebral irritation, with anxiety, mania, hallucinations, hydrophobia, convulsions, progressing to paralysis, coma and death. Sometimes there is an ascending flaccid paralysis and sensory disturbance. There is no effective treatment and the disease is notifiable.

The virus has a variety of animal hosts, in many different countries of the world except Australasia and Antarctica. In Europe, foxes are the predominant host, but the dog, cat and the horse and many wild animals like deer, badgers and martens are infected. In the USA the number of rabid animals has increased in the last half century, the majority being skunks, racoons and bats.

Apart from a few cases of rabies having been acquired through infected corneal grafts, person to person transmission has not been reported, despite the fact that the virus may be present in the tissue fluids of an infected person and the incubation period can vary widely: from nine days to two or more years, although the usual range is between two to eight weeks.

A vaccine is available and so is a rabies specific immunoglobulin. Details of these are found in the section on Immunisation, together with recommendations as to the people to whom these products should be given and under what circumstances.

Sexually Transmitted Diseases

All patients with sexually transmitted diseases should, if possible, be referred to special clinics, because of the need for accurate diagnosis, the exclusion of multiple infection, appropriate treatment, adequate follow-up and contact tracing. This applies to school children as well as adults and they should be reassured about the expertise and the confidentiality with which they will be treated. Only brief descriptions will be given here.

Gonorrhoea

Gonorrhoea is caused by infection with the gonococcus, Neisseria gonorrhoeae. The incubation period is short, usually two to four days, and the presenting symptoms and signs in the male are urethritis, dysuria and a urethral discharge. In the female, the disease is often symptomless, but there may be dysuria and a vaginal discharge. Complications in the male include epididymitis and in the female, bartholinitis and pelvic inflammatory disease, which can lead to infertility. Contact with the gonococcus in the birth canal can cause ophthalmia neonatorum. Treatment with penicillin is very effective, unless the organism has developed penicillin resistance.

Non Specific Urethritis

Non-specific urethritis is a common sexually transmitted disease, probably caused by Chlamydia trachomatis. The incubation period is two to three weeks and the symptoms of discharge and dysuria are usually less severe than in the case of gonorrhoea. Complications involve prostatitis, epididymitis and Reiter's syndrome. (A condition with eye and joint involvement.)Treatment is more difficult than in the case of gonorrhoea and a fairly long course of tetracycline or erythromycin is usually necessary.

Syphilis

Syphilis, a disease of historical importance and protean manifestations, is now uncommon in the UK. The causal agent is Treponema pallidum, with an incubation period of nine to 90 days. The primary lesion is a painless genital chancre. Six to eight weeks later, the signs of secondary syphilis occur, with a characteristic rash and influenza like symptoms. Diagnosis is by discovering treponemes in scrapings from the chancre, examined microscopically by dark-ground illumination. Serological tests for syphilis become positive at a later stage. The diagnosis, treatment and follow-up must be undertaken by an STD clinic.

Genital Herpes

Genital herpes, caused by the herpes simplex virus Type II, resembles herpes simplex of the lip. The incubation period is four to five days after which, a cluster of vehicles appear on the genitalia. These usually rupture and form painful erosions which heal in about ten days unless secondarily infected. Recurrences may occur but are usually less severe than the initial attack. Systemic treatment is now available (but expensive) in the form of aciclovir or famaclovir tablets. Aciclovir cream is used for localised secondary attacks.

Genital warts

Genital warts, or condylomata acuminata, are viral warts transmited sexually. The incubation period is about three months. Treatment with podophylin and similar agents is best carried out in hospital.

Trichomonas Vaginalis

Trichomonas vaginalis is caused by a flagellated protozoon which is usually sexually acquired. In the female it is manifested by a frothy, malodorous, greenish-white, vaginal discharge, which causes irritation and soreness. There may be dysuria and the male partner may have a penile rash. Diagnosis is confirmed microscopically and on culture. Treatment with metronidazole, (for both partners simultaneously), is almost always effective.

Other Sexually Transmitted Diseases

Scabies and pediculosis pubis may be transmitted sexually and are described in the section on skin infections below. Candidiasis (vaginal thrush, due to yeast organisms) is not usually caused by sexual activity, but may be transmitted sexually. Predisposing factors include diabetes mellitus, oral contraceptives, broad spectrum antibiotics and pregnancy. The symptoms are itchy vaginal discharge and balanitis, and the diagnosis is confirmed by microscopy and culture. Treatment, again of both partners simultaneously, in the form of local applications of nystatin, clotrimazole, miconazole or econazole creams is recommended, with preparations like oral diflucan, again for both partners simultaneously, in resistant cases.

Skin Infections and Infestations
Impetigo Contagiosa

Impetigo is a superficial infection of the skin, initally causing vesicles, which later become encrusted with sero-purulent plaques. The causal organisms are Steptococcus pyogenes or Staphylococcus aureus, either singly or together. Diagnosis is by clinical inspection and by culture of a swab taken from the lesion. Impetigo is acquired by contact with a case or with a carrier. The incubation period is short and the lesions are highly infectious until healed.

Contacts of streptococcal impetigo may develop throat infections. Acute nephritis still commonly occurs in some tropical countries and in young people more often follows streptococcal skin infection than upper respiratory infection.

Prevention requires attention to personal hygiene as well as the prompt diagnosis and treatment of established cases. Young children and severe cases should be excluded from school in the acute stage. This is particularly necessary during an outbreak of streptococcal infection.

Treatment should be with an antibiotic cream or ointment such as fusidic acid, mupirocin or chlortetracycline, depending on the sensitivities of the organisms. Systemic antibiotics – penicillin or erythromycin for streptococcal infections – may be needed in severe cases.

Erysipelas

Erysipelas is an acute infection of the skin caused by streptococcus pyogenes. There is fever and an acutely inflamed erythematous swelling of the skin with a sharply defined border. The commonest site is the face. Erysipelas can occur at any age but it is commonest in the elderly, when there may be an associated confusional state. The infection responds to penicillin and erythromycin.

Scabies

Scabies is a contagious skin disease, rarely transmitted from animals, caused by penetration of the skin by the mite, Sarcoptes scabiei. The characteristic burrows are to be found most commonly on the front of the wrist, the ulnar side of the hand, the webs of the fingers, the anterior axillary folds of skin, the umbilicus and the genitalia. The face is spared. Sometimes the skin over the end of the burrows is raised into a small vesicle. Itching occurs most persistently at night, in bed, when the patient is warm. Cases may present simply as 'the itch' with a sparse rash.

The diagnosis is made on the clinical appearance of the burrows and the recognition of the mite, alternatively called an acarus, microscopically. Transmission is generally by close and prolonged contact. The infection is usually contracted in bed from an infected companion or spread via clothing or bedding.

Scabies is treated by the application of a scabicide, which should be used by all members of the household simultaneously. Benzyl benzoate application, 1%, gamma benzene hexochloride cream, or monosulfiram. (tetmasol) 25% in an alcoholic base, diluted with 2 or 3 parts of water, is applied from the neck down, following a hot bath during the course of which, the burrows are gently rubbed open with a soft brush. After treatment, which may have to be repeated, the patients may be permitted to return to school promptly.

Pediculosis (Lice)

Pediculosis is an infestation of the head, the hairy parts of the body, or the clothing, by blood-sucking lice. These are Pediculus capitis (the head louse), Pediculus corporis (the body louse) and Pediculus pubis (the crab louse). By far the commonest of these in schools is the head louse, which has greatly increased in the past few years to the point where it is almost endemic.

The head louse exists in three forms – egg (or nit), nymph and adult. The egg is yellowish and grey white and measures 0.8 to 1. 0 mm long. It is attached to the hair close to the scalp by a cement-like substance and incubated by body heat. Following an incubation period of about a week, the young nymph emerges and remains in the nymph stage for five to nine days before reaching sexual maturity. The nymph resembles an adult louse but does not have a fully developed reproductive capacity.

The adult female louse is about 3mm long. Its body is composed of three parts, a head, a thorax with three pairs of legs, and a segmented abdomen. At the end of each leg is a hook-like claw and an opposing thumb, by means of which the louse maintains its hold on hair.

Symptoms

The bite of the louse causes irritation, and the principal symptom of infestation is itching. Children who are seen scratching their heads repeatedly often prove to have head lice. Scratching produces secondary infection of the scalp, resulting in posterior cervical and sub occipital lymphadenitis.

Diagnosis

Adults and nymphs of head lice are found on the hair, on the scalp and along hair partings. They tend to be more prevalent on the back of the neck and behind the ears. Generally, a single individual will harbour only 10 – 20 head lice so there are very few crawling forms on any individual. Nits are laid close to the scalp, so any found more than 1cm from the scalp are almost certainly hatched or dead.

Period of Communicability

Head lice are spread only by direct contact. Body lice can be spread by infected clothing or bedding, and crab lice are usually spread by sexual contact. Transmission can occur at any time whilst live lice are present.

Prevention

A national campaign to eliminate head lice by inspection and treatment of all school children in 1977 failed completely. Encourage vigorous and frequent hair washing and combing.

Treatment

Malathion and carbaryl are recommended as the best treatment for lice. The lotion should be applied to dry hair, rubbed well into the scalp and removed by washing after 12 hours. Repeat the procedure at seven to nine days. Gamma benzene hexachloride has fallen out of favour because of the supposed emergence of resistant strains of lice. It is advisable to change the chemical from time to time because of resistance and advice may be obtained from the Community Nursing Services. Each member of the family should be treated at the same time to prevent the lice from being passed backwards and forwards between them. Routine hair inspections are now considered to be a waste of nursing time. In the case of body lice, heating to 55 degrees C for 40 minutes will kill lice and eggs in clothing and other fomites.

Return to School.

Pupils may return to school after effective treatment.

Ringworm

This is a general term applied to certain mycotic infections of the keratinized areas of the body, i. e skin, hair and nails. The lesions are caused by dermatophytes, some of which are found in domestic and wild animals who act as sources of infection for man. Dogs are often the sources of infection for children. Microsporon canis is the commonest cause of ringworm in dogs and cats and is easily transmitted to man.

Cattle ringworm causes inflammatory lesions in man in the characteristic scalp condition known as kerion.

Where there is clinical uncertainty, confirmation of the diagnosis of ringworm should be sought by microscopy and culture of scrapings or nail clippings.

Tinea pedis (Athlete's Foot)

There are two types of this common infection, the acute inflammatory condition and the more usual chronic dry type. The acute type arises in the toe clefts, usually between the 4th and 5th toes and may spread over the feet causing a vesiculo-pustular eruption. The principal symptom of the dry type is itching.

Tinea cruris

Tinea of the groin appears predominantly in males and must be distinguished from simple intertrigo. Usually bilateral, it starts as a round, scaly, itchy patch on the upper medial aspect of the thigh spreading peripherally from the groin and having an active advancing edge which is red and slightly scaly. Unlike intertrigo, which is often painful, tinea cruris usually itches.

Tinea corporis (Body Ringworm)

Most species of Tricophyton and microsporon can involve areas of smooth skin, usually producing red-ringed lesions with small peripheral vesicles and a scaly centre.

Tinea unguum (Ringworm of the Nails)

Fungus infections of the toe and finger nails produce a characteristic dystrophy of the nails which apart from being unsightly in some instances, and chronic, is symptom free.

Tinea capitis (Scalp Ringworm)

Scaly patches of different sizes with broken hairs are characteristic of scalp ringworm. The disease can spread to the eyelids, neck and trunk. The diagnosis can be made using Wood's lamp, as fluorescence occurs in most cases of scalp ringworm.

Prevention

Tinea pedis in particular, is fairly easily spread by wet surfaces and towels. Pupils with acute tinea pedis should be excluded from swimming and communal towels should be avoided. No other exclusion from school is necessary; children should be encouraged to dry thoroughly the clefts between the toes after bathing or washing and treatment should be started early.

Treatment

A variety of topical fungicides can be used for all types of ringworm, supplemented when necessary by oral griseofulvin. (Beware of the interaction with oral contraceptives.) Whitfield's ointment, (ung acid benz. co.), has stood the test of time and is still effective, but it has now been superseded by more elegant preparations containing clotrimazole, econazole or miconazole. Twice daily applications of one of these products will clear most cases ot tinea pedis, corporis and cruris. Acute weeping tinea pedis is best treated in the early stages by soaking feet in a 1 in 8000 solution of potassium permanganate for several minutes up to thrice daily.

Scalp ringworm and some cases of nail ringworm, should be treated with griseofulvin tablets (see earlier warning regarding oral contraceptives) in a dose of 0.5-1g. daily (10 mg/Kg for a child). In the case of nail ringworm, especially of the toe nails, the treatment needs to be prolonged and this must be considered in deciding whether to embark on treatment at all. Local treatment of extensive tinea corporis can be supplemented by oral griseofulvin for 2-3 weeks. (See earlier warning.)

Candidiasis (Thrush)

Thrush is caused by yeast organisms, usually Candida albicans, although other species may produce illness. Oral thrush is mainly a disease of infants, although some cases of stomatitis and pharyngitis in older children and adults are due to candida infection. Primary infection also causes vulvo-vaginitis (see Medical Problems of Childhood and Adolescence), intertrigo (including nappy rash) and chronic paronychia. People with diabetes mellitus, the immunodeficient and patients on broad spectrum antibiotics are particularly at risk. Serious systemic illness due to candida, sometimes occurs in patients with severe underlying diseases. Treatment of cutaneous candidiasis, which is the only kind occurring in healthy school children, is with topical amphotericin, nystatin or one of the broad spectrum fungicides mentioned in the section on ringworm above.

Warts
These are dealt with in 'Medical Problems of Childhood and Adolescence'.

Worm Infestations
Of the many worm infestations in man few occur in Europe except as exotic rarities and this section will deal only with those varieties which occur in western school children.

Threadworms
These are the commonest of worm infestations in the UK. Also, they are known as pinworms or enterobius vermicularis. They may be symptomless, or cause sleep disturbance through anal or vulvo-vaginal itching. The adult worm lays her eggs at night in the perianal area. The male worm is 2-5mm in size, white and thread-like in appearance and the female is 8-13 mm long.

Diagnosis
The diagnosis is made by recognition of the worms in the peri-anal area or on the stools, or collection of ova on a perianal swab or adhesive tape.

Incubation Period
Three to six weeks.

Communicability
The infection is transmitted by the faecal-oral route and re-infection is common. This may maintain the infection in a family group until effective treatment is instituted.

Prevention
Prevention requires a high standard of hygiene, including short finger nails, the use of a nail brush and measures to prevent sufferers from scratching their perianal regions whilst asleep.

Treatment
Piperazine in tablet form or as an elixir is effective, and should be given daily for a week. All members of the family should be treated simultaneously. Alternatively, mebendazole may be used in a single dose of 100mg.

Roundworms
Roundworm infestation (ascariasis) is spread by the faecal-oral route or indirectly via ova. After ingestion, larvae escape from the eggs in the duodenum, and migrate to the lungs where further development occurs. Then they enter the bronchi, ascend the trachea, are swallowed, before reaching the intestine, where they can attain a length of 20-25 cm. Symptoms may be

caused by an allergic reaction, with an eosinophilia, or by intestinal obstruction due to the worms. The diagnosis is made by identification of the live worms in the faeces or vomit, or of the ova by microscopy.

Treatment
Treatment is by piperazine or mebendazole

Tapeworms
Tapeworms have a complicated life cycle involving other animal or fish hosts. They are segmented and segments may be recognised in the stools. Treatment is with niclosamide.

Schistosomiasis (Bilharzia)
Schistosomes have an intermediate stage in water snails and infection may be acquired by bathing in rivers in the tropics or the Middle East. There are three different species with different geographical distribution and symptom complexes. Schistosoma haematobium causes bladder inflammation leading to haematuria and chronic cystitis. Schistosoma mansoni and Schistosoma japonica both cause chronic colonic irritation and subsequent pulmonary fibrosis. The diagnosis may be suggested by an eosinophilia and should be confirmed by serology and the identification of ova in the faeces, urine or tissue biopsy.

Assessment and management of established cases is very specialised and is best left to hospitals for tropical diseases.

References
1. Haemophilus influenzae infection (1996) *Immunisation against Infectious Disease.* p77 HMSO London

2. Doull. I. (1995) Corticosteroids in the management of croup. *Br. Med. J.* 311: 1244.

3. Geddes A. M. (1983) Q Fever. *Brit. Med J.* 287. 927

4. Hoskins T. W., Davies J. R., Smith A. J., Miller C. L. and Allchin A. (1979) Assessment of inactivated influenza A vaccine after three outbreaks of influenza A at Christ's Hospital. *Lancet,* 1, 33-34.

5. Payler D. K. and Purdham P. A. (1984) Influenza A prophylaxis with amantadine in a boarding school. *Lancet,* 1, 502.

6. Kennedy, D. H. (1990) Measles. *The Practitioner.* October 1990 p. 896.

7. Brook, G. (1990) Parvovirus, RSV and CMV infections. *The Practitioner.* October 1990. p. 918.

8. Brown D., Ramsay R., Richards A. and, Miller, E. (1994) Salivary diagnosis of measles: A study of notified cases in the United Kingdom, 1991-93. *Brit. Med. J.* 308. 1015.

9. McQuay, H., J., Moore, A.J. (1997) Antidepressants and chronic pain – Effective analgesia in neuropathic pain and other syndromes. Editorial *Br Med. J.* 314: 763.

10. Amir, J. Hare, L. Smetana, Z. Varsano, Izhak (1997) Treatment of herpes simplex gingivostomatitis with aciclovir in children: a randomised double blind placebo controlled study. *Br. Med J* 314 1800

11. Smith, H. (1990) Mumps. *The Practitioner* October 1990 p. 903.

12. Flegg, P. J. (1991) Recent advances in viral hepatitis. *Update,* 1 April 1991 p. 629.

13. Hepatitis A. (1996) *Immunisation against Infectious Disease.* p 85. HMSO London.

14. Hepatitis B (1996) *Immunisation against Infectious Disease*. p 95. HMSO London

15. Choo, Q. L., Weiner, A. J., Overby, L. R., Houghton, M., Bradley, D. W. (1990) Hepatitis C virus : the major causative agent of viral non-A, non-B hepatitis. (Review). *Br. Med. Bull.* 46 423

16. Tibbs, C., Davies, M. and Williams, R. (1995) Hepatitis C *Update* 1st Sept. 1995. p 165

17. Zuckerman, A. J. (1984) The elusive hepatitis C virus. *Br. Med. J.* . 300. 871

18. Aids and HIV Infection. *CDC UK Monthly Report.* Vol 6 No 51. (1996) PHLS London.

19. Hoskins, T. W. (1996) Personal Communication.

20. Evans, J. (1995) Care of HIV infected children in school. *MOSA Proceedings and Report* No 42 p14.

21. Meningococcal Infection (1996) *Immunisation against Infectious Disease*. p147 HMSO London.

22. Levin, M. (1995). Meningococcal Disease. *MOSA Proceedings and Report* No 42. p. 13.

23. Meningococcal Infection (1996) *Immunisation against Infectious Disease*. p.149. HMSO London

24. Meningococcal Disease (1996) *Ibid.* p. 151.

25. Tuberculosis (1996) *Ibid.* p. 219.

26. Ferguson, I., R. (1991) Leptospirosis Update. *Br. Med. J.*, 302, 128.

27. Gorbach, S., L. (1997) Treating diarrhoea. *Br. Med. J.,* 7096. 1776.

28. Christie, A. B. (1980) *Infectious Diseases: Epidemiology and Clinical Practices*. 3rd. Edition. p. 118 . (Edinburgh: Churchill-Livingstone.)

29. Brown, G. (1997) Fighting malaria. *Br. Med. J.* 7096: 1717

30. W.H.O. (1996) *Fact Sheet. Malaria Revised* December 1996. No94. WHO Geneva.

31. Conlon, C. (1990) Imported malaria. *Practitioner*, 234, 841.

32. Bradley, D. J., and Warhurst, D. C. (1995) Malaria prophylaxis: guidelines for travellers from Britain. *Br. Med. J.*; 310: 709.

Further Reading

1. De Cock, K. (1997) Guidelines for managing HIV infection. Editorial *Br. Med. J.*;7099:1

2. HIV and AIDS Guide for the Education Services.

   AIDS VIDEO PACKS available free from DfEE Publications, P.O. Box 5050, Sudbury, Suffolk CO10 6LQ. Tel: 0845 602 2260.

APPENDIX A
TABLE OF NOTIFIABLE DISEASES

The following diseases are notifiable to the local Director of Public Health via the Consultant in Communicable Diseases.

ACUTE ENCEPHALITIS	MEASLES	SCARLET FEVER
ACUTE POLIOMYELITIS	MENINGITIS	SMALLPOX
ANTHRAX	MENINGOCOCCAL SEPTICAEMIA (without MENINGITIS)	TETANUS
CHOLERA	MUMPS	*TUBERCULOSIS
DIPHTHERIA	OPHTHALMIA NEONATORUM	TYPHOID FEVER
DYSENTERY (AMOEBIC OR BACILLARY)	PARATYPHOID FEVER	TYPHUS
FOOD POISONING (OR SUSPECTED FOOD POISONING)	PLAGUE	VIRAL HAEMORRHAGIC FEVER (inc Lassa fever & Marburg disease)
LEPROSY	RABIES	WHOOPING COUGH
LEPTOSPIROSIS	RELAPSING FEVER	YELLOW FEVER
MALARIA	RUBELLA	

*TUBERCULOSIS is required to be notified in order to check the spread of infection and to bring about the proper management of the individual patient and immediate contacts. A person who should be notified as 'suffering from tuberculosis', therefore, is a person who, because of tuberculosis infection, may infect others; or a person who is suffering from an active tuberculous lesion which calls for medical treatment or for some form of modification of the patient's normal course of living.

To this list should be added any disease made notifiable in the area by an order made under Section 147 of the Public Health Act 1936 as amended by and construed in accordance with Section 52 of the Health Services and Public Health Act 1968 and as amended by Schedule 14 and Schedule 29, paragraph 4, to the Local Government Act 1972.

Incubation and Exclusion Periods For The Commoner Communicable Diseases

Disease	Incubation period (days)	Return to school (subject to clinical recovery)
Chickenpox	11-21 (commonly 16)	6 days after appearance of rash
Measles	10-15 (commonly 10) to onset of illness and 14 to appearance rash.	7 days after appearance of rash
Rubella	14-21 (commonly 18)	4 days after appearance of rash
Whooping cough (Pertussis)	7-10	21 days from onset of paroxysmal cough.
Mumps	12-26 (commonly 18)	After all swellings have subsided, usually 7-10 days.

No routine quarantine of contacts is advised for these diseases.

Appendix B

New Pupil Medical Examination (Male)

NAME				DoB		Age	y m

B.P.	Initial	5m lying	Date	URINALYSIS		PEFR	
Systolic				Protein		Actual	
Diastolic				Glucose		Predict	

Date		Initials	

Major Illnesses, Operations, Investigations	
Allergies, Drug Idiosyncracies	
Asthma, Hay Fever, Rashes	
Current Medical Problems	
Current Medication	

ENT	
Chest, Heart	
Abdomen	
Hernia?	
Scoliosis?	
Musc/Skel	
Pubic Hair Stage		Sexual Dev't: Appropriate
Genitals Stage		Delayed

CONCLUSION:

ACTION:

Dr: Date:

New Pupil Medical Examination (Female)

NAME		DoB	Age y m

B.P.	Initial	5m lying	Date	URINALYSIS		PEFR	
Systolic				Protein		Actual	
Diastolic				Glucose		Predict	

Date		Initials	

Major Illnesses, Operations, Investigations	
Allergies, Drug Idiosyncracies	
Asthma, Hay Fever, Rashes	
Current Medical Problems	
Current Medication	
Menarche	Periods

ENT	
Chest, Heart	
Abdomen	
Hernia?	
Scoliosis?	
Musc/Skel	
Pubic Hair Stage	Sexual Dev't: Appropriate
Breast Stage	Delayed

CONCLUSION:

ACTION:

Dr: Date:

Appendix C

Height/Weight Growth Charts Boys 5 years to 18 years

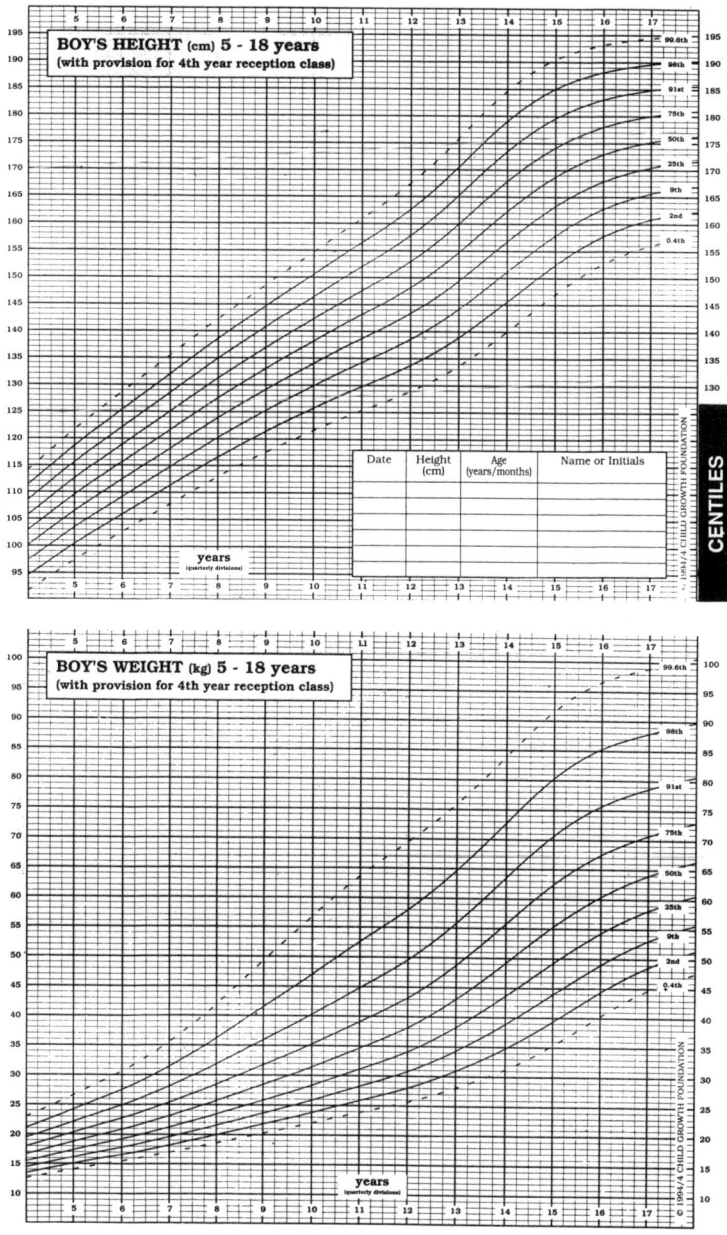

These height and weight charts are reproduced by kind permission of the Child Growth Foundation.

Note that the range of 9-centile charts produced for the UK are obtainable from Harlow

Height / Weight Growth Charts Girls 5 years to 18 years

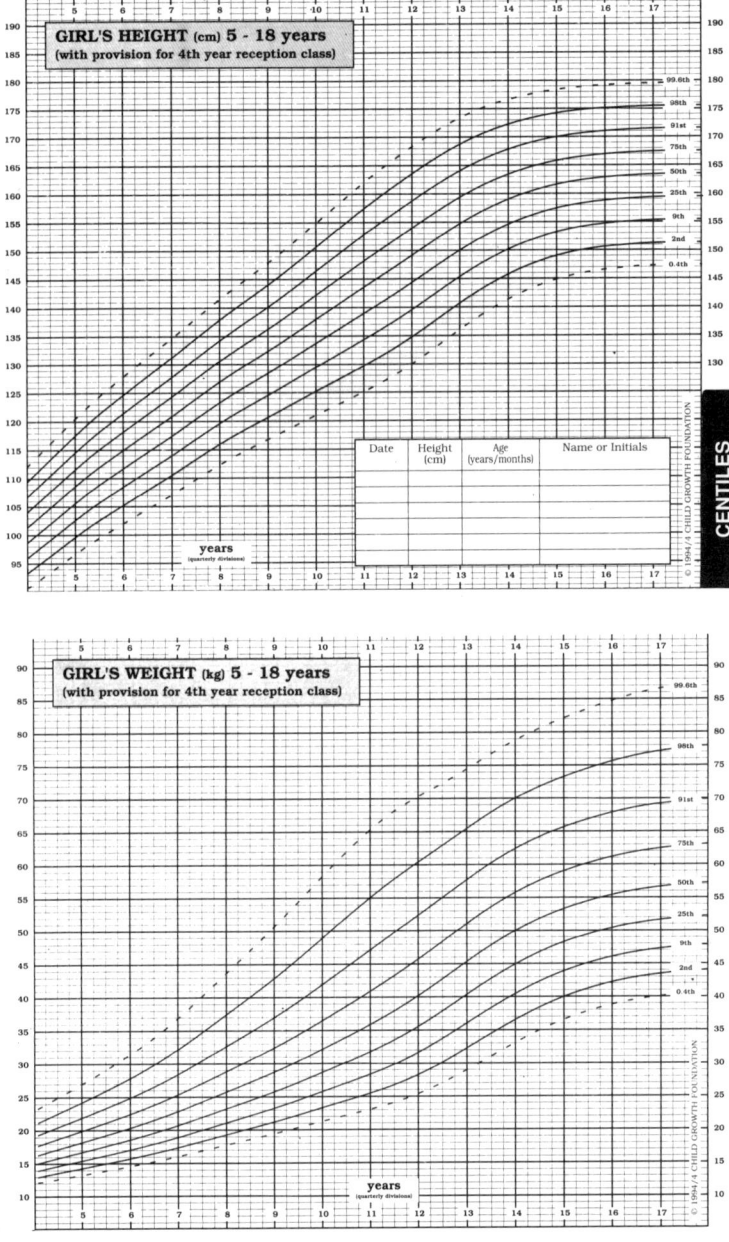

These height and weight charts are reproduced by kind permission of The Child Growth Foundation.

Note that the range of 9-centile charts produced for the UK are obtainable from Harlow Printing.

APPENDIX D

Swimming Pool Disinfectants

Chlorine-based Disinfectants

Two alternatives to chlorine gas are recommended and are in common use. The choice is between one of the chlorinated isocyanurates (such as Fi-chlor granules or tablets) and sodium hypochlorite (so-called liquid chlorine).

When the chlorinated isocyanurates are in solution, an equilibrium reaction is established between the donor molecule, cyanuric acid and hypochlorous acid. This has the effect of prolonging the action of the disinfectant. This equilibrium reaction is particularly useful in open-air swimming pools as it has the effect of protecting free chlorine residuals against sunlight which quickly destroys them. The isocyanurates are convenient to use and store but are more expensive than sodium hypochlorite. The large demand for chlorine by high bathing loads may result in unacceptably high levels of cyanuric acid, which therefore need to be monitored. This is easily done by a bath side check with the necessary test gear. Sodium hypochlorite is inexpensive, but if it is to be used as the only disinfectant a storage tank is needed, and the hypochlorite deteriorates if stored for too long.

A convenient system is to use an isocyanurate for normal pool conditions, and to boost the free chlorine residual by means of a dosing pump and carboys of sodium hypochlorite when high bathing loads occur. Some schools successfully use calcium hypochlorite. A minor disadvantage is that it is not fully soluble, and therefore has to be dosed via a settling tank and then a reservoir. It also has the disadvantage that pool staff sometimes dislike handling the powder.

Non-chlorine based Disinfectants

In general, bromine based disinfectants are more expensive and have a weaker disinfectant action than equivalent chlorine-based compounds. They also have long-term and short-term side-effects. There is no easy method for estimating sodium bromide, which is one of the end products of the action of bromine disinfectants and is a cumulative CNS and skin poison. The equivalent chlorine end-product is sodium chloride which is harmless.

Chlorobromodimethylhydantoin (Aquabrome) is associated with rashes, especially in older females. Skin problems may be very unusual in the young school population, but severe when they do occur. No information is available on the toxicity of the donor molecule of Aquabrome, dimethylhydantoin, and it cannot be estimated outside specialised laboratories. It is a member of the hydantoin group of chemicals which includes phenytoin. The chlorinated isocyanurates, which are used in the same way as Aquabrome, do not have these disadvantages.

Pools treated with Baquacil tend to be cloudy and to foam and to have high bacterial counts. Baquacil is expensive and also non-algicidal, so that a powerful algicide is always needed in addition. It is generally unsuitable for school pools.

Sources of Technical Advice

It is difficult to obtain advice which is not commercially biased although day to day advice and supplies of disinfectant can be obtained from a local swimming pool firm. When a new pool is planned or if an old pool has unusual problems, it is suggested that advice is obtained from one of the companies specialising in water treatment plant for large public pools. The following points may be helpful in avoiding problems.

Specialists should be involved early in the planning stages, and the plant installed should be designed for the maximum bathing load rather than the size of the pool. There is no substitute for pressure sand filters: the small high rate variety are not suitable for school pools because of their potential heavy bathing load. Disinfectants should always be injected before the filter as this is where infection may build up. When sodium hypochlorite is being used, the acid usually necessary for pH correction should be injected after the filter so that chlorine gas is not produced by direct mixing of acid and alkali. Dosing pumps must be fitted with cut-out devices so that they do not continue to inject chlorine into the pool when the main pump has failed. Dilution with fresh water is important. The practice of conserving warm water which has been used to backwash filters and returning it to the pool is hygienically unsound. Similarly, backwashing filters with mains water is not recommended as this reduces dilution of the pool.

Methods of Working for Swimming Pool Staff

Free combined chlorine levels should be tested and recorded daily. This should be increased to three times a day when there are heavy bathing loads. When samples are being taken for bacteriological analysis, disinfectant and pH levels should be recorded at the same time from the same part of the pool. E. coli and coliforms should usually be absent from samples. The occasional presence of coliforms (not E. coli) is acceptable as long as the colony counts are not more than 10, and not more than 100 colonies per ml at 24 hours incubation at 37 degrees F. Filters should be operated for at least one hour before, one hour after and during bathing sessions. During times of high bathing loads, the plant should be operated for 24 hours a day. As pool contamination is mainly responsible for eye irritation and chlorinous odours, it may be necessary to limit bathing loads during very hot weather: also it is very important to encourage the use of toilets before swimming. Pool surrounds should be kept visibly clean, and irrigated with disinfectant solution containing approximately 200ppm of chlorine, or according to the maker's instructions; it is not necessary to use disinfectants. Shampoos, soap and disinfectants should not be allowed to circulate back into the pool. School staff should refer to the disinfectant manufacturer's literature as well as to the Department of the Environment booklets on the safe operation of pools disinfected by various methods.

References and Advice

Pool Water Guide. This is the standard book of reference for pool operators. Price £24. 00. Available from: Pool Water Treatment Advisory Group, P. O. Box. 19, Diss. Norfolk. IP22 3ES

Advice is available from:The Technical Secretary, PWTAG, at the above address.

POOL WATER SAFETY 1996
Published by The Sports Council and the Health and Safety Executive.
Available from HMSO or The Sports Council.

Appendix E

Dental Care in Schools

1. Current recommendations are that both day and boarding pupils should as far as possible, continue to receive continuing dental care of a routine nature in their home town during holidays and periods of absence from the school. So far as is possible this should continue to be encouraged.

2. All schools, both those in the maintained and private sectors, should be encouraged to form a close working relationship with an appropriately qualified dental practitioner who is prepared to take on provision of care following dental trauma. It is likely that the school may wish to form a contractual relationship with this practitioner.

3. So far as is possible, schools should be encouraged to invoke a policy of good dental health, including advice concerning the reduction of sugary foods and fizzy drinks available at different times of the day.

4. Schools are encouraged to have an appropriate policy concerning the protection of a child's teeth from trauma, however induced.

Further useful information
Dietary Sugars and Human Disease. Report from the Panel on Dietary Sugars of The Committee on Medical aspects of Food policy. (COMA) HMSO 1989 (Reports on Health and Social subjects. 37.)

An Oral Health strategy for England and Wales, Department of Health 1994.

The Scientific Basis of Dental Health Education, Health Education Council 1996.

Notes on Dental Health Edited by Anthony S. Blinkhorn and Elizabeth J. Kay. Published by Eden Bianchi Press, 2, Ashwood avenue, West Didsbury, Manchester M20 8ZB

PREVENT A CHILD LOSING HIS SMILE If an 'adult' tooth is knocked out all is not lost! An A 4 size poster in colour, detailing First aid Advice if a tooth is knocked out, is available (free) from the University of Manchester Dental School, Higher Cambridge Street, Manchester M15 6FH

'Reduce the consumption and especially the frequency of intake of sugar-containing foods and drink, clean the teeth and gums thoroughly every day with a fluoride toothpaste, drink fluoridated water, and attend for regular dental check-ups'

Healthy Tuckshops
To foster a whole school approach to healthy eating, snack sales could include the following healthier options:

Sandwiches, Rolls, Toast, Sugar-free cakes, Oatcakes, Sugar- free scones and biscuits

Bread sticks, Pitta bread, Pizza slice, High-fibre low salt crisps, Fresh fruit and vegetables Sugar-free-low fat yoghourt, Sugar-free low-fat cottage cheese, Milk, Mineral water, Sugar-free tea and coffee

Sugar-free confectionery.

Incorporating MOSA Policy Guidelines February 1996.

APPENDIX F

Colour Vision and Eye Care in Sports

Defective Colour Vision

This is most important, especially when considering choices of career since approximately 8% of boys and1% of girls are colour deficient. Often the girls are carriers and pass on the deficiency to their sons and grandsons. The extent of the colour deficit varies between individuals and from only slight to severe. The type and severity of the deficit can be determined by examination. There is no treatment which will improve improve the condition. Required standards of colour vision vary from time to time and are published in the Annual Reference Handbook of The Association of Optometrists, Bridge House, 233-234 Blackfriars Road, London SE1 8NW. (Tel:0171 261 9661), who have kindly given permission for the reproduction of the following table.

NB. The table can only be a very general guide. For more precise information about visual requirements for specific careers ask your optometrists or careers officer. In many cases a final decision rests with the medical authority dealing with entry to a particular career, e. g. Police, RAF, Employer, etc

Profession	Official Eye Test	Conditions	Glasses/Contact lenses allowed
Drivers:			
Private	YES	Must pass specified vision test;	YES
PCV	YES	have no significant loss of visual	YES
LGV	YES	field; no double vision, no severe night vision disability and PCV and LGV drivers must have adequate vision in both eyes.	YES
Merchant Navy	YES	Good standard of vision in each eye; binocular vision; normal colour vision.	YES
Civil Aviation	YES	Good standard of vision in each eye; normal visual fields, some colour vision requirements.	YES
RAF	YES	Good standard of vision; generally good colour vision.	YES
Teacher	YES	Basic standard of vision in at least one eye.	YES

Fire Brigade	YES	Good standard of vision without glasses – limits on optical error present; adequate colour vision; good night vision.	NO on operational duties
Electrician	Varies with type of work	Adequate standard of vision for type of work; adequate colour vision.	YES
VDU Operator	YES as 'user' under *H & SW Act.	Adequate standard of vision at middle and near distances; no binocular vision disabilities likely to cause symptoms.	YES some need additional glasses for specific focal distances.
Police	YES	Good standard of vision: binocular vision; adequate colour vision (different forces vary)	YES (in most forces)
Accountant	NO	Adequate vision in at least one for sustained near vision.	YES

*Health and Safety at Work Act.

Guidelines for Lenses

Should be made from impact-resistant plastic or, preferably, polycarbonate.

Glass lenses should be avoided, but if used must be toughened.

Indoor use lenses should not be tinted and should be specially coated to reduce reflection from the lights.

Polycarbonate, tougher than other materials, MUST be used for squash, and other active ball / racquet sports.

Some Recommendations

Sport	Spectacles	Contact Lenses
*Tennis	Yes or goggles	All, but soft best.
Table Tennis	Yes	All, but soft best.
Squash	Squash goggles only.	All, under goggles.
Snooker	Special frames.	Rarely work well.
*Fishing	Polarised	All, with polarised sun-glasses if bright.
*Association Football	No	Soft.
*Rugby Football	No	Soft or scleral.
*American Football	Goggles	Soft or scleral.
*Water Sports	Ventilated goggles	Sclerals best,
Swimming	Goggles	Soft only with care, best under goggles.
Scuba Diving	Diving mask	Soft with mask.
*Horse Riding	Yes	All, but soft best.
*Hang—gliding & Parachuting	Yes, under goggles	Soft, under goggles.

*Target Shooting	Special frames	All.
*Clay Shooting	High frame	All, but soft best.
*Athletics	Yes	All.
*Jogging	Yes	All.
Wrestling and Judo	No	Soft or scleral.
Darts	Yes	All, but beware of atmosphere.
Fencing	Yes, or goggles	All.
*Hockey	Goggles best	All.
*Cricket & Basketball	Yes, or goggles	All.
Volleyball	Yes, or goggles	Soft.
Badminton	Yes, or goggles	All, but soft best.
*Ski-ing	Yes, under mask	All, under mask.
*Abseiling	Yes, or goggles	Sclerals.

*An ultra violet absorber is recommended in all appliances, spectacle or contact lenses for outdoor sports. Sun spectacles, to BS 2724, may be of benefit in bright sunlight.

Eye Care in Sports
The Association of Optometrists (address above) and the Sports Vision Association (at the same address) have kindly supplied the following information about eye care in sports. Spectacles are contraindicated in contact sports or if they are likely to get wet or steamed up. (Special lens coating treatments and anti mist sprays are now available.) Contact lenses are the practical solution to these problems and soft contact lenses are the best for most vigorous sports, even if people are unable to wear them for normal daily use. However, contact lenses provide very little eye protection and they should be worn, where necessary or appropriate in conjunction with protective goggles. Certain sports are best performed with the protection of special frames or goggles. Squash, for instance, requires goggles which protect the temples and bridge of the nose as well as the eyes.

Guidelines for Frames
Lightweight, yet strong enough to resist strong impact.
Could be fitted with side pieces that curl securely behind the ears.
Could be fitted with elasticated sports band.
Metal frames should be fitted with a padded bridge.
Specially designed goggles are preferable.

Further Information
Sports Vision Edited by D. F. C. Loran and C. J. Mac Ewen.

Sports vision is a relatively new but fast expanding area of multi-disciplinary eye care involving not only optometrists but also dispensing opticians, ophthalmologists, athletes, sports organisations and coaches. This book deals with optimising safe and efficient vision in sport.

Published by Butterworth Heinemann.

Orders to Reed Book Services Ltd., PO BOX 5 Rushden. Northants. NN10 6YX.

MEDICAL REPORT ON AND EXAMINATION OF STAFF MEMBER

Logo of School

School Address

Headmaster's Name.

Tel & Fax Numbers
Date.

Dear Doctor,

An appointment is being made for the post of. . . . .
at . . . . School.

It is hoped that you will be able to make a medical report (from the medical records and from your knowledge of . . . .) and undertake a medical examination.

. . . . should be offered a sight of the report. You may decline to let . . . . see all or part of the report if you consider that this will be inappropriate. In these circumstances you should ask for . . . . 's consent before releasing the report.

The report and the medical examination report should be sent direct to the School Medical Officer. They will be treated in the strictest confidence and none of the contents will be disclosed to the school.

You are obliged to keep a copy of the report for 6 months.

On receipt of the report a fee of £. . . . . . will be forwarded to you, which will be payable by the participating school.

Thank you for your help.

Yours sincerely,

Signature.

Typed name.

The report should be forwarded in the S. A. E. provided.

Logo of School   School Address

                                  Telephone & Fax Numbers

Headmaster's Name

Date.

To the Appointee

Before I confirm your appointment, it is necessary to obtain a medical report from your doctor, as stated in the Job Description. To obtain this we require your written consent and you should therefore, sign the form set out below. You have the right to refuse consent for such a report, though if you do, I may not be able to proceed further with your appointment.

You have the right to see the report before it is sent, and to request its alteration. Your doctor has then to inform the School Medical Officer that the report has been altered.

Your doctor may decline to let you see the report if he/she considers that to let you see it would be inappropriate. In this circumstance, your consent would be required before it could be released to the School Medical Officer.

The report is totally confidential to the School Medical Officer. None of the contents of the report will be released by him, but he may advise the Headmaster regarding your appointment.

Each doctor must retain a copy of the report he prepares for 6 months, and you may request to see it during that time.

Signature.

Type Name.

I have been advised of my rights and the Access to Medical Reports Act 1988—I understand the School is requesting a report from my Doctor to be sent in the strictest confidence to the Medical Officer of (Insert the name of the School).

Signed. . . . .

Date. . . . .

Two copies to be signed: one to be kept and one to be forwarded in the medical report to the G. P.

1. Medical Report Required For:

   Full Name. . . . .   Date of Birth. . . . .

   Address. . . . .

   Occupation. . . . .

   Marital Status. . . . .

2. a)   How long have you been the medical attendant?

   b)   How far do the records which you hold go back?

   c)   When was medical advice last sought and why?

   d)   Is there anything apparent from your records, examinations or from your
        personal knowledge of the person, which indicates to you that the person about
        whom information is being sought

        i) takes non-prescribed drugs by inhalation, orally or par-enterally?

        ii) has any particular vulnerability to the acquired immunodeficiency syndrome?

        iii) has any relevant history of anxiety or depression?

3. Please give particulars of any serious illnesses or accidents which have required treatment
   or advice from yourself or other medical advisers.

DATE	NATURE OF CONDITION	TREATMENT	DURATION OF ILLNESS AND TIME OFF WORK

   (Please continue on a separate sheet of paper and staple to this if necessary.)
   a)   Have any of the above left any sequelae?
        (If so, please give details).

   b)   Is any treatment by drugs or otherwise being given at present?
        (if so, please give details).

4. What do you know of the smoking, drinking or other habits of the person about whom
   information is being sought?

5.   Please give details of any urine tests, X-rays, ECGs or other investigations.

DATE   NATURE OF INVESTIGATIONS   RESULT

6.   Please give details of any blood pressure readings. (If on treatment, please indicate any pre-treatment level).

DATE:

SYSTOLIC:

DIASTOLIC:

7.   Additional information relevant to a person employed in a school.

8.   Has . . . . seen this report?   Yes/No.

9.   Has any information been omitted either at your or the examinee's insistence? Yes/No.

Medical Examiner's Report

. . . .
. . . .

I.   Height (without shoes)   (cm) ft. ins   2. Chest; full inspiration   (cm) ins
                                                    complete expiration   (cm) ins
     Weight (in outdoor clothing) (Kg)st. lbs. Abdominal girth at umbilicus (cm) ins

3.   Cardiovascular System
     list any abnormality of heart, pulse or blood vessels.

                                             . . . .
                                             Systolic Diastolic (5th phase)

                                             . . . .
     Blood Pressure   initial
     if initially abnormal, please repeat   reading . . . .
     after five minutes.   . . . .

4.   Lungs
     Peak flow reading appreciated, if
     available and relevant

5.   Abdominal Examination

6.   Central Nervous System

7.   (a)   What is the build and general   (a)
           appearance?

     (b)   Does your examination support all
           the declarations made by the applicant?   (b)

8.   Urine Testing including quantity of
     albumen or sugar if positive.   albumen   sugar.

Additional Notes: Please indicate whether or not you feel that any abnormal findings are significant.

Please see the attached schedule.

Date. . . . .   Name. . . . .
                                                              (IN BLOCK CAPITALS PLEASE.)
(Please advise full name of account
to whom the cheque should be
made payable.   Signature. . . . .

                                                              Address. . . . .
                                                              . . . .
                                                              . . . .

It would be appreciated if this report could be returned as soon as possible in the S. A. E . provided.

APPENDIX H

SPECIMEN JOB DESCRIPTION FOR SCHOOL NURSE

JOB TITLE: School Nurse.

QUALIFICATION: RGN Minimum. Registration with the UKCC and a current PIN. Membership of the Royal College of Nursing is recommended.

PAY GRADE; F or G
RESPONSIBLE TO: Board of Governors
ACCOUNTABLE TO: School Medical Officer, Headteacher.
She is professionally accountable as an autonomous practitioner and both she and her employer should be familiar with the UKCC Codes of Professional Conduct and terms of PREP.

AREAS OF RESPONSIBILITY
1. Supervisory responsibility and policy making (Senior Nurse).

2. Assessment, management and continuing responsibility for a defined caseload, including record keeping.

3. Responsibility for carrying out all duties delegated by the School Medical Officer.

4. Responsibility for own continuing education.

5. Setting and maintaining standards in a team.

6. Measurement, evaluation and audit.

7. Child surveillance programme.

8. Treatments.

9. Counselling.

10. Health Education, Health Promotion.

11. Stock Control

12. Liaison with external agencies.

13. Administration.

14. Health and Safety.

1. SUPERVISORY RESPONSIBILITY AND POLICY MAKING

With the school MO and Headmaster, ensuring that standards of care are set and maintained by all staff. Capital expenditure, equipment maintenance and staff organisation i. e. off duty.

2. ASSESSMENT, MANAGEMENT AND CONTINUING RESPONSIBILITY FOR A DEFINED CASELOAD

Each nurse is professionally responsible as an autonomous practitioner. She should have read and understood the following documents:

i)   Guidelines For Professional Practice. UKCC 1996.
ii)   Code of Professional Conduct. UKCC 1992.
iii)   The Scope of Professional Practice. UKCC 1992.
iv)   Standards of Records and Record Keeping. UKCC 1993.
v)   Standards for the Administration of Medicine. UKCC 1992.
vi)   Confidentiality. UKCC Advisory Paper.
vii)   Exercising Accountability. UKCC Advisory Paper.

3. RESPONSIBILITY FOR CARRYING OUT ALL DUTIES DELEGATED BY THE SCHOOL MO.

These should be to agreed levels of competence and the nurse as an autonomous practitioner has the right to refuse to carry out those duties for which she feels inadequately trained.

4. RESPONSIBILITY FOR OWN CONTINUING EDUCATION.

The nurse has a duty to maintain her level of training in all areas of her practice. PREP (Post Registration And Practice 1st April 1995) is a legal requirement. She must retain an effective registration and hold a current UKCC PIN.

5. SETTING AND MAINTAINING STANDARDS OF CARE WITHIN A TEAM.

Writing of protocols which should be agreed by all and not imposed by one. Updating of guidelines to staff e. g. kitchen, Houseparent Handbooks.

6. MEASUREMENT EVALUATION AND AUDIT

This will require the keeping of records in such a way as to facilitate easy and accurate retrieval of information, often in line with methods used in the GP practice.

7. CHILD SURVEILLANCE PROGRAMME

The surveillance of children in full time education, assessing the general standard of health and detecting any deviation from the normal likely to affect their development and their capacity to learn.

This is usually started by means of the medical examination on entry to the school and continued by routine monitoring at appropriate intervals.

8. TREATMENTS

First Aid provision for any casualties during school hours.
Treatments under the direction of the school MO.
Nursing treatments which meet the agreed levels of competence.
Aid and chaperon school MO during clinical procedures, surgeries, medical examinations, etc.

9. COUNSELLING SKILLS

Children with physical, emotional or sexual problems which interfere with their normal life will need help. Counselling should be undertaken by the nurse only where appropriate training has been completed. However, staff, pupils, parents and guardians will at all times need sympathetic guidance on the management of pupil problems.

10. HEALTH EDUCATION

Maintain a library of up to date material on a wide range of appropriate health issues. e, g, books, videos, leaflets.

Keep up to date with current Health Promotion initiatives.

11. STOCK CONTROL

Maintain treatment room stock, hygiene and tidiness.
Be aware of recommended storage and disposal guidelines.
Be aware of current infection control guidelines.

12. LIAISON WITH EXTERNAL AGENCIES

Primary Health Care Team
Surgery staff, Practice nurse, Reception Staff and Pharmacist.
Appointments and admission Staff for consultants, orthodontists and dentist.
Community staff where appropriate.
Social Services, where appropriate.

13. ADMINISTRATION

Maintain medical records, ensure confidential, safe and legal storage.
Keep nursing records to a high standard ensuring the accurate and rapid retrieval of information.
(Standards For Records and Record Keeping and Data Protection Act.)
Maintenance of general office procedures in line with those in the GP practice.
Set up and organise school medical examinations.

14. HEALTH AND SAFETY

Involvement with Health and Safety issues within the school affecting staff, children, or the environment.

Keeping records of and reporting of all accidents.

Maintaining up to date records on all hazardous substances used and stored in school or the school grounds.

SCHOOL NURSES

LEVEL OF COMPETENCE FOR IMMUNISATION AND VACCINATION SCHOOL NURSES' SELF ASSESSMENT FORM

Adapted from: Nurses, Midwives and Health Visitors Advisory Council, Policy and Standards Group.
Competencies for Immunisation and Vaccination
by
Hilary Fairfield, Primary Care Facilitator, Wiltshire NHS Trust 1994.

Rate yourself on a scale of 1-5 where:
 1 = little or no competence
 5 = competent enough to accept accountability.

1 2 3 4 5

KNOWLEDGE
 (1) Identify and describe your own professional accountability.

 (2) Identify relevant national policies.

 (3) Be familiar with practice protocol.

 (4) State the correct method of patient identification.

 (5) Describe the physiology of the immune system.

 (6) Identify relevant local / national epidemiological trends

 (7) State the correct information for:

    (a) prescription documentation.

    (b) methods of recording administration.

 (8) For each individual vaccine, state the correct information about:

    (a) appropriate storage,

    (b) contraindications for use.

    (c) side-effects.

    (d) reconstitution

    (e) injection site

1 2 3 4 5

(f) route of administration

(g) appropriate advice to patient / carer

9. Identify and describe the following:

(a) allergic reaction

(b) anaphylaxis

10. State the appropriate treatment for the following:

(a) allergic reaction

(b) anaphylaxis

11. Select and apply relevant research as an aid to practice

12. Identify and utilise appropriate information resources

SKILL

1. Assess the fitness of the individual for immunisation or vaccination

2. Use acceptable interpersonal skills in approaching, advising and educating the patient, carer, other members of the PHCT

3. Administer each vaccine according to the practice protocol :

(a) identification of patient

(b) reading and interpreting prescriptions

(c) calculation of vaccine doses

(d) administration of the vaccines

(e) completion of relevant documentation

(f) safe disposal of unused vaccines and equipment

4. Observe patient for adverse reaction during and following procedures

5. Effectively perform resuscitation procedures where appropriate

ATTITUDES

1. Accept own accountability during immunisation and vaccination

2. Maintain competency

3. Accept own limitations and know when to seek advice

4. Where appropriate, adopt the role of patient advocate

5. Acknowledge and maintain the rights and values of the individual

Now consider areas where you have not scored '5'

Consider how you can increase your competency in these areas,
e.g.   reading journals and articles
       using a practice nurse mentor
       discussion with colleagues

APPENDIX K

SPECIMEN CONTRACT
(SCHOOL DOCTOR)

THIS AGREEMENT is made the . . . . .day of . . . . One Thousand Nine Hundred

and. . . . .   BETWEEN. . . . . SCHOOL

whose registered office is at. . . . .

. . . . (hereinafter called 'the Company') of the one part

and Dr. . . . . of. . . . .

. . . . (hereinafter called 'the

Doctor') of the other part.

WHEREAS:
The Company is the proprietor of
in the County of
(hereinafter called 'the School') and is desirous of obtaining the service of a Physician as Medical
Officer to the School and the Doctor has agreed to serve the Company in such capacity upon
the terms and conditions following.

NOW IT IS HEREBY AGREED as follows:
1.   THE Company hereby engages the Doctor as Medical Officer to the School and the
        Doctor will to the best of his skill and knowledge serve the Company in such capacity
        from the first day of   until such engagement shall be determined as hereinafter
        provided.

2.   FOR the consideration hereinafter appearing the Doctor hereby undertakes:-

        (a)   to accept as a patient under and in accordance with the National Service Acts any
                pupil attending the School as a boarder and to receive the National Health
                Service Fees or other appropriate fee.

        (b)   to be responsible for the medical supervision of the School Sanatorium and to
                advise on the appointment of nursing staff and the general direction of their
                professional duties. PROVIDED that in the absence of personal default on the
                part of the Doctor he shall not be liable for default or misconduct on the part of
                any member of the Staff or person who shall fail to comply with the Doctor's
                instructions nor shall the Doctor be liable for any failure by the staff to keep the
                Sanatorium in a proper state of cleanliness.

(c) to visit the School Sanatorium or elsewhere on the School premises as often as reasonably required by the School during the School terms and whenever reasonably requested to do so during the School holidays, and to medically attend when required any pupil at the School who is his patient.

(d) in co-operation with the Headmaster, to provide for the appropriate medical care of all day pupils during the time they are within the precincts of the School and until they are able to return home under parental care and the supervision of their own family doctor.

(e) to conduct in such a manner as the Doctor shall think proper such examinations of pupils or Staff outside the National Health Service as he may consider desirable or as may be requested by the Governors or by the Headmaster of the School and to advise the Headmaster and/or the Governors as to any administrative action which in his judgment should be taken in the interests of hygiene.

(f) to advise the Headmaster and the Governors on matters of health.

(g) to liaise with housemasters, housemistresses and other staff concerning the physical and mental health and fitness of individual pupils, with parental permission.

(h) to undertake the periodic medical examination of pupils, including screening for vision, hearing, height and weight.

(i) to provide epidemiological surveillance, including maintenance of sickness and injury records additional to clinical notes forming part of the National Health Service records

(j) to supervise the maintenance of immunisation programmes to ensure that, with parental permission where necessary, all pupils are immunised in accordance with current practice recommended by the Department of Health including tetanus, poliomyelitis, BCG, mumps, measles and rubella vaccination.

(k) to advise on the prevention of accidents and sports injuries, and also to ensure that all legal duties are dispatched regarding the requirements of all the regulations applicable to schools under the facility of the enabling legislation of The Health and Safety at Work Act. (1974).

(l) to make available at his own expense a qualified deputy satisfactory to the Headmaster of the School to act for him in cases where he is prevented from acting in person or by unavoidable absence and for the purposes of this Sub Clause any partner of the Doctor shall be deemed satisfactory to the Headmaster.

(m) to be and to remain throughout the tenure of this Contract of Service a member or representative member (as the case may be) of The Medical Defence Union Limited, Medical Protection Society or other professional indemnity organisation and to be prepared to furnish annually for the information of the governors a certificate of membership showing the payment of the appropriate annual subscription at the date to one of the organisations mentioned.

(n) to attend on any pupils or staff at any Local Hospital within the practice area of the Doctor when the occasion arises.

(o) to submit an annual report if required to do so.

3.   IN consideration of the Undertakings at Clause 2, Sub-Clauses (b) to (o) inclusive but excluding Sub-Clause (a) the School will pay the Medical Officer a fee of per annum such fee to be revised in   and annually thereafter so long as this agreement remains in force, the fee payable by equal monthly instalments in arrears. The Company will make payable to the Doctor the same concessions by way of remission or partial remission of the School fees in respect of any children of his who shall be attending the School as shall from time to time be accorded to members of the teaching staff.

4.   The Doctor shall have the right to call in a Specialist or authorise treatment involving extra expenditure in an emergency though normally if possible, he will first obtain the authority of the parents of the pupil concerned or of the Headmaster of the School or of the pupil's Housemaster and shall be indemnified by the Company against any consequential loss or expense.

5.   THE Agreement shall be terminated at any time by either party giving to the other one full term's notice to take effect at the end of any School term PROVIDED that and it is HEREBY AGREED that if the Doctor is unable to continue the duties and obligations of this Agreement the Company shall have the right to determine this Agreement forthwith. For the purpose of the clause the School's terms shall be deemed to end respectively on 31st December, 30th April and 31st August as the case may be.

6.   WITHOUT prejudice to the right of either party to determine this Agreement as provided in clause 5 thereof it is hereby agreed that the Company shall not be required to continue the Doctor's engagement (subject nevertheless to the provisions of clause 5 hereof) beyond the normal retirement age of sixty five years.
        AS WITNESS the hands of the parties hereto on the day and year first before written.

Signed for and on behalf of the Company. . . . .

Signed for and on behalf of the Doctor. . . . .

APPENDIX L

MEDICAL QUESTIONNAIRE ON ENTRY OF PUPIL

The following questionnaire is designed to cover the salient points of importance in the pupil's medical history. Medical officers may wish to adapt it to their individual needs, adding where necessary, further questions on family and social history and such other information as may be needed for administrative purposes.

Name of pupil (BLOCK LETTERS, surname first and underline Christian name by which known at home)

. . . .

Date and place of birth. . . . .

Has he/she had the following infections? If so, please give approximate dates:

Mumps. . . . . .Whooping cough. . . . . Chickenpox. . . . .

Rheumatic fever. . . . . .Measles. . . . .

Has he/she been immunised against any of the following conditions?

	Primary course Tick as appropriate	Booster dates

Diphtheria
Haemophilus Influenzae (Hib)
Tetanus

Pertussis
(Whooping
cough)

Poliomyelitis
BCG

	Yes	No	Dates of all immunisation given

Measles

Rubella
(German
Measles)

Mumps

Typhoid

Cholera

Yellow fever

Haemophilus
influenzae (Hib)

Influenza

Tuberculosis (BCG)

Any other disease

Please give details of illness and treatment:

	Yes	No
Asthma		

Eczema

Hay Fever

Bone or joint disease

Fits or convulsions

Discharging ears

Deafness

Frequent sore throats

Nasal obstruction

Psychological problems

Please give details of any other illness, operation or hospital investigation:

Please give details of any known allergy, including sensitivity to drugs:

Has he/she lived overseas? If so, please state country and give details of any infection with tropical disease:

Please give details of any known exposure to active pulmonary tuberculosis:

Does he/she wear spectacles or contact lenses?

When was the eyesight last tested?

If so, with what result?

Has he/she had an audiometry test?
If so, please give date and result (pass or fail)

Does he/she wet the bed or have poor bladder or bowel control?
Please give details

Is there any feature in the family history which might have a bearing on his /her health, including any family history of psychiatric illness, coronary heart disease, high blood pressure or diabetes in the immediate family?

Is there any feature of his/her physical or mental health of which you feel the school doctor should be aware, or which you would like to discuss with him?

Do you consider that he/she is fit to take part in all the normal school games and activities?

Is he /she at present under any form of medical treatment? (If yes, a letter from the specialist or family doctor would be helpful).

Signature of parent or guardian
Address, telephone no, Date etc.

Advice to parents of boarding school pupils

The following is suggested as a specimen note to parents of children in boarding school.

Holiday treatment

If your son or daughter should need treatment during the holidays, they may go with their National Health number to your family doctor, or any other NHS general practitioner offering general medical services, who may accept them as temporary patients.

If your son or daughter has an operation, accident, severe illness, immunisation or special treatment during the holidays, it is necessary to inform the school medical officer on or (preferably) before their return to school. The information should be given in a letter from the parent, supported if necessary by a report from the family doctor, and including details of medicines and treatment recommended, if these are to continue.

Infectious diseases

If, during the holidays, your son or daughter is exposed to anyone suffering from an infectious disease (e. g. chickenpox or mumps) they may return to school when the term begins, but the medical officer should be informed if your child has not already had the disease. Only in the unlikely event of contact with diphtheria, poliomyelitis, typhoid or paratyphoid fever, bacillary dysentery, meningococcal infection, hepatitis A or B or HIV infection should the pupil be kept at home until you have consulted the school medical officer.

Tropical diseases

It is important that the school medical officer should be informed if a pupil has been exposed to the risk of malaria or other tropical disease.

Consent form

The following is suggested as a specimen consent form allowing the medical officer to carry out immunisations and the headteacher to act in *loco parentis* in an emergency. For convenience, instruction on private treatment and participation in an accident insurance scheme are included on the same form. The exact wording of course, is a matter for individual schools to decide.

I agree that the school medical officer may carry out such immunisations against tetanus, measles, poliomyelitis, mumps and rubella (German measles) or other infections, as he deems necessary.

I understand that in an emergency every effort will be made to obtain my consent to an operation and/or the administration of an anaesthetic, but if this proves impossible I hereby authorise the headmaster or the headmistress or their senior deputy to act in *loco parentis*.

I wish to participate in the school's accident insurance scheme, and will pay such premiums as are currently in force.

In the event of referral of my child to a consultant, I should like this to be done under the National Health Service/as a private patient. (Delete as appropriate).

Date   Signed
                                         Parent or Guardian.

Index

This index is in word-by-word alphabetical order, and includes the main body of text and the appendices.